AF333079

In Vitro Neurotoxicology

METHODS IN PHARMACOLOGY AND TOXICOLOGY

In Vitro Neurotoxicology

Principles and Challenges

Edited by

Evelyn Tiffany-Castiglioni

Department of Veterinary Anatomy and Public Health
Texas A&M University College of Veterinary Medicine
and Center for Environmental and Rural Health,
College Station, TX

Foreword by

Mannfred A. Hollinger

University of California
Davis, CA

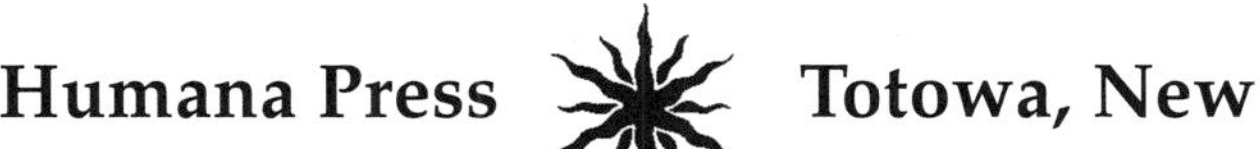

Humana Press Totowa, New Jersey

Production Editor: Tracy Catanese

Cover Illustration: Figure 2 from Chapter 7, "Cell-Type-Specific Responses of the Nervous System to Lead" by Evelyn Tiffany-Castiglioni.

Cover design by Patricia F. Cleary.

For additional copies, pricing for bulk purchases, and/or information about other Humana titles, contact Humana at the above address or at any of the following numbers: Tel.: 973-256-1699; Fax: 973-256-8341; E-mail: humana@humanapr.com or visit our website: http://humanapress.com

This publication is printed on acid-free paper. ∞
ANSI Z39.48-1984 (American National Standards Institute) Permanence of Paper for Printed Library Materials.

Photocopy Authorization Policy:

Printed in the United States of America.   10 9 8 7 6 5 4 3 2 1

1-59259-651-7 (e-book)

Library of Congress Cataloging-in-Publication Data

Tiffany-Castiglioni, Evelyn.
    In vitro neurotoxicology : principles and challenges / edited by Evelyn Tiffany-Castiglioni.
       p. cm. -- (Methods in pharmacology and toxicology)
    Includes bibliographical references and index.
    ISBN 1-58829-047-6 (alk. paper)
     1. Neurotoxicology. 2. Toxicity testing--In vitro. I. Title. II. Series.

  RC347.5.T54 2003
  616.8'047--dc21

                                              2003049933

Dedication

To Robert S. Tiffany, Jr. and Frances James Tiffany
In Memoriam

Foreword

Researchers in pharmacology and toxicology are constantly searching for relevant in vitro methods in order to obtain valid data without the use of whole animals with their attendant costs and ethical questions. This is particularly true for workers interested in neurotoxicology, where we continue to discover new neurotoxic effects of drugs and other xenobiotics. Over the years, a number of creative and useful methods have emerged. For someone entering the field of neurotoxicology, the decision regarding type of method most appropriate for his or her work can be a daunting one. For example, the time and effort required to search the literature and evaluate candidate systems can require weeks, if not months.

In Vitro Neurotoxicology: Principles and Challenges, edited by Dr. Evelyn Tiffany-Castiglioni, is a masterful contribution to the field of neurotoxicology. With each passing year the need for new and improved in vitro methods to help further our understanding of neurotoxicology will increase. This volume brings us up to date.

Mannfred A. Hollinger
Professor Emeritus
University of California
Davis, CA

Preface

Neurotoxicity assessment with in vitro systems is the focus of both increasing expectations and heightened challenges. Such systems prospectively offer a means to improve screening efficiency for potential neurotoxicants, a method for better understanding mechanisms of toxicant action, a decreasing use of animals, and a means to obtain data from human samples. On the other hand, in vitro systems have not yet been used in consistent, broadly applied formats that would validate and exploit their value for neurotoxicity testing. Inherent problems, such as test chemical concentration and delivery, lack of heterogeneous cell–cell interactions, immaturity of cell types available, phenotypic variations induced by culture techniques, and insensitivity of endpoints tested, significantly impede the use and interpretation of in vitro assays. In addition, standardized metrics and methods for comparing results across studies and laboratories, as well as benchmark criteria for linking in vitro to in vivo studies, are often lacking.

The purpose of *In Vitro Neurotoxicology: Principles and Challenges* is to synthesize principles and concepts of in vitro neurotoxicology that will facilitate the development of significantly improved methods and systems for in vitro neurotoxicity testing, with emphasis on their relevance to in vivo systems. An outstanding list of contributors has been assembled, including well-respected leaders in the field and new investigators who are exploring emerging frontiers in the area of genomic toxicology. Contributors have taken a fresh look at their own and others' work, critically and comparatively analyzed it across experimental systems and toxicants, and formalized essential principles for in vitro neurotoxicity testing. In most cases, chapters are arranged around major themes or central ideas, rather than around individual toxicants or specific in vitro models. Most chapters are collaborative efforts that address a theme and employ examples comprised of multiple experimental systems and endpoints. The chapters emphasize several neurotoxicants that are of prominent human health concern and about which metabolism and dose–responses are best understood, both in vivo and in vitro: lead, mercury, organophosphorus insecticides, polychlorinated biphenyls and dioxin, ethanol, and endogenous proteins.

There are already several excellent articles and monographs that describe materials and techniques applicable to in vitro neurotoxicology, such as cell lines, methods of primary cell culture, brain slice preparations, and in vitro assays for viability and function. Rather than repeating the contents of these previous works, *In Vitro Neurotoxicology: Principles and Challenges* provides an Appendix containing a critically reviewed list of related works. The list, carefully selected and annotated by the contributors, includes important review articles, books on in vitro toxicology, neurotoxicology, and in vitro neurotoxicology, and chapters from methods manuals. The Appendix collects in one place references to most of the major reviews and seminal work related to in vitro neurotoxicology that have appeared in the past ten years.

Evelyn Tiffany-Castiglioni

Contents

Contributors

MELVIN E. ANDERSEN • *Associate Professor, Department of Environmental and Radiological Sciences, College of Veterinary Medicine and Biomedical Sciences, Colorado State University, Ft. Collins, CO*

MICHAEL ASCHNER • *Professor, Department of Physiology and Pharmacology, Wake Forest University School of Medicine, Winston-Salem, NC*

GERALD J. AUDESIRK • *Professor, Department of Biology, University of Colorado at Denver, Denver, CO*

STANLEY BARONE, JR. • *Research Biologist, Cellular and Molecular Toxicology Branch, Neurotoxicology Division/NHEERL/ORD US Environmental Protection Agency, Research Triangle Park, NC*

RUTH E. BILLINGS • *Research Associate, Department of Environmental and Radiological Sciences, College of Veterinary Medicine and Biomedical Sciences, Colorado State University, Ft. Collins, CO*

CAROLYN BROCCARDO • *Research Assistant, Department of Environmental and Radiological Sciences, College of Veterinary Medicine and Biomedical Sciences, Colorado State University, Ft. Collins, CO*

LUCIO G. COSTA • *Professor, Department of Environmental and Occupational Health Sciences, University of Washington, Seattle, WA*

ROBERT K. DEARTH • *Technician I, Department of Veterinary Anatomy and Public Health, College of Veterinary Medicine, Texas A&M University, College Station, TX*

W. LES DEES • *Professor, Department of Veterinary Anatomy Public Health, College of Veterinary Medicine, Texas A&M University, College Station, TX*

DAVID C. DORMAN • *Director of the Division of Biological Sciences, CIIT Centers for Health Research, Research Triangle Park, NC*

HEATHER D. DURHAM • *Professor, Department of Neurology and Neurosurgery, McGill University, Montreal Neurological Institute, Montreal, Quebec, Canada*

MARION EHRICH • *Professor, Virginia-Maryland Regional College of Veterinary Medicine, Blacksburg, VA*

CHRISTINE T. FRENCH • *Research Assistant, Department of Environmental and Radiological Sciences, College of Veterinary Medicine and Biomedical Sciences, Colorado State University, Ft. Collins, CO*

MARY E. GILBERT • *Assistant Professor, Neurotoxicology Division, US Environmental Protection Agency, Research Triangle Park, NC*

WILLIAM H. HANNEMAN • *Assistant Professor, Head of Toxicology Section, Department of Environmental and Radiological Sciences, College of Veterinary Medicine and Biomedical Sciences, Colorado State University, Ft. Collins, CO*

JILL K. HINEY • *Research Assistant Professor, Department of Veterinary Anatomy and Public Health, College of Veterinary Medicine, Texas A&M University, College Station, TX*

PAUL HONEGGER • *Professeur Associe, Institute of Physiology, University of Lausanne, Lausanne, Switzerland*

SID HUNTER • *Toxicologist, Reproductive Toxicology Division, US Environmental Protection Agency, Research Triangle Park, NC*

PRASADA R. S. KODAVANTI • *Research Toxicologist, Neurotoxicology Division, US Environmental Protection Agency, Research Triangle Park, NC*

STEPHEN M. LASLEY • *Professor, Department of Biomedical and Therapeutic Sciences, University of Illinois College of Medicine, Peoria, IL*

MARIE E. LEGARE • *Assistant Professor, Department of Environmental and Radiological Health Science, College of Veterinary Medicine and Biomedical Sciences, Colorado State University, Ft. Collins, CO*

TAMI S. MCMULLIN • *Research Assistant, Department of Environmental and Radiological Sciences, College of Veterinary Medicine and Biomedical Sciences, Colorado State University, Ft. Collins, CO*

MICHAEL W. MILLER • *Professor, Department of Neuroscience and Physiology, State University of New York-Upstate Medical University, Syracuse, NY*

FLORIANNE MONNET-TSCHUDI • *Maitre Assistant, Institute of Physiology, University of Lausanne, Lausanne, Switzerland*

WILLIAM R. MUNDY • *Research Toxicologist, Neurotoxicology Division, US Environmental Protection Agency, Research Triangle Park, NC*

YONGCHANG QIAN • *Research Assistant Professor, Department of Veterinary Anatomy and Public Health, College of Veterinary Medicine, Texas A&M University, College Station, TX*

BENOÎT SCHILTER • *Nestlé Research Centre, Vers-chez-les Blanc, Lausanne, Switzerland*

URSULA SONNEWALD • *Professor, Department of Clinical Neuroscience, Norwegian University of Science and Technology, Trondheim, Norway*

VINOD K. SRIVASTAVA • *Research Assistant Professor, Department of Veterinary Anatomy and Public Health, College of Veterinary Medicine, Texas A&M University, College Station, TX*

EVELYN TIFFANY-CASTIGLIONI • *Professor and Head, Department of Veterinary Anatomy and Public Health, Associate Dean for Undergraduate Education, College of Veterinary Medicine, Texas A&M University, College Station, TX*

RONALD B. TJALKENS • *Assistant Professor, Department of Veterinary Anatomy and Public Health, College of Veterinary Medicine, Texas A&M University, and Center for Environmental and Rural Health, College Station, TX*

LORI D. WHITE • *Biologist, Cellular and Molecular Toxicology Branch, Neurotoxicology Division, NHEERL/ORD US Environmental Protection Agency, Research Triangle Park, NC*

MARIE-GABRIELLE ZURICH • *Premiere Assistante, Institute of Physiology, University of Lausanne, Lausanne, Switzerland*

1

In Vitro Neurotoxicology

Introduction to Concepts

Evelyn Tiffany-Castiglioni

1. UTILITY OF IN VITRO SYSTEMS

The history of neuroscience is punctuated by oracular disclosures from in vitro systems. In 1907, a pivotal tissue culture study by Harrison proved that Ramón y Cajal's theory on the developmental origin of nerve fibers was correct. Cajal had proposed in 1890, based on microscopic analysis of static histologic tissue sections, that the immature neuronal cell body sends out an axon that elongates freely, bearing a motile growth cone at its tip. Competing theories held that free growth of neurites did not occur, but that the neurites formed from the fusion of elements produced by other cells or from the stretching of a protoplasmic bridge between central and peripheral cell bodies of a multinucleated cell *(1)*. These theories could not be tested by the histologic methods of the time, because axonal growth by a living neuron could not be directly observed. Harrison *(2)* pioneered a culture system for long-term microscopic observation of neuronal differentiation in living tadpole neural tube tissue. His observation that neurites grow out from cell bodies has been hailed as "one of the most revolutionary results in experimental biology" *(3)*.

Some 50 yr later, tissue culture provided the means for an advance of similar magnitude by Levi-Montalcini, Hamberger, and Cohen *(4,5)*, the discovery of nerve growth factor (NGF). NGF became the paradigm for the discovery of other growth and differentiation factors. These investigators used an in vitro chick ganglion bioassay to detect NGF in a variety of sources

From: *Methods in Pharmacology and Toxicology: In Vitro Neurotoxicology: Principles and Challenges*
Edited by: E. Tiffany-Castiglioni © Humana Press Inc., Totowa, NJ

1

suspected to harbor this heretofore undefined polypeptide. Neurons in the chick ganglion explants perceived the subtle presence of NGF in extracts of the S-180 mouse sarcoma, snake venom, and the male mouse submaxillary gland and extended neurites toward it. Thus, Levi-Montalcini's Nobel Prize address was published in the journal of the Tissue Culture Association *(6)*, with the recognition by its editor, Gordon Sato, that the award to Levi-Montalcini and Cohen was "an affirmation of the growing importance of cell culture in biological research."

Contemporary neuroscience has also profited extensively from tissue culture models, examples of which are the glial guidance theory for neuronal migration and the emerging appreciation of glial–neuronal signaling. The glial guidance theory, whereby radial glial cell processes provide a scaffold for the directed migration of postmitotic neurons during development, was hypothesized from painstaking morphological studies at both the light and electron microscopic levels by Rakic *(7–9)*. The theory gained support and mechanistic explication from the in vitro work of Hatten and colleagues *(10–12)*, who devised a cell culture system for the videomicroscopic examination of the migration of living cerebellar granule cells along the cytoplasmic "monorails" of radial glia. Among their many discoveries with this in vitro system has been the identity of cell–cell adhesion molecules, such as astrotactin *(13,14)*, with which neurons and glia interact to form a complex histoarchitecture. The emerging story of bidirectional communication between glia and neurons, including the requirement of astrocytes for synapse formation by neurons, is similarly founded upon cell culture work. Astrocytes apparently integrate and modulate neuronal synaptic transmission through intrinsic signaling properties discovered in cell culture models. Astrocytes exhibit Ca^{2+} excitability, functional neurotransmitter receptors that regulate intracellular Ca^{2+} concentrations, the ability to propagate $[Ca^{2+}]$ oscillations to neighboring cells through gap junctions, and the release of neuroactive transmitters to neurons (reviewed in refs. *15–17*). A major focus of current neurobiology is to confirm these tantalizing properties in intact tissues.

The achievements of in vitro neurotoxicology, to date, have been more modest, but its potential is still untold. With many technical improvements in imaging and molecular biology, in vitro neurotoxicology has become a major focus for understanding basic mechanisms of toxicant action. In time, it may form the basis for reliable, high-throughput screening systems for the neurotoxicity of new and untested chemicals. In order to develop in vitro neurotoxicology to a higher level of utility, its strengths must be exploited and its weaknesses overcome. Like oracles and like the classic experiments of Harrison, Levi-Montalcini, and Hatten, cell and tissue culture studies of neurotoxicity are, by themselves, abstract. They must be critically designed and interpreted in the context of biological complexity. In vitro studies offer the greatest insights to biology when they are performed in complement with in vivo experimentation.

The central theme of this book is that neuroscience and neurotoxicology exhibit a significant degree of alignment in the common ground of in vitro models. Alignment is visible in two areas. First, both disciplines recognize the need for valid in vitro models in which the biological significance of the end points measured and limitations of the model are well understood. Validity will be addressed in several chapters of this volume by comparisons between observations made in vivo and in vitro. Furthermore, contributing authors present underlying concepts and detailed commentary about the use of complementary in vivo/in vitro strategies. Second, the range of neurological diseases with a toxicologic component is expanding. Neurotoxicology may provide preliminary road maps for exploring the basis of some neurodevelopmental and neurodegenerative diseases. Evidence that neurotoxicology has advanced basic biomedical knowledge is beginning to emerge. Three selected examples in this volume are the concept of astroglia as depots for lead and possibly other metals in the central nervous system, the elucidation of factors involved in onset of puberty in females, and the exploration of endogenous proteins as neurotoxicants.

As an introduction to the ensuing chapters, this chapter will briefly describe several background topics: common neurotoxicants and their target cells, acute and accumulated damage from exposure to neurotoxicants, biological concepts in in vitro neurotoxicology and their interrelationships, trends in in vitro neurotoxicology, and general research needs.

2. NEUROTOXICANTS AND THEIR CELLULAR TARGETS

Common neurotoxicants selected for the focus of this book are organophosphorus pesticides, lead (Pb), methyl mercury, halogenated aromatic hydrocarbons (HAHs), and ethanol. Organophosphorus (OP) compounds represent the largest group of chemical insecticides in use throughout the world today *(18)*. In addition, OP compounds comprise a major portion of the US military stockpile of chemical nerve agents that include Tabun, sarin, soman, and VX. OPs cause potent neurotoxicological effects in humans and animals. Although the immediate, acute neurotoxic action of OPs is the inhibition of acetylcholinesterase (AChE), some OPs also produce a neurodegenerative disorder known as organophosphate-induced delayed neurotoxicity (OPIDN) with Wallerian-type degeneration of the axon and myelin *(19)*. Growing experimental and epidemiologic evidence suggests that OPs are developmental neurotoxicants as manifested by developmental delays and impaired cognitive function *(20–25)*. OPs will be a focus of Chapter 2 on risk assessment and Chapter 5 on apoptosis.

Lead ranks second of 275 substances on the ATSDR/EPA Priority List of Hazardous Substances for 2001 *(26)*. Despite an encouraging decline in both the number and severity of lead poisoning cases over the past 20 yr by the reduction of lead levels in gasoline and paint, lead continues to be a pervasive contaminant in the environment with significant health risks, causing developmental neurotoxicity in children manifested by cognitive deficits and increased aggression *(27,28)*. In addition, long-term occupational exposure to lead may be a risk factor in the development of Parkinson's disease *(29–32)*. The latter studies are suggestive but not conclusive, as they are small case studies or population-based case studies. The effects of lead and other toxicants on cellular homeostasis will be addressed in Chapter 4. In Chapters 7–9, the effects of lead on glia, neuritogenesis, and synaptic function, respectively, will be examined.

Mercury is another neurotoxic metal, with methylmercury (MeHg), inorganic mercury (Hg^+ and Hg^{+2}), and elemental mercury (Hg^0) of long-standing concern and ethyl mercury under recent scrutiny for possible health risks. MeHg is produced by bacteria exposed to inorganic mercury and concentrates in the aquatic food chain in edible fish *(33)*. MeHg is more likely to enter the primate nervous system than is inorganic mercury *(34)*. Toxic effects are most notable if exposure occurs when the nervous system is still developing. Cell division and migration are impaired in the prenatal human brain *(35,36)*, resulting severe brain damage from high exposure *(37,38)*, and deficits in motor and visuospatial function from lower exposure in children *(39–42)*. The ethyl mercury-containing preservative thiomersal (thimerosal) has been in use in the United States since the early 1930s. In 1999, the safety of this compound when administered to infants was questioned by the American Academy of Pediatrics and the United States Public Health Service and it is no longer used by manufacturers for vaccines administered in the United States *(43)*. However, the first reported study that specifically examined mercury levels in American infants given vaccinations containing thiomersal suggests that this metal is eliminated rapidly from blood via stools *(44)*. Larger studies that measure end points in addition to mercury clearance are needed. In Chapters 5, 6, and 8, contributors will address the effects of methylmercury on apoptosis, neurotransmitter metabolism, and neurite extension, respectively.

Other neurotoxicants to be considered are high-molecular-weight HAHs, such as polychlorinated biphenyls (PCBs) and polychlorinated dibenzodioxins (PCDDs). These lipophilic compounds persist in the environment and accumulate in the food chain, with potential risks to human health, including immunotoxicity and cancer *(45,46)*. Intellectual impairment has been reported in children exposed to PCBs *in utero (47)*. Gestational and lactational exposure also alters neurobehavior and neurodevelopment in monkeys *(48)* and rats *(49)*. Although PCBs and PCDDs apparently elicit most of their toxic and biochemical effects through signal transduction involving the aryl hydrocarbon receptor (AhR) *(45)*, alternative mechanisms have been suggested in cell culture *(50–53)* and brain slice studies *(54)*. In addition, HAHs may alter cognitive function by indirect effects upon the endocrine system *(55)*. The example of 2,3,7,8-tetrachlorodioxin-*p*-dioxin, a paradigmatic planar HAH and strong AhR agonist, is used in Chapter 3 to illustrate emerging ideas in toxicogenomics.

Ethanol is a teratogen and a neuroendocrine disruptor. Ethanol consumption during pregnancy is associated with reduced neurogenesis, cell death, decreased neuronal migration, impaired axonal and dendritic arboraization, and abnormal astroglial development in the fetus and neonate *(56–58)*. Fetal alcohol syndrome is characterized by cognitive functional deficits, reduced brain weight, and other congenital malformations *(59)*. Furthermore, alcohol use and abuse by human adolescents may disrupt endocrine function. The possibility for alcohol use to alter the secretion of puberty-related hormones in human adolescents has not been evaluated, but studies in rats have shown that ethanol ingestion delays female puberty and alters levels of puberty-related hormones *(60–62)*. Ethanol ingestion also suppresses the increased secretion of puberty-related hormones in the developing female rhesus monkey and affects the development of a regular menstrual pattern *(63)*. Contributors will consider the induction of apoptosis by ethanol in Chapter 5 and will address the effects of ethanol on cell–cell interactions in aggregating cell cultures in Chapter 10. The complementary use of in vitro and in vivo techniques to provide important insights into the effects of ethanol (ETOH) on the neuroendocrinology of puberty will be addressed in Chapter 11.

Each of the above-mentioned exogenous toxicants has been studied extensively in vivo and in vitro. These neurotoxicants can therefore serve as models for the design and interpretation of future studies with other neurotoxicants. Endogenous proteins are also implicated in neurodegerative diseases, among them the β-amyloid protein in Alzheimer's disease *(64–66)* and α-synuclein in Parkinson's disease *(67,68)*. Therefore, the toxicity of the endogenous proteins in the brain will be addressed in Chapter 12.

The contributors to this book will examine the molecular, pathological, and functional responses of the major cells of the mammalian nervous system to common neurotoxicants, with emphasis on the central nervous system (brain and spinal cord). All types of brain cell can be primary or secondary targets for damage by neurotoxic substances, particularly when viewed in a temporal context. Neurons, which are of neuroectodermal origin, are the signaling cells of the nervous system. Neurons are responsible for the perception of sensory stimuli and the coordination of cellular, tissue, and organismal responses to stimuli from the environment. Among the possible effects of neurotoxicants on neurons are apoptosis or necrosis of neuronal stem cells in both the developing and mature brain, impaired neuronal migration (a secondary effect of damage to radial glia), and impaired synaptogenesis or synaptic function. Some manifestations of neuronal effects are developmental or late-onset cognitive, a sensory or motor dysfunction. Toxic effects on neurons will be addressed in Chapters 5–10.

Neuronal function and nervous tissue structure require the participation of neuroglia, or glia. The three main types of neuroglia in the central nervous system are astroglia, oligodendroglia, and microglia. Astroglia and oligodendroglia, like neurons, are of neuroectodermal origin. Astroglia participate in neurotransmitter metabolism and respond to stress and injury. Radial glia and Bergmann glia, two specialized types of astroglia, provide scaffolding for neuronal migration during development. Astroglia and radial glia may respond to toxicants by disruption of radial glial scaffolding in the developing nervous system, gliosis or glial activation, altered metabolism (e.g., activation of protective mechanisms against oxidative damage to brain), and, possibly, glial tumor formation. Oligodendroglia myelinate axons in the central nervous system. Their counterparts in the peripheral nervous system are Schwann cells. Toxic effects on oligodendroglia may include demyelination, apoptosis succeeded by proliferation, and loss of oligodendroglial progenitor cells. Toxic effects on astroglia, oligodendroglia, and Schwann cells will be addressed in Chapters 6, 7, and 10. Microglia, which are the only glia of mesenchymal origin, mediate inflammatory responses in the central nervous system *(69)*. Microglia have received little attention as primary targets for neurotoxicants but have been viewed as reactive cells. Activated microglia may have a pathogenic role in neurodegenerative diseases, such as dopaminergic cell injury in Parkinson's disease, based on elevated levels of cytokines, a plausible but largely untested hypothesis *(70)*. Recently, several studies have appeared that investigate the underappreciated importance of microglia in neurotoxic processes. Two of these studies *(71–73)* are identified in Table 1, which surveys in vitro systems of increasing complexity and provides selected references of their use for in vitro neurotoxicology in the past few years. Also, the use of aggregating cell cultures that contain neurons, oligodendroglia, astroglia, and microglia for the comparative analysis of several neurotoxicants, including OPs, trimethyl tin, and methylmercury, is described in Chapter 10.

Cells of the central nervous system directly interact with other cell types, notably the endothelial cells that compose the blood–brain barrier. The blood–brain barrier should be considered in two respects when discussing neurotoxicity: the transport of toxicants across it to the brain parenchyma and the direct effects of toxicants on the integrity of the barrier. Although the dependence of cerebral endothelial cells on astrocytes for differentiation of signals is well established *(114–116)*, the blood–brain barrier itself has rarely been the direct subject of neurotoxicity studies in vitro. This situation may be improved by the development in several laboratories of selectively permeable blood–brain barrier models in culture *(117)*. One promising but technically difficult and costly approach is to culture cells intraluminally or extraluminally on microporous hollow fibers in a perfusion system. Both astroglia alone *(118)* and astroglia with endothelial cells have been cultured in these types of vessels *(119)*.

3. PARADIGM OF ACCUMULATED DAMAGE

Toxic damage to the brain must be considered in a temporal context to include both acute and cumulative damage. Unless reversible, the processes that occur after toxic exposure as the cell, tissue, or organism degenerates from a state of health to a state of irreversible damage or death form a chronological continuum. The value of thinking about toxic effects in the context of time is that one can separately consider the effects of several variables on the outcome: dose (lethal or sublethal; one time or repeated), developmental age at time(s) of exposure, secondary effects resulting from primary damage, and plasticity and repair in the nervous system. Acute effects occur shortly after exposure to a neurotoxicant and are by definition severe enough to be observed in the organism. In general, acute toxicity refers to cytotoxicity, massive brain damage, and perhaps death from high exposure to the toxicant. Thus, the acute effects of high methylmercury exposure on the developing brain are encephalopathy, neuronal necrosis, seizures, and death or severe brain damage *(37,38)*. Cumulative damage, on the other hand, reflects incremental, sublethal effects of neurotoxicants on target cells and tissues. The cumulative, often latent, effects of neurotoxicants are more poorly understood, and likely more prevalent, than the acute effects.

The temporal context is more important in the immature than the mature nervous system because the former must establish a complex histoarchitecture

Table 1

Examples of In Vitro Neurotoxicity Studies with Models of Increasing Complexity

Model Type	Example	Selected study	Ref.
Cell lines			
Neuroblastoma	SK-N-SH-SY5Y human neuroblastoma cells	Induction of apoptosis by organophosphorus insecticides	74
	SK-N-SH-SY5Y human neuroblastoma cells differentiated with nerve growth factor (NGF)	Inhibition of neurite outgrowth by mipafox but not by paraoxon; disruption of Ca homeostasis by paraoxon	75
	SK-N-SH-SY5Y human neuroblastoma cells	Utility of this cell line for the study of SNARE protein function in norepinephrine release and insensitivity of cell line to botulism toxins	76
Pheochromocytoma	PC-12 rat pheochromocytoma cells differentiated with NGF	Inhibition of neurite outgrowth by mipafox but not by chlorpyrifos oxon	77
	PC-12 rat pheochromocytoma cells differentiated with NGF	Inhibition of differentiation by chlorpyrifos	78
	PC-12 rat pheochromocytoma cells differentiated with NGF	Cocaine inhibition of neuronal differentiation independent of ras signaling	79
	PC-12 rat pheochromocytoma cells primed or unprimed with NGF	Alteration of neural differentiation and Sp1 DNA binding by lead	80
	PC-12 rat pheochromocytoma cells primed or unprimed with NGF	Inhibition of neurite outgrowth by mipafox but not by sublethal levels of methyl mercury	81
	PC-12 rat pheochromocytoma cells primed or unprimed with NGF	Effects of prolonged exposure to nanomolar concentrations of methylmercury on voltage-sensitive sodium and calcium currents in PC-12 cells	82
Neuronal cell line	SN4741 nigral dopaminergic clonal cell line derived from transgenic mouse embryos containing the targeted expression for SV40Tag	Neuroprotection against 1-methyl-4-phenylpyridinium, glutamate, and nitric oxide-induced neurotoxicity by exogenous brain-derived neurotrophic factor	83
	SN4741 nigral dopaminergic cell line	Induction of the endoplasmic reticulum-localized protein chaperone glucose regulated protein 78 kDa (GRP78) and caspases by manganese	84
Glioma	C6 rat glioma	Induction of GRP78 by lead	85
	C6 rat glioma	Inhibition of cAMP-induced differentiation by 2,3,7,8-tetrachlorodibenzo-*p*-dioxin (TCDD)	86

Astrocytoma	1321 N1 human astroctyoma	Inhibition of carbachol-induced proliferation via M3 muscarinic acetylcholine receptors by ethanol; specific signaling pathways	87
	C6 rat glioma, 1321 N1 human astroctyoma, neonatal rat primary astroglia	Evaluation of multiple astrocytic systems for ability to identify substances known to be gliotoxic in vivo	88
Immortalized microglial cells	N9 murine microglial cell line	Potentiation of nitric oxide production by N9 cells by manganese, but not other transition metals	71
Primary cell cultures			
Neuron-enriched cultures	Developing cultures of rat primary cortical neurons	Demonstration that a toxicant (PCBs) can affect multiple aspects of calcium signaling from the plasma membrane to the nucleus.	89
	Fetal rat cerebellar granule cells	Translocation of protein kinase C (PKC) isoforms α and ε by nonplanar but not planar PCB	90
	Dissociated cerebellar cells of 10-d-old mice	Enhancement of lead entry into cerebellar neurons by lipopolysaccharide and interleukin-6	91
	Fetal rat hippocampal neurons	Increased branching of axons and dendrites by nanomolar concentrations of nicotine but not its metabolite cotinine	92
	Fetal rat hippocampal neurons	Demonstration by patch clamping that nominal nanomolar concentrations of Pb^{2+} decreased tetrodotoxin-sensitive, Ca^{2+}-dependent glutamate and GABA release	93
	Embryonic chick forebrain neurons	Inhibition of axonal morphogenesis by methylmercury not due to cell death or microtubule disassembly	94
Pituitary cells	Primary rat anterior pituitary cells	Stimulation of adrenocorticotropic hormone secretion by TCDD via aryl hydrocarbon (Ah) receptor	95
Astroglia	Neonatal rat primary astroglial cultures	Microarray analysis of differential gene expression in lead-exposed astroglia	96
	Transiently transfected rat primary astroglial cultures	Increased resistance to methylmercury-induced cytotoxicity in neonatal rat primary astrocyte cultures and astrocytoma cells overexpressing metallothionein (MT)-I	97
	Transiently transfected rat primary astroglial cultures	Increased protection against acute methylmercury cytotoxicity in MT-I and -II null astrocytes by transient transfection with foreign MT-I	98

continues

Table 1 (*Continued*)
Examples of In Vitro Neurotoxicity Studies with Models of Increasing Complexity

Model Type	Example	Selected study	Ref.
Oligodendroglia	Neonatal rat oligodendrocyte progenitor cells	Inhibition by lead of proliferation and differentiation of oligodendrocyte lineage cells in vitro through a mechanism requiring PKC activation	99
	Neonatal rat primary cultures	Cytotoxicity of β-amyloid peptide to oligodendroglia	100
Schwann cells	Neonatal rat sciatic nerve primary cultures	Greater sensitivity of Schwann cells than astrocytes to lead-induced cytotoxicity	101
Adrenal medullary cells	Permeabilized chromaffin cells	Use of free-ion concentrations to support multiple binding sites for Pb^{2+} on the C PKC enzyme, indicating that Pb^{2+} is a partial agonist capable of both activation and inhibition.	102
Transfected primary cells	Xenopus oocytes expressing various rat nicotinic aceylcholine receptor subunits	Analysis of species- and receptor-type diversity in neurotoxic responses to the insecticide WL 145004 and lead	103
Systems with heterogeneous cell interactions			
Heterologous conditioned medium	Cerebellar rat granule cells cultured in conditioned medium from C6 cells transfected with glial maturation factor (GMF)	Demonstration that conditioned medium from C6 cells overexpressing but not secreting GMF protected cerebellar granule cells from ethanol toxicity	104
	Cultures of primary neonatal rat astroglia in conditioned medium of other cells	Stimulation of intracellular lead accumulation by conditioned medium from SY5Y cells but not cerebellar endothelial cells	105
Bicameral cultures	Cocultures of rat astroglial primaries and SH-SY5Y human neuroblastoma cells in a Millipore® semi-permeable membrane system	Selective accumulation of Pb by astroglia compared to SY5Y cells from shared medium containing Pb	105
Mixed-cell cultures	Primary neonatal rat hippocampal neurons and astroglia	Disruption of gap junctional communication from astroglia to neurons by 2,3,7,8-TCDD	53
	Primary neonatal rat cotical astroglial and fetal hippocampal neuronal cultures	Inhibition of uptake of cystine into astrocytes but not neurons by methylmercury	106
	Rat primary mesencephalic mixed neuron/glia cultures	Pivotal role of microglia in the selective degeneration of dopaminergic neurons in cultures treated with the herbicide rotenone	72

	Mixed postnatal rat primary glial cultures	Role of proinflammatory cytokines in the trimethyl tin-induced glial response through experimental modulation	73
Aggregating cultures	Reaggregates of dispersed cells from fetal rat brain	Maturation-dependent effects of chlorpyrifos and parathion and their oxon derivatives on acetylcholinesterase activity	107
Nervous tissue explants	Embryonic rat cerebral cortex	Inhibition by ethanol of neuronal migration and abnormal distribution of neuronal cell adhesion molecule	108
Brain slices	Adolescent to adult rat hippocampal slices	Congener-specific suppression of CA1 field excitatory postsynaptic potential by halogenated aromatic hydrocarbons	54
Isolated cells			
Acutely isolated neurons	Rat retinal ganglion cells	Demonstration that rod mitochondria are the target site for Ca^{2+}- and Pb^{2+}-induced apoptosis and that these ions bind to the internal metal binding site of the permeability transition pore	109
Acutely isolated astrocytes	Rat astrocytes from postnatal age 1–35 d	Closer resemblance of acutely isolated cells than primary cultures to *in situ* preparations with regard to metabotropic glutamate receptor expression	110
Ex vivo preparations from toxicant-treated animals			
Radial glia	Radial glial primary cultures from ethanol treated and control 13-d-old rat fetuses	Delay of expression of glial fibrillary acidic protein by prenatal ethanol exposure (in vivo/ex vivo correlation)	111
Brain slices	Hippocampal slices from rats exposed during gestation or lactation to lead	Enhancement of phorbol ester-stimulated PKC translocation	112
	Hippocampal slices from adult rats exposed during development to lead	Increased inhibitory actions of acute ethanol exposure in vitro on slices from lead-treated rats	113

with neural connections that are reinforced by synaptic activity. The histoarchitecture depends on interactions between neurons and glia for neuronal migration. Therefore, the developing nervous system is exquisitely sensitive to damage by several well-known neurotoxicants, such as lead *(27)*, methylmercury *(43)*, and ethanol *(120)*, with various types of damage accruing in each critical period of development. The temporal context also includes repair through nervous tissue regeneration and/or plasticity and resistance or adaptation through the induction of cellular protective mechanisms.

Figure 1 illustrates a chronological continuum for radiation-induced toxicity in the adult brain. Radiation was chosen because its cellular effects are somewhat more temporally distinct than the patterns seen with many other toxic exposures. Classically, radiation-induced injury to the central nervous system progresses through three phases: acute, early delayed, and late delayed (reviewed in ref. *121*). Acute and early-delayed injury may be severe, but are typically considered reversible in medical radiotherapy protocols. Late-delayed effects are irreversible and are characterized by demyelination and necrosis of white matter, which implies primary damage to oligodendroglia and the vascular system. Figure 1 shows a progression of the nervous system from health to permanent damage or death. Early effects of exposure to X-rays may include death of immature and proliferating cells, such as oligodendroglia progenitors, astroglia and radial glia, and neuronal progenitors. These effects are extremely significant in the developing brain in which cells are actively proliferating. Our appreciation of the importance of loss of progenitor cells in the adult brain may grow as our knowledge of the role of these cells in neural regeneration and plasticity increases. It is plausible that progression may be slowed or reversed by the induction of protective, adaptative, or repair mechanisms within the brain tissue. A later effect of toxic damage to the brain may be the activation of astroglia and microglia, producing scarring and oxidative damage from cytokines. Temporally, the last cumulative effect of radiation damage on the adult brain may be sublethal, functional damage to terminally differentiated cells, including mature neurons and mature astroglia.

The speed at which damage begins and progresses through the continuum depends on interactions of many factors, such as toxicant, dose, developmental stage of the nervous system, and relative vulnerability of various cell types. Various toxic insults would have different patterns of progression through this sequence. For example, oligodendroglia and neurons are more sensitive to lead than are astroglia, and astroglia apparently have the ability to resist or adapt to high amounts of intracellular lead *(122)*. On the other hand, ethanol and radiation produce very similar patterns of damage to the fetal brain *(111,120,123,124)*.

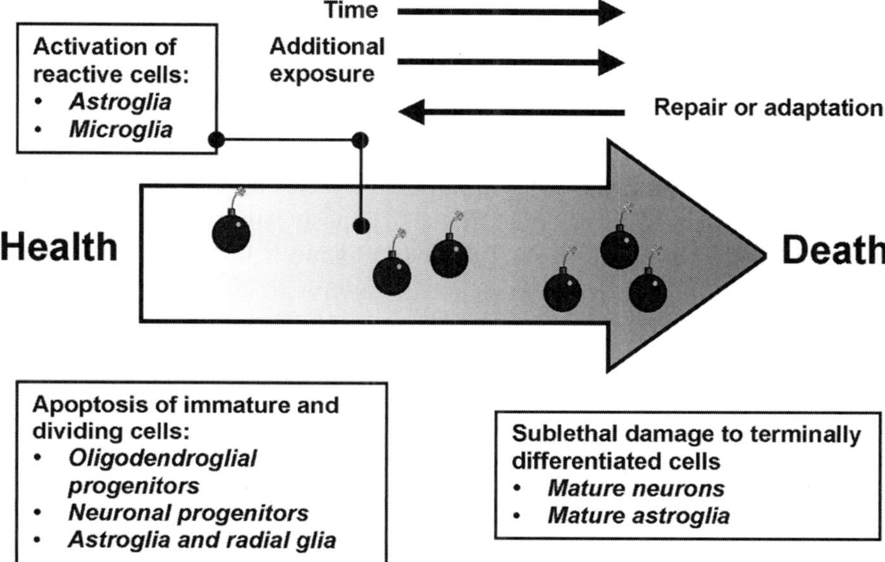

Fig. 1. Chronological continuum of neurotoxic events in the mammalian nervous system following X-ray exposure. The large arrow represents progressive damage (accumulation of bomb symbols) from a state of nonexposure or health to permanent injury or death. Driving the arrow forward are time (because of cumulative degenerative effects subsequent to the initial damage) and additional exposure. Driving the arrow backward is repair or plasticity. Immediate effects of X-irradiation are DNA damage and apoptosis of proliferating cells, such as neuronal and glial progenitor cells, in both the immature and mature brain, as well as dividing glia in the immature brain. A subsequent reactive response to cell death or damage is gliosis and microglial activation. A possible cumulative effect of radiation damage to the mature brain is damage of neural networks that exceeds the capacity of neuronal plasticity and redundancy to confer full restoration of function. This model could be adapted for other types of neurotoxic exposure.

4. INTERACTING FACETS OF IN VITRO NEUROTOXICOLOGY

The underlying principles of in vitro neurotoxicology can be expressed as the interactions of four fundamental factors or facets: exposure (concentration, duration of exposure, and pattern of exposure, as well as coexposure with other toxic insults), target of damage (molecules, cells, tissues, and secondary targets), physiology (functional significance of target cells, interactions of the toxic insult with the cell surface, cytoplasm, and DNA), and the toxic insult itself (e.g., heavy metals or pesticides). These factors are depicted as the faces of a flattened tetrahedron in Fig. 2. Although each of these four factors is extremely important in itself as an underlying concept of neurotoxicology, the convergence of each facet with the other three is equally important. One might think of the six edges of the tetrahedron as illustrative of additional critical issues: end points, mechanisms, bioavailability, bioaccumulation, susceptibility, and metabolism. Thus, the intersection of exposure and target is end points, and the intersection of target and physiology is mechanisms. The following brief discussion of these two intersections will serve to highlight their significance in the context of in vitro neurotoxicology.

Structural, functional, genetic, and biochemical end points can be measured in vitro in both early and latent phases of neurotoxicity, but only within the limitations of the in vitro system used. In vitro systems do not lend themselves well to long-term studies that would parallel the life-span of the exposed organism or half-life of the toxic substance in brain tissue. The useful life of various in vitro preparations ranges from hours to several weeks *(125)*. For example, viable tissue slices can be maintained for a period of hours and primary cell cultures for days to weeks. Immortalized cell cultures have been maintained for decades, such as C6 rat glioma cells *(126,127)* and SY5Y human neuroblastoma cells *(128,129)*. Belying their name, however, such cultures do not provide an opportunity for long-term exposures to toxic chemicals. Because of their short population doubling times, immortalized cell lines require frequent passaging, which temporarily disrupts both cell attachment and cell–cell interactions and adds a confounding factor to long-term studies. Examples of neural cultures with extended longevity are aggregating cell cultures *(130)*, and hollow fiber perfusion cultures *(118)*, which can be maintained functionally intact for 2 or 3 mo.

Clarification of the meaning of the term "mechanism" in culture systems can illustrate how intricately it is tied to other facets of neurotoxicology. Shown in Fig. 2 is a definition of mechanism as the intersection between target and physiology, which is a contextually rich framework in which to consider this concept. Mechanism is not merely the molecular or cellular entities acted upon by the toxic substance; it is also the associated perturbations in physiology. Examples include the disruption of normal synaptic overproduction and pruning by exposure during development, impairment of plasticity and repair, and altered synaptic function. Each of these physiological processes has molecular components amenable to examination. In the case of synaptic function, these include the molecular interactions involved in presynaptic neurotransmitter release, postsynaptic receptor function, and postsynaptic intracellular signaling. Each of these effects could be studied in a detailed fashion in vitro with validation in vivo. Therefore, mechanism is a critical link for validation of in vitro results.

The manner in which the above 10 interacting facets (*see* Fig. 2) of in vitro neurotoxicology translate into concepts is a work in progress that will be considered in depth throughout this book. The basic principle of toxicology that the dose makes the poison, as formulated by the early 16th-century physician Paracelsus, can be directly applied at the level of molecular and cellular processes in vitro. A preliminary list of essential concepts reflecting this utility of in vitro toxicology is as follows:

- Each toxicant has unique chemical properties that govern its toxicity, such as solubility in biological environments and affinity for specific biomolecules.
- The toxicity of an agent is modulated by its bioavailability to target cells, as well as by the inherent phenotypic and genotypic sensitivity of the target cells to the agent.
- The operative dose is modified chemically by the solubility and binding properties of the toxicant in the extracellular and intracellular milieus.
- The operative dose is modified biologically by the degree of biodegradation, cytosolic buffering, and/or metabolism of the toxicant.
- Target cells interact dynamically to form structural and functional components of complex nervous tissues. Therefore, toxic actions upon them are likely to produce secondary effects on the cells with which they interact.

5. TRENDS IN IN VITRO NEUROTOXICOLOGY

Much current work with in vitro systems for neurotoxicity testing lies in maximizing their potential for yielding valid mechanistic responses. Experimental systems for the mechanistic understanding of toxicant-induced damage to the nervous system are often reductionist in nature in order to increase the specificity and sensitivity of end points measured. In vitro models offer many advantages for neurotoxicity assessment that have been described in detail elsewhere *(131,132)*. Among these advantages are the option to study a single cell type of interest in the absence of other cell types, ease of direct observation and measurement of cellular responses to toxicants, a defined extracellular environment, and direct interactions of the toxicant with test cells. Furthermore, in vitro systems may offer the economic benefit of a reduced requirement for test chemicals, although in general this potential benefit has not yet been realized.

On the other hand, conceptual weaknesses are inherent in reductionist systems. In vitro systems lack the capacity to assess behavioral end points, which is the major outcome of concern to neurotoxicologists. Lacking this ability, the value of in vitro systems lies in their potential capacity to respond mechanistically to a toxicant in a manner similar to that occurring from in

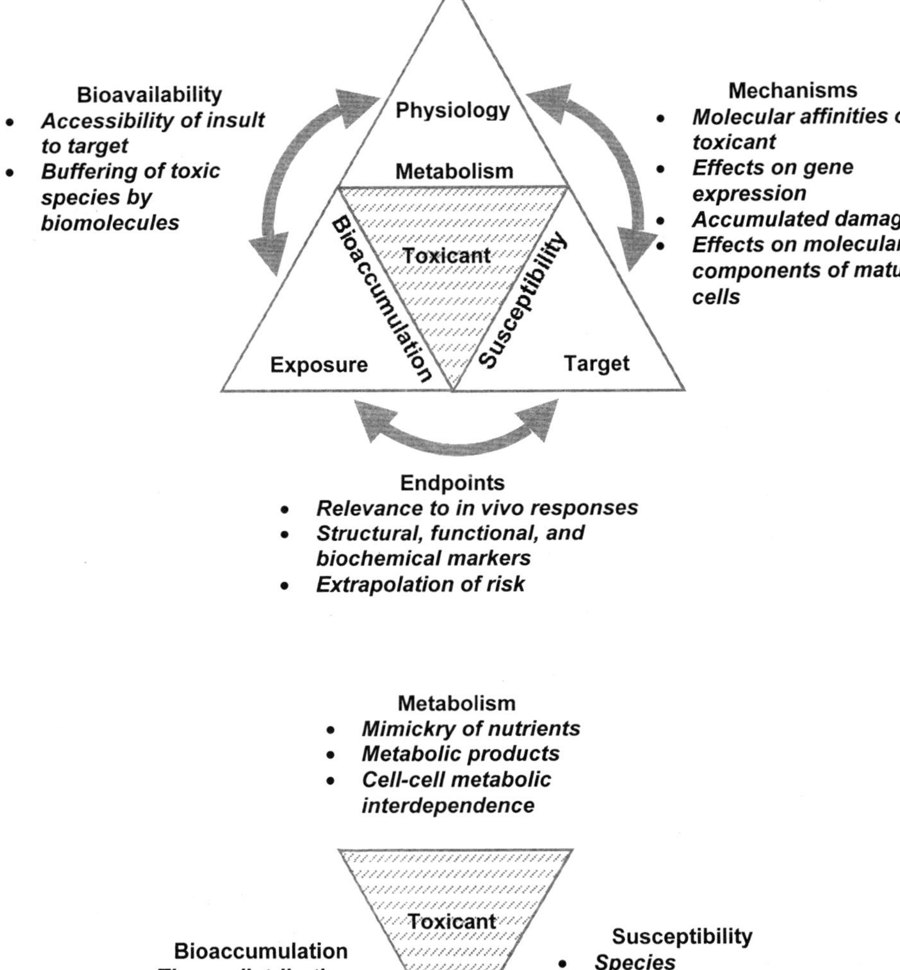

Fig. 2. Converging facets of in vitro toxicology. Four major concepts or issues concerning in vitro toxicology are depicted in this drawing as faces of a flattened tetrahedron: *toxicant* (OP, heavy metal, PCB, ethanol, etc.) *exposure* (concentration, route, pattern, coexposure with other toxicants), *target* (molecules, cells, tissues, organs; primary vs secondary targets), and *physiology* (interactions of the toxicant with cell–cell communication, cell surface receptors, cytoplasmic organelles, ions, signaling pathways, and nucleic acids). A tetrahedron has six edges where each face intersects with the other three. The interfaces between each two

vivo exposure. Furthermore, in vitro systems have limited (although expandable) capacities for mimicking heterogeneous cell–cell interactions, systemic endocrine control, or metabolism of xenobiotics. Additionally, appropriate age and developmental stage of the nervous system at the time of exposure have been extremely difficult to approximate in culture, to the point of disregarding the effects of experience and learning on the developing nervous system. Technical improvement should be possible in most of these areas. Improvement can also come from continuous re-evaluation of the concept of toxicity testing in vitro. In this regard, well-designed complementary in vivo/in vitro approaches offer the promise to accelerate progress toward both an understanding of the mechanistic effects of neurotoxicity and the development of in vitro models for extrapolating risk.

Four major trends in in vitro neurotoxicology address these needed improvements and will be discussed in greater detail by other chapters in this volume. The first trend is the refinement of end points. One of the critical decisions in the design of in vitro assays is the selection of appropriate end points, which must be relevant to in vivo responses. Whereas older studies focused on cytotoxicity, newer studies are increasingly mechanism driven, with careful selection of functional end points that are relevant to in vivo effects of the toxicant. This approach is expected to allow the fine dissection of biochemical mechanisms of toxicity. A second trend reflects the use of more histotypic, tissuelike culture systems for certain types of study. This trend counterbalances three decades of work on clonal cell lines that has dominated much of modern in vitro toxicology. Clonal cell lines have been the system of choice for many studies because they are well characterized, easy to culture, and homogeneous in their responses to toxicants. Such cell lines still have considerable value for specific applications, as will be described in several chapters. However, wide morphological and functional heterogeneities exist in both neurons and glia, so that toxic chemicals do not uniformly affect each member of a class of cells. Researchers are returning to the use of biologically more complex models, such as heterologous cell cultures, explants, and ex vivo tissue slices from toxicant-exposed animals. Their use is supported by improvements in analytical techniques that make

---

juxtaposed faced are labeled to illustrate six additional concepts of in vitro neurotoxicology: *bioavailability* of the toxicant, biological *end points* that change as a result of toxic exposure, *mechanisms* of toxic action, *bioaccumulation* of the toxicant, *susceptibility* of the target to toxic damage, and *metabolism* of the toxic agent. Each of these concepts is mentioned briefly in the text and will be addressed in detail in subsequent chapters.

single cells accessible to measurement, such as interactive laser cytometry *(89,133,134)*. Table 1 provides examples of both simple and complex biological models used for in vitro neurotoxiciology in recent years.

The third and fourth trends are sophisticated extensions of reductionist systems that will demand interdisciplinary innovation to achieve. The third trend is a renewed emphasis on validation. Two problems have been pervasive regarding validation of in vitro systems. One is the delivery of toxicologically relevant concentrations of chemicals to target cells at appropriate times. The other is that the developmental relevance of some in vitro systems, such as cell culture, is very limited at this time. Attempts are being made through toxicodynamics, improved culture methods, and methodical comparisons with in vivo systems to deal with these issues *(135,136)*. The fourth trend is toward new applications for in vitro neurotoxicity testing. Although in vitro screening of possible or suspected neurotoxicants remains an important goal of in vitro neurotoxicologists, other applications are also becoming apparent, especially the development of mechanism-based therapies for toxic exposure. Cell and tissue culture systems may expedite the development and testing of pharmacologic or molecular therapies to ameliorate the effects of neurotoxicants on brain cell function.

6. GENERAL RESEARCH NEEDS

The following is a list of essential research objectives for in vitro neurotoxicology. This list is applicable to organophosphorus compounds, heavy metals, radiation, ethanol, aromatic hydrocarbons, and endogenous neurotoxic proteins in a general sense, although subsequent chapters in the book will illustrate toxicant-specific contemporary approaches and needs. Major areas are as follows:

- Mechanistic integration of any known behavioral effects of the toxicant with its molecular and cellular substrates
- Molecular, physiologic, and morphologic effects of neurotoxicants on synaptogenesis, neuronal plasticity, and regeneration
- Complete chronological effects of neurotoxicants on tumorigenesis in brain
- Differences in sensitivity between immature and mature cells of all types (neurons, oligodendroglia, astroglia, and microglia) to neurotoxicants
- Interactions among neurotoxicants

Each of these areas is quite broad and most of them are still in early stages of investigation. Furthermore, progress in these areas is heavily dependent on progress in basic and applied neuroscience and will be facilitated by close interdisciplinary collaborations. Addressing these and similar issues should provide significant advances in identifying, treating, and preventing diseases and functional impairments associated with neurotoxic exposures.

Neurotoxicology has already made contributions that advance basic biomedical knowledge, as will be discussed in this book. In the future, in vitro systems will offer insight into how genetic polymorphisms affect susceptibility to diseases induced by environmental contaminants. As a platform for examining genetic susceptibility, in vitro neurotoxicology may become not only a central approach for risk assessment but also for understanding commonalities between neurodegenerative diseases caused by chemicals in the environment and those caused by endogenous proteins.

ACKNOWLEDGMENTS

The author's work is supported by National Institutes of Health grants P42 ES04917, P30 ES09106, and T32 ES07273 and by ATSDR grant U61/ATU684505. I gratefully acknowledge helpful comments by Dr. Marion Ehrich, Dr. Stephen Lasley, Dr. A. Joseph Castiglioni, and Dr. Michael Aschner on earlier drafts of this manuscript. I also thank these investigators and Dr. William Mundy, Dr. Stanley Barone, and Dr. Gerald Audesirk for recommendations on Table 1.

REFERENCES

1. Ramón y Cajal, S. (1991) *Recollections of My Life* (Craig, E. H. and Cano, J., transl.), The MIT Press, Cambridge, MA.
2. Harrison, R. G. (1907) Observations on the living developing nerve fiber. *Anat. Rec.* **1,** 116–118.
3. Shephard, G. M. (1994) *Neurobiology*, 3rd ed. Oxford University Press. New York.
4. Levi-Montalcini, R., Meyer, H., and Hamburger, V. (1954) In vitro effects of mouse sarcomas 180 and 37 on the spinal and sympathetic ganglia of the chick embryo. *Cancer Res.* **14,** 49–57.
5. Cohen, S., Levi-Montalcini, R., and Hamburger V. (1954) A nerve growth-stimulating factor isolated from sarcomas 37 and 180. *Proc. Natl. Acad. Sci. USA* **40,** 1014–1018.
6. Levi-Montalcini, R. (1987) The nerve growth factor thirty-five years later. *In Vitro Cell. Dev. Biol.* **23,** 227–238.
7. Rakic, P. (1971) Neuron-glia relationship during granule cell migration in developing cerebellar cortex. A Golgi and electronmicroscopic study in Macacus Rhesus. *J. Comp. Neurol.* **141,** 283–312.
8. Rakic, P. (1972) Mode of cell migration to the superficial layers of fetal monkey neocortex. *J. Comp. Neurol.* **145,** 61–83.
9. Rakic, P. (1978) Neuronal migration and contact guidance in the primate telencephalon. *Postgrad. Med. J.* **54(Suppl. 1),** 25–40.

10. Edmondson, J. C. and Hatten, M. E. (1987) Glial-guided granule neuron migration in vitro: a high-resolution time-lapse video microscopic study. *J. Neurosci.* **7(6)**, 1928–1934.
11. Hatten, M. E. (1993) The role of migration in central nervous system neuronal development. *Curr. Opin. Neurobiol.* **3**, 38–44.
12. Hatten, M. E. (1999) Central nervous system neuronal migration. *Annu. Rev. Neurosci.* **22**, 511–539.
13. Edmondson, J. C., Liem, R. K., Kuster, J. E., and Hatten, M. E. (1988) Astrotactin: a novel neuronal cell surface antigen that mediates neuron-astroglial interactions in cerebellar microcultures. *J. Cell. Biol.* **106**, 505–517.
14. Adams, N. C., Tomoda, T., Cooper, M., Dietz, G., and Hatten, M. E. (2002) Mice that lack astrotactin have slowed neuronal migration. *Development* **129(Suppl.)**, 965–972.
15. Carmignoto, G. (2000) Reciprocal communication systems between astrocytes and neurones. *Prog. Neurobiol.* **62**, 561–581.
16. Bezzi, P. and Volterra, A. (2001) A neuron-glia signalling network in the active brain. *Curr. Opin. Neurobiol.* **11**, 387–394.
17. Araque, A., Carmignoto, G., and Haydon, P. G. (2001) Dynamic signaling between astrocytes and neurons. *Annu. Rev. Physiol.* **63**, 795–813.
18. National Research Council, Committee on Alternative Chemical Demilitarization Technologies (CACDT). (1993) *Alternative Technologies for the Destruction of Chemical Agents and Munitions*, Board on Army Science and Technology, Commission on Engineering and Technical Systems, National Academy of Sciences, Washington, DC.
19. Ecobichon, D. J. (1991) Toxic effects of pesticides, in *Casarett and Doull's Toxicology: The Basic Science of Poisons* (Amdur, M.O., Doull, J., and Klaassen, C.D., eds.), Pergamon, New York, pp. 565–622.
20. Pope, A. M., Heavner, J. E, Guarnieri, J. A., and Knobloch, C.P. (1986) Trichlorfon-induced congenital cerebellar hypoplasia in neonatal pigs. *J. Am. Vet. Med. Assoc.* **189**, 781–783.
21. Berge, G. N., Fonnum, F., and Brodal, P. (1987) Neurotoxic effects of prenatal trichlorfon administration in pigs. *Acta Vet. Scand.* **28**, 321–332.
22. Czeizel, A. E., Elek, C., Gundy, S., et al. (1993) Environmental trichlorfon and cluster of congenital abnormalities. *Lancet* **341**, 539–542.
23. Chanda, S. M. and Pope, C. N. (1996) Neurochemical and neurobehavioral effects of repeated gestational exposure to chlorpyrifos in maternal and developing rats. *Pharmacol. Biochem. Behav.* **53**, 771–776.
24. Loewenherz, C., Fenske, R. A., Simcox, N. J., Bellamy, G., and Kalman, D. (1997) Biological monitoring of organophosphorus pesticide exposure among children of agricultural workers in central Washington State. *Environ. Health Perspect.* **105**, 1344–1353.
25. Hjelde, T., Mehl, A., Schanke, T. M., and Fonnum, F. (1998) Teratogenic effects of tricholorfon (Metrifonate) on the guinea-pig brain. Determination of the effective dose and the sensitive period. *Neurochem. Int.* **32**, 469–477.

26. ATSDR (2001) *CERCLA List of Priority Hazardous Substances.* ATSDR Information Center, Division of Toxicology, Agency for Toxic Substances and Disease Registry, US Department of Health and Human Services, Atlanta, GA.

27. Markowitz, M. (2000) Lead poisoning: a disease for the new millennium. *Curr. Probl. Pediatr.* **30,** 62–70.

28. Tong, S., von Schirnding, Y. E., and Prapamontol, T. (2000) Environmental lead exposure: a public health problem of global dimensions. *Bull. World Health Organ.* **78,** 1068–1077.

29. Duckett, S., Galle., P, and Kradin, R. (1977) The relationship between Parkinson syndrome and vascular siderosis: an electron microprobe study. *Ann. Neurol.* **2,** 225–229

30. Kuhn, W., Winkel, R., Woitalla, D., Meves, S., Przuntek, H., and Müller T. (1998) High prevalence of parkinsonism after occupational exposure to lead-sulfate batteries. *Neurology* **50,** 885–1886

31. Gorell, J. M., Rybicki, B. A., Johnson, C. C., and Peterson, E. L. (1999) Occupational metal exposures and the risk of Parkinson's disease. *Neuroepidemiology* **18,** 303–308.

32. Gorell, J. M., Johnson, C. C., Rybicki, B. A., et al. (1999) Occupational exposure to manganese, copper, lead, iron, mercury and zinc and the risk of Parkinson's disease. *Neurotoxicology* **20,** 239–248.

33. ATSDR (1999) *Toxicological Profile for Mercury,* Agency for Toxic Substances and Disease Registry, US Department of Health and Human Services, Atlanta, GA.

34. Charleston, J. S., Body, R. L., Mottet, N. K., Vahter, M. E., and Burbacher T. M. (1995) Autometallographic determination of inorganic mercury distribution in the cortex of the calcarine sulcus of the monkey *Macaca fascicularis* following long-term subclinical exposure to methylmercury and mercuric chloride. *Toxicol. Appl. Pharmacol.* **132,** 325–333.

35. Miura, K. and Imura N. (1987) Mechanism of methylmercury cytotoxicity. *Crit. Rev. Toxicol.* **18(3),** 161–168.

36. Rodier, P. M., Aschner, M., and Sager, P. R. (1984) Mitotic arrest in the developing CNS after prenatal exposure to methyl mercury. *Neurobehav. Toxicol. Teratol.* **6,** 379–385.

37. Choi, B. H., Lapham, L. W., Amin-Zaki, L., and Saleem T. (1978) Abnormal neuronal migration, deranged cerebral cortical organization, and diffuse white matter astrocytosis of human fetal brain: a major effect of methylmercury poisoning *in utero. J. Neuropathol. Exp. Neurol.* **37,** 719–733.

38. Matsumoto, H., Koya, G., and Takeuchi, T. (1965) Fetal Minamata disease: a neuropathological study of two cases of intrauterine intoxication by a methylmercury compound. *J. Neuropathol. Exp. Neurol.* **24,** 563–574.

39. Myers, G. J., Marsh, D. O., Davidson, P. W., et al. (1995) Main neurodevelopmental study of Seychellois children following *in utero* exposure to methylmercury from a maternal fish diet: outcome at six months. *Neurotoxicology* **16,** 653–664.

40. Grandjean, P., Weihe, P., White, R. F., and Debes, F. (1998) Cognitive performance of children prenatally exposed to "safe" levels of methylmercury. *Environ. Res.* **77,** 165–172.
41. Grandjean, P., White, R. F., Nielsen, A., Cleary, D., and de Olivereira Santos E. C. (1999) Methylmercury neurotoxicity in Amazonian children downstream from gold mining. *Environ. Health Perspect.* **107,** 587–591.
42. Dolbec, J., Mergler, D., Sousa-Passos C. J., Sousa, de-M. S., and Lebel, J. (2000) Methylmercury exposure affects motor performance of a riverine population of the Tapajos river, Brazilian Amazon. *Int. Arch. Occup. Environ. Health* **73,** 195–203.
43. Clarkson, T. W. (2002) The three modern faces of mercury. *Environ. Health Perspect.* **110,** 11–23.
44. Pichichero, M. E., Cernichiari, E., Lopreiato, J., and Treanor, J. (2002) Mercury concentrations and metabolism in infants receiving vaccines containing thiomersal: a descriptive study. *Lancet* **360,** 1737–1741.
45. Safe, S. H. (1990) Polychlorinated biphenyls (PCBs) dibenzo-*p*-dioxins (PCDDs), dibenzofurans (PCDFs) and related compounds: environmental and mechanistic considerations which support the development of toxic equivalency factors (TEFs). *CRC Crit. Rev. Toxicol.* **21,** 51–88.
46. Swanson, G. M., Ratcliffe, H. E., and Fischer, L. J. (1995) Human exposures to polychlorinated biphenyls (PCBs): a critical assessment of the evidence for adverse health effects. *Regul. Toxicol. Pharmacol.* **21,** 136–150.
47. Jacobson, J. L. and and Jacobson, S. W. (1996) Intellectual impairment in children exposed to polychlorinated biphenyls in utero. *N. Engl. J. Med.* **335,** 783–789.
48. Schantz, S. L., Ferguson, S. A., and Bowman, R. E. (1992) Effects of 2,3,7,8-tetrachlorodibenzo-*p*-dioxin on behavior of monkeys in peer groups. *Neurotox. Teratol.* **14,** 433–446.
49. Schantz, S. L., Moshtaghian, J., and Ness, D. K. (1995) Spatial learning deficits in adult rats exposed to ortho-substituted PCB congeners during gestation and lactation. *Fundam. Appl. Toxicol.* **26,** 117–126.
50. Hanneman, W. H., Legare, M. E., Barhoumi, R., Burghardt, R. C., Safe, S., and Tiffany- Castiglioni, E. (1996) Stimulation of calcium uptake in cultured rat hippocampal neurons by 2,3,7,8-tetrachlorodibenzo-*p*-dioxin. *Toxicology* **112(1),** 19–28.
51. Barhoumi, R., Mouneimne, Y., Phillips, T. D., Safe, S. H., and Burghardt, R. C. (1996) Alteration of oxytocin-induced calcium oscillations in clone 9 cells by toxin exposure. *Fundam. Appl. Toxicol.* **33(2),** 220–228.
52. Kodavanti, P. R. S. and Tilson, H. (2000). Neurochemical effects of environmental chemicals: in vitro and in vivo correlations on second messenger pathways. *Ann. NY Acad. Sci.* **919,** 97–105.
53. Legare, M. E., Hanneman, W. H., Barhoumi, R., Burghardt, R. C., and Tiffany-Castiglioni, E. (2000) 2,3,7,8-Tetrachlorodibenzo-p-dioxin alters hippocampal astroglia-neuronal gap junctional communication. *Neurotoxicology* **21,** 1109–1116.

54. Hong, S. J., Grover, C. A., Safe, S. H., Tiffany-Castiglioni, E., and Frye, G. D. (1998) Halogenated aromatic hydrocarbons suppress CA1 field excitatory postsynaptic potentials in rat hippocampal slices. *Toxicol. Appl. Pharmacol.* **148,** 7–13.

55. Schantz, S. L. and Widholm, J. J. (2001) Cognitive effects of endocrine-disrupting chemicals in animals. *Environ. Health Perspect.* **109,** 1197–1206.

56. Clarren, S. K. and Smith, D. W. (1978) The fetal alcohol syndrome. *N. Engl. J. Med.* **298,** 1063–1067.

57. Miller, M. W. (1992) The effects of prenatal exposure to ethanol on cell proliferation and neuronal migration, in *Development of the Central Nervous System: Effects of Alcohol and Opiates* (Miller M., ed.), Alan R. Liss, New York, pp. 47–69.

58. Guerri, C., Sáez, R., Portolés, M., and Renau-Piqueras, J. (1993) Derangement of astrogliogenesis as a possible mechanism involved in alcohol-induced alterations of central nervous system development. *Alcohol Alcohol.* **2(Suppl.),** 203–208.

59. Jones, K. L., Smith, D. W., Ulleland, C. N., and Streissguth, A. P. (1973) Pattern of malformation in offspring of chronic alcoholic mothers. *Lancet* **1,** 1267–1271.

60. Bo, W. J., Krueger, W. A., Rudeen, P. K., and Symmes, S. K. (1982) Ethanol-induced alterations in the morphology and function of the rat ovary. *Anat. Rec.* **202,** 255–260.

61. Dees, W. L. and Skelley, C. W. (1990) Effects of ethanol during the onset of female puberty. *Neuroendocrinology* **51,** 64–69.

62. Dees, W. L., Skelley, C. W., Hiney, J. K., and Johnston, C. A. (1990) Actions of ethanol on hypothalamic and pituitary hormones in prepubertal female rats. *Alcohol* **7,** 21–25.

63. Dees, W. L., Dissen, G. A., Hiney, J. K., Lara, F., and Ojeda, S. R. (2000) Alcohol ingestion inhibits the increased secretion of puberty-related hormones in the developing female rhesus monkey. *Endocrinology* **141,** 1325–1331.

64. Masters, C. L., Multhaup, G., Simms, G., Pottgiesser, J., Martins, R. N., and Beyreuther, K. (1985) Neuronal origin of a cerebral amyloid: neurofibrillary tangles of Alzheimer's disease contain the same protein as the amyloid of plaque cores and blood vessels. *EMBO J.* **4,** 2757–2763.

65. Yankner, B. A., Dawes, L. R., Fisher, S., Villa-Komaroff, L., Oster-Granite, M. L., and Neve, R. L. (1989) Neurotoxicity of a fragment of the amyloid precursor associated with Alzheimer's disease. *Science* **245,** 417–420.

66. Behl, C. (1997) Amyloid beta-protein toxicity and oxidative stress in Alzheimer's disease. *Cell Tissue Res.* **290,** 471–480.

67. Polymeropoulos, M. H., Lavedan, C., Leroy, E., et al. (1997) Mutation in the alpha-synuclein gene identified in families with Parkinson's disease. *Science* **276,** 2045–2047.

68. Spillantini, M. G. and Goedert, M. (2000) The alpha-synucleinopathies: Parkinson's disease, dementia with Lewy bodies, and multiple system atrophy. *Ann. NY Acad. Sci.* **920,** 16–27.

69. Aschner, M., Allen, J. W., Kimelberg, H. K., LoPachin, R. M., and Streit, W. J. (1999) Glial cells in neurotoxicity development. *Annu. Rev. Pharm. Toxicol.* **39,** 151–173.

70. Le, W-D., Rowe, D., Xie, W., Ortiz, I., He, Y., and Appel, S. H. (2001) Microglial activation and dopaminergic cell injury: an in vitro model relevant to Parkinson's Disease. *J. Neurosci.* **2,** 8447–8455.

71. Chang, J. Y. and Liu, L-Z. (1999) Manganese potentiates nitric oxide production by microglia. *Mol. Brain. Res.* **68,** 22–28.

72. Gao, H.-M., Hong, J.-S., Zhang, W., and Liu, B. (2002) Distinct role for microglia in rotenone-induced degeneration of dopaminergic neurons. *J. Neurosci.* **22,** 782–790.

73. Harry, G. J., Tyler, K., d'Hellencourt, C. L., Tilson, H. A., and Maier, W. E. (2002) Morphological alterations and elevations in tumor necrosis factor-α, interleukin (IL)-1α, and IL-6 in mixed glia cultures following exposure to trimethyltin: modulation by proinflammatory cytokine recombinant proteins and neutralizing antibodies. *Toxicol. Appl. Pharm.* **180,** 205–218.

74. Carlson, K., Jortner, B. S., and Ehrich, M. (2000) Organophosphus compound-induced apoptosis in SH-SY5Y human neuroblastoma cells. *Toxicol. Appl. Pharmacol.* **168,** 102–113.

75. Hong, M. S., Hong, S. J., Barhoumi, R., et al. (2003). Neurotoxicity induced in differentiated SK-N-SH-SY5Y human neuroblastoma cells by organophosphorus compounds. *Toxicol. Appl. Pharmacol.* **186,** 110–118.

76. Purkiss, J. R., Friis, L. M., Doward, S., and Quinn, C. P. (2001) Clostridium botulinum neurotoxins act with a wide range of potencies on SH-SY5Y human neuroblastoma cells. *Neurotoxicology* **22,** 447–453.

77. Li, W. F. and Casida, J. E. (1998) Organophosphorus neuropathy target esterase inhibitors selectively block outgrowth of neurite-like and cell processes in cultured cells. *Toxicol. Lett.* **98,** 139–146.

78. Das, K. D. and Barone, S. J. (1999). Neuronal differentiation in PC12 cells is inhibited by chlorpyrifos and its metabolites: Is acetylcholinesterase inhibition the site of action? *Toxicol. Appl. Pharmacol.* **160,** 217–230.

79. Zachor, D. A., Moore, J. F., Brezauzek, C. M., Theibert, A. B., and Percy, A. K. (2000) Cocaine inhibition of neuronal differentiation in NGF-induced PC12 cells is independent of ras signaling. *Int. J. Dev. Neurosci.* **18,** 765–772.

80. Crumpton, T. L., Atkins, D., Zawia, N., and Barone, S., Jr. (2001) Lead exposure in pheochromocytoma (PC12) cells alters neural differentiation and Sp1 DNA-binding. *Neurotoxicology* **22,** 49–62.

81. Parran, D. K., Mundy, W. R., and Barone, S., Jr. (2001) Effects of methylmercury and mercuric chloride on differentiation and cell viability in PC12 cells. *Toxicol. Sci.* **59,** 278–290.

82. Shafer, T. J., Meacham, C. A., and Barone, S. (2002). Effects of prolonged exposure to nanomolar concentrations of methylmercury on voltage-sensitive sodium and calcium currents in PC12 cells. *Dev. Brain Res.* **136,** 151–164.

83. Son, J. H., Chun, H. S., Joh, T. H., Cho, S., Conti, B., and Lee, J.W., (1999) Neuroprotection and neuronal differentiation studies using substantia nigra dopaminergic cells derived from transgenic mouse embryos. *J. Neurosci.* **19,** 10–20.

84. Chun, H. S., Lee, H., and Son, J. H. (2001). Manganese induces endoplasmic reticulum (ER) stress and activates multiple caspases in nigral dopaminergic neuronal cells, SN4741. *Neurosci. Lett.* **316,** 5–8.

85. Qian, Y, Harris, E. D., Zheng, Y., and Tiffany-Castiglioni, E. (2000) Lead (Pb) targets GRP78, a molecular chaperone, in C6 rat glioma cells. *Toxicol. Appl. Pharmacol.* 163, 260–266.

86. Takanaga, H., Kunimoto, M., Adachi, T., Tohyama, C., and Aoki, Y. (2001) Inhibitory effect of 2,3,7,8-tetrachlorodibenzo-p-dioxin on cAMP-induced differentiation of rat C6 glial cell line. *J. Neurosci. Res.* **64,** 402–409.

87. Guizzetti, M. and Costa, L. G. (2002) Effect of ethanol on protein kinase Cζ and p70S6 kinase activation by carbachol: a possible mechanism for ethanol-induced inhibition of glial cell proliferation. *J. Neurochem.* **82,** 38–46.

88. Mead, C. and Pentreath, V. M. (1998) Evaluation of toxicity indicators in rat primary astrocytes, C6 glioma and human 1321N1 astrocytoma cells: can gliotoxicity be distinguished from cytotoxicity? *Arch. Toxicol.* **72,** 372–380.

89. Inglefield, J. R., Mundy, W. R., and Shafer, T. J. (2001) inositol 1,4,5-trisphosphate receptor- sensitive Ca^{2+} release, store-operated Ca^{2+} entry, and camp responsive element binding protein phosphorylation in developing cortical cells following exposure to polychlorinated biphenyls. *J. Pharmacol. Exp. Ther.* **297,** 762–773.

90. Yang, J.-H. and Kodavanti, R. S. (2001) Possible molecular targets of halogenated aromatic hydrocarbons in neuronal cells. *Biochem. Biophys. Res. Commun.* **280,** 1372–1377.

91. Dyatlov, V. A., Dyatlov, O. M., Parsons, P. J., Lawrence, D. A., and Carpenter, D. O. (1998) Lipopolysaccharide and interleukin-6 enhance lead entry into cerebellar neurons: application of a new and sensitive flow cytometric technique to measure intracellular lead and calcium concentrations. *Neurotoxicology* **19,** 293–302.

92. Audesirk, T. and Cabell, L. (1999). Nanomolar concentrations of nicotine and cotinine alter the development of cultured hippocampal neurons via non-acetylcholine receptor-mediated mechanisms. *Neurotoxicology* **20,** 639–646.

93. Braga, M. F. M., Pereira, E. F. R., and Albuquerque, E. X. (1999) Nanomolar concentrations of lead inhibit glutamatergic and GABAergic transmission in hippocampal neurons. *Brain Res.* **826,** 22–34.

94. Heidemann, S. R., Lamoureux, P., and Atchison, W. D. (2001) Inhibition of axonal morphogenesis by nonlethal, submicromolar concentrations of methylmercury. *Toxicol. Appl. Pharmacol.* **174,** 49–59.

95. Bestervelt, L. L., Pitt, J. A., and Piper, W. N. (1998) Evidence for Ah receptor mediation of increased ACTH concentrations in primary cultures of rat anterior pituitary cells exposed to TCDD. *Toxicol. Sci.* **46,** 294–299.

96. Bouton, C. M. L. S., Hossain, M. A., Frelin, L. P., Laterra, J., and Pevsner, J. (2001) Microarray analysis of differential gene expression in lead-exposed astrocytes. *Toxicol. Appl. Pharmacol.* **176,** 34–53.

97. Yao, C. P., Allen, J. W., Conklin, D. R., and Aschner, M. (1999) Transfection and overexpression of metallothionein-I in neonatal rat primary astrocyte cultures and in astrocytoma cells increases their resistance to methylmercury-induced cytotoxicity. *Brain Res.* **818,** 414–420.

98. Yao, C. P., Allen, J. W., Mutkus, L. A., Xu, S. B., Tan, K. H., and Aschner, M. (2000) Foreign metallothionein-I (MT-I) expression by transient transfection in MT-I and -II null astrocytes confers increased protection against acute methylmercury cytotoxicity. *Brain Res.* **855,** 32–38.

99. Deng, W. and Poretz, R. D. (2002) Protein kinase C activation is required for the lead-induced inhibition of proliferation and differentiation of cultured oligodendroglial progenitor cells. *Brain Res.* **929,** 87–95.

100. Xu, J., Chen, S., Ahmed, S. H., et al. (2001) Amyloid-β peptides are cytotoxic to oligodendrocytes. *J. Neurosci.* **21,** 1–5.

101. Tang, H. W., Yan, H. L., Hu, X. H., Liang, Y. X., and Shen, X.Y. (1996) Lead cytotoxicity in primary cultured rat astrocytes and Schwann cells. *J. Appl. Toxicol.* **16,** 187–196

102. Tomsig, J.L., and Suszkiw, J.B. (1995) Multisite interactions between Pb^{+2} and protein kinase C and its role in norepinephrine release from bovine adrenal chromaffin cells. *J. Neurochem.* **64,** 2667–2773.

103. Vijverberg, H. P. M., Zwart, R., Van Den Beukel, I., Oortgiesen, M., and Van Kleef, R. G. D. M. (1997) *In vitro* approaches to species and receptor diversity in cellular neurotoxicology. *Toxicol. In Vitro* **11,** 491–498.

104. Pantazis, N. J., Zaheer, A., Dai, D., Zahee,r S., Green, S. H., and Lim, R. (2000) Transfection of C6 glioma cells with glia maturation factor upregulates brain-derived neurotrophic factor and nerve growth factor: trophic effects and protection against ethanol toxicity in cerebellar granule cells. *Brain Res.* **865,** 59–76.

105. Lindahl, L. S., Bird, L., Legare, M. E., Mikeska, G., Bratton, G. R., and Tiffany-Castiglioni, E. (1999) Differential ability of astroglia and neuronal cells to accumulate lead: dependence on cell type and on degree of differentiation. *Toxicol. Sci.* **50,** 236–243.

106. Shanker, G., Allen, J. W., Mutkus, L. A., Aschner, M. (2001) Methylmercury inhibits cysteine uptake in cultured primary astrocytes, but not in neurons. *Brain Res.* **914,** 159–165.

107. Monnet-Tschudi, F., Zurich, M.-G., Schilter, B., Costa, L. G., and Honegger, P. (2000) Maturation-dependent effects of chlorpyrifos and parathion and their oxygen analogs on acetylcholinesterase and neuronal and glial markers in aggregating brain cell cultures. *Toxicol. Appl. Pharmacol.* **165,** 175–183.

108. Hirai, K., Yoshioka, H., Kihara, M., Hasegawa, K., Sawada, T., and Fushiki, S. (1999) Effects of ethanol on neuronal migration and neural cell adhesion molecules in the embryonic rat cerebral cortex: a tissue culture study. *Dev. Brain Res.* **118,** 205–210.

109. He, L., Poblenz, A. T., Medrano, C. J., and Fox, D.A. (2000) Lead and calcium produce rod photoreceptor cell apoptosis by opening the mitochondrial permeability transition pore. *J. Biol. Chem.* **275,** 12,175–12,184.

110. Kimelberg, H. K., Cai, Z., Schools, G., and Zhou, M. (2000) Acutely isolated astrocytes as models to probe astrocyte functions. *Neurochem. Int.* **36,** 359–367.

111. Vallés, S., Sancho-Tello, M., Miñana, R., Climent, E., Renau-Piqueras, J., and Guerri, C. (1996) Glial fibrillary acidic protein expression in rat brain and in radial glia culture is delayed by prenatal ethanol exposure. *J. Neurochem.* **67,** 2425–2433.

112. Chen, H-H., Ma, T., and Ho, I. K. (1999) Protein kinase C in rat brain is altered by developmental lead exposure. *Neurochem. Res.* **24,** 415–421.

113. Grover, C. A. and Frye, G. D. (1996) Ethanol effects on synaptic neurotransmission and tetanus-induced synaptic plasticity in hippocampal slices of chronic in vivo lead-exposed adult rats. *Brain Res.* **734,** 61–71.

114. Goldstein, G. W. (1988) Endothelial cell-astrocyte interactions: a cellular model of the blood-brain barrier. *Ann. NY Acad. Sci.* **529,** 31–39.

115. Sobue, K., Yamamoto, N., Yoneda, K., et al. (1999) Induction of blood–brain barrier properties in immortalized bovine brain endothelial cells by astrocytic factors. *Neurosci. Res.* **35,** 155–164.

116. Wolburg, H., Neuhaus, J., Kniesel, U., et al. (1994) Modulation of tight junction structure in blood–brain barrier endothelial cells: effects of tissue culture, second messengers and cocultured astrocytes. *J. Cell. Sci.* **107,** 1347–1357.

117. Gumbleton, M. and Audus, K. L. (2001) Progress and limitations in the use of in vitro cell cultures to serve as a permeability screen for the blood–brain barrier. *J. Pharm. Sci.* **90,** 1681–1698.

118. Tiffany-Castiglioni, E., Neck, K.F., and Caceci, T. (1986) Glial culture on artificial capillaries: electron microscopic comparison of C6 rat glioma cells and rat astroglia. *J. Neurosci. Res.* **16,** 387–396.

119. Stanness, K. A., Westrum, L. E., Fornaciari, E., et al. (1997) Morphological and functional characterization of an in vitro blood-brain barrier model. *Brain Res.* **771,** 329–342.

120. Guerri, C., Pascual, M., and Renau-Piqueras, J. (2001) Glia and fetal alcohol syndrome. *Neurotoxicology* **22,** 593–599.

121. Tofolin, P. J. and Fike, J. R. (2000) The radioresponse of the central nervous system: a dynamic process. *Radiat. Res.* **153,** 357–370.

122. Tiffany-Castiglioni, E. (1993) Cell culture models for lead toxicity in neuronal and glial cells. *Neurotoxicology* **14(4),** 513–536.

123. Roper, S. N., Abraham, L. A., and Streit, W. J. (1997) Exposure to in utero irradiation produces disruption of radial glia in rats. *Dev. Neurosci.* **19,**521–528.

124. Gressens, P. (2000) Mechanisms and disturbances of neuronal migration. *Pediatr. Res.* **48,** 725–730.

125. Freshney, R. I. (2000) *Culture on Animal Cells: A Manual of Basic Technique*, 4th ed., Wiley–Liss, New York.

126. Bissell, M. G., Eng, L.F., Herman, M. M., Bensch, K. G., and Miles, L. E. (1975) Quantitative increase of neuroglia-specific GFA protein in rat C-6 glioma cells in vitro. *Nature* **255,** 633–634.

127. Lee, K., Kentroti, S., Billie, H., Bruce, C., and Vernadakis, A. (1992) Comparative biochemical, morphological, and immunocytochemical studies between C-6 glial cells of early and late passages and advanced passages of glial cells derived from aged mouse cerebral hemispheres. *Glia* **6,** 245–257.

128. Biedler, J. L., Helson, L., and Spengler, B. A. (1973) Morphology and growth, tumorigenicity, and cytogenetics of human neuroblastoma cells in continuous culture. *Cancer Res.* **33,** 2643–2652.

129. Perez-Polo, J. R., Werrbach-Perez, K., and Tiffany-Castiglioni, E. (1979) A human clonal cell line model of differentiating neurons. *Dev. Biol.* **71,** 341–355.

130. Zurich, M. G., Honegger, P., Schilter, B., Costa, L. G., and Monnet-Tschudi, F. (2000) Use of aggregating brain cell cultures to study developmental effects of organophosphorus insecticides. *Neurotoxicology* **21,** 599–606.

131. Harry, G.J., Billingsley, M., Bruinink, A., et al. (1998) In vitro techniques for the assessment of neurotoxicity. *Environ. Health Perspect.* **106(Suppl.),** 131–158.

132. Gad, S.C. (2000) Neurotoxicology in vitro, in *In Vitro Toxicology*, 2nd ed., (Gad, C. G., ed.), Taylor and Francis, New York, pp. 188–221.

133.   Barhoumi, R., Mouneimne, Y., Ramos, K. S., et al. (2000) Analysis of benzo[a]pyrene partitioning and cellular homeostasis in a rat liver cell line. Toxicol. Sci. 53, 264–270.

134. Barhoumi, R., Mouneimne, Y., Awooda, I., Safe, S.H., Donnelly, K.C., and Burghardt, R.C. (2002) Characterization of calcium oscillations in normal and benzo[a]pyrene-treated Clone 9 cells. *Toxicol. Sci.* **68,** 444–450.

135. Chanda, S. M., Mortensen, S. R., Moser, V. C., and Padilla, S. (1997) Tissue-specific effects of chlorpyrifos on carboxylesterase and cholinesterase activity in adult rats: An *in-vitro* and *in vivo* comparison. *Fund. Appl. Toxicol.* **38,** 148–157.

136. Carpenter, D. O., Hussain, R. J., Berger, D. F., Lombardo, J. P., and Park, H-Y. (2002) Electrophysiologic and behavioral effects of perinatal and acute exposure of rats to lead and polychlorinated biphenyls. *Environ. Health Perspect.* **110(Suppl.),** 377–386.

2

Predictive Value of In Vitro Systems for Neurotoxicity Risk Assessment

Marion Ehrich and David C. Dorman

1. INTRODUCTION: NEUROTOXICITY RISK ASSESSMENT

Risk assessment has been broadly defined as the characterization of the adverse health effects of human exposures to environmental hazards and can be divided into four major steps: hazard identification, dose–response assessment, exposure assessment, and risk characterization *(1)*. Hazard identification is defined as determining whether human exposure to an agent can cause an increased incidence of an adverse health effect (e.g., neurotoxicity). Dose–response assessment is the process of characterizing the relationship between the administered or effective dose of an agent and the incidence of an adverse health effect in exposed populations, estimating the incidence of the effect as a function of human exposure to the agent. A dose–response assessment should account for exposure intensity and duration, developmental age, and other factors that may modify the response (e.g., gender, diet). Exposure assessment is the process of measuring or estimating the intensity, frequency, and duration of human exposure to an agent found in the environment or an agent that may be released into the environment. Risk characterization integrates these preceding steps by estimating the incidence of a health effect under various conditions of human exposure.

These four steps form the basis of risk assessment. They are independent of the nature of the adverse health effect (e.g., neurotoxicity vs carcinogenesis), although underlying assumptions (e.g., threshold vs nonthreshold effects) may influence the approaches used.

From: *Methods in Pharmacology and Toxicology: In Vitro Neurotoxicology: Principles and Challenges*
Edited by: E. Tiffany-Castiglioni © Humana Press Inc., Totowa, NJ

Neurotoxicity is defined as any adverse effect on the chemistry, structure or function of the nervous system during development or at maturity induced by chemical or physical influences *(2)*. For a chemical to be regarded as a neurotoxicant, effects on the nervous system should be direct rather than indirect, adverse rather than adaptive, and toxicological rather than pharmacological. Chemically induced neurotoxic effects are of special concern because neurotoxicological syndromes may be delayed and are often progressive or irreversible and prevention is far less costly than treatment *(3,4)*. Only recently have regulatory agencies focused their attention on developing guidelines for the conduct of neurotoxicity risk assessments *(5)*.

Requirements for animal testing of pesticides and some commercial chemicals for neurotoxicity are promulgated worldwide by a number of regulatory agencies. For example, the US Environmental Protection Agency administers the Federal Insecticide, Fungicide and Rodenticide Act (FIFRA) and the Toxic Substances Control Act (TSCA). Testing for specific end points indicative of neurotoxicity may also be recommended by the Food and Drug Administration for certain food additives that demonstrate positive results in a very basic, initial neurotoxicity screen *(6)*. It is estimated that only a small fraction of the 70,000 chemicals currently in commerce have been adequately assessed for neurotoxicity *(7)*; thus, there is a need to develop cost-effective screens to assess chemicals for potential neurotoxicity.

Bioassays remain the principal method to identify possible human health risks posed by exposure to chemicals and other potential neurotoxicants. The primary advantage of using animals for hazard identification and risk characterization is that all potential targets for injury (e.g., the many types of cell, tissue, neurochemical) are included in the test system *(4,8)*. This is especially important because neurotoxicants can affect a variety of different organs and tissues and they can induce alterations in chemistry, function, structure, or behavior (*see* Fig. 1). End points of interest in bioassays often include histopathology to assess morphologic damage and batteries of functional, neurobehavioral, neurochemical, and neurophysiological tests to examine the operational integrity of the nervous system *(9)*. Because there are physiological and anatomical similarities among mammals, the finding of a positive response in vivo is taken as evidence that an agent may also pose a risk for exposed humans. This integrated in vivo approach is valuable for a detailed characterization of both the effects and possible mechanisms of suspected neurotoxicants under specific exposure conditions. In vivo methods are relatively well developed and the data are used to determine no observable adverse effect levels (NOAELs), uncertainty factors, and benchmark doses.

The use of animals in toxicity testing is often the subject of intense scrutiny and criticism by the general public. The toxicology community continually

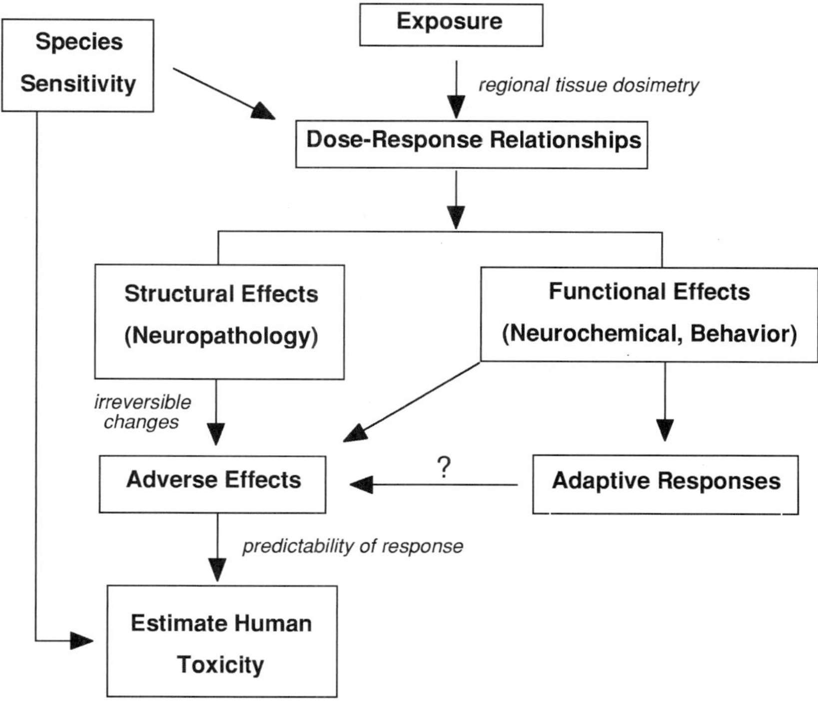

Fig. 1. Critical elements in characterizing neurotoxicity risk from exposure to a chemical. (Reprinted with permission from ref. *9*.)

strives to replace the use of animals in research, to reduce the numbers of animals to the minimum necessary to obtain valid results where replacement was impossible, and to refine all experimental procedures to minimize adverse effects on animals. The use of in vitro test systems is a logical alternative to the use of animals and can often complement and enhance in vivo data. In vitro tests can be sensitive, replicable, valid, and cost-effective. They are amenable to studies done over a wide range of concentrations and over multiple periods of time. Exposure to the test chemical can be tightly controlled and human materials can be used. In vitro data can provide important structure–activity data concerning the relative potency of different chemicals and contribute to choices for chemicals to study in vivo. In addition, in vitro data can be used to identify the mode of action of a chemical and identify critical factors that determine species- or tissue-specific differences in response. Studies of relationships between in vitro and in vivo data have helped to identify these and other factors that contribute to and modify toxicity *(2–4,7,8,10–14)*. It is well recognized that the risk assessment process is improved if data concerning the chemical's mechanism(s) of action are included. However, it remains speculative whether in vitro data can replace any in vivo data used for the risk assessment of a neurotoxicant. Indeed, in vitro data are rarely considered in the risk assessment process because current statutory guidelines do not classify changes observed in vitro as indicative of an adverse response *(7,10,11,15–17)*.

As with any technology, in vitro systems have distinct limitations. In vitro test systems have a reduced cellular complexity, therefore, the responses observed in vitro may not be representative of those observed in the substantially more complex intact nervous system *(see* Fig. 2). One important structural difference of most neural cell culture systems is the lack of a functional equivalent to the so-called blood–brain barrier. This blood–brain barrier excludes the movement of certain chemicals or their metabolites into the intact nervous system, thereby attenuating the observed neurotoxic response. Additionally, isolated in vitro systems often lack the hepatic and extrahepatic metabolic systems that are normally present in the intact animal to activate or detoxify the agent under investigation. Thus, in vitro systems have only a limited capacity to metabolize selective toxicants. Current choices are often between simple systems that are significantly divergent to the in vivo situation but are easy to manipulate and complex systems that are technically difficult to establish and use. In spite of these limitations, in vitro models are proving useful for the screening of chemicals for neurotoxic potential. In vitro model systems may provide an economical first-tier evaluation that will help to guide more extensive whole-animal studies.

2. SYSTEMS FOR EVALUATION OF NEUROTOXICITY IN VITRO: MECHANISTIC MODELS AND SCREENING TESTS

A number of reports suggest that in vitro tests for neurotoxicity would be more useful in providing mechanistic information than they would be for general screening purposes for agents of unknown toxicity. This suggestion is based on the complexity and multiple targets of the nervous system and the comparative simplicity of in vitro test systems *(2–4,8,18)*. Although the development of screening tests may appear formidable to some, the suggestion has been made that end points indicative of cytotoxicity (i.e., cell viability) could be more sensitive in cells of the nervous system exposed to neurotoxicants than cells of extraneural origin. This assumption, based on the premise of tissue selectivity, may have value when appropriate comparisons are made. However, although potent cytotoxins can be neurotoxicants, they are likely to be toxic to other tissues as well (e.g., liver, kidney, lung) *(2,12,15,16)*.

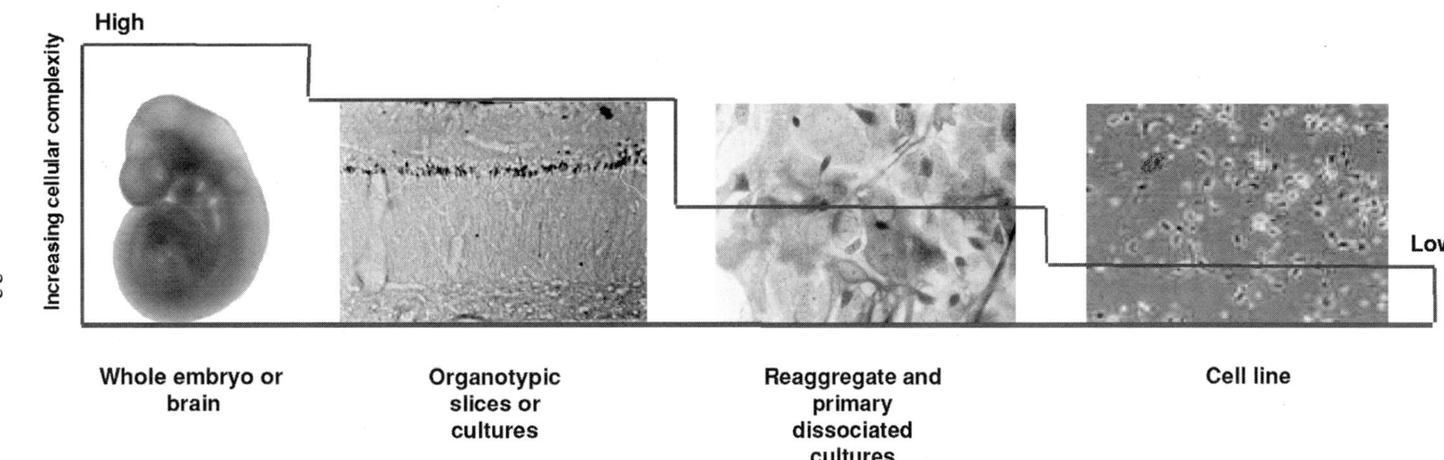

Fig. 2. Types of in vitro systems used in neurotoxicology research. Cultures composed of individual cell lines have the least structural complexity and predictability to man.

Like their in vivo counterparts, in vitro neurotoxicity screens require the use of test systems and end points that are sensitive, efficient, and neural-specific. The systems should provide low numbers of false negatives or positives *(2)*. The sole reliance on a single experimental model, whether it be in vivo or in vitro, with a limited number of biological markers is not generally considered sufficient for estimation of risk. For this reason, a tiered system for in vitro neurotoxicity screening has been proposed *(15)*. The tiered system was designed to include cytotoxicity and cell-specific effects determined in simple and more complex in vitro systems in the first and second tiers and mechanistic studies in the third tier. An initial study, using a neuronal cell line and multiple end points (some neural-specific, some not), suggested that the number of end points was not sufficient to use a single clonal cell line as a screening system for neurotoxicity *(19)*. This contrasts with results of another large study examining cytotoxicity in non-neural cells, which suggested that cell viability appeared to be a valid indicator of general toxicity *(20)*. Regardless of end points, however, concentration–response and time–response studies need to be included into any in vitro test screen *(10,20,21)*. It has also been suggested that in vitro screens should include human neural cells to allow evaluation of interspecies differences in response *(1,3,14,16,18,22)*.

Many neurotoxicants have unknown and/or multiple mechanisms of action *(4,11,23,24)*. The use of in vitro test systems often yields valuable mechanistic data on chemical-induced neurotoxicities and thus offers an attractive alternative to the use of animals for this type of research. Mechanistic studies can be designed to evaluate multiple mechanisms of action and can be modified to the toxic agent of concern. End points can include general glial or neuronal measures, neurotransmitter systems, and indicators of the biochemical and electrical responses of neural cells. Reversibility and irreversibility of effects, protective mechanisms and repair, and ability to affect cell proliferation and differentiation can be determined. Characterization of the cellular and molecular substrates and pathways that follow exposure to neurotoxicants can be evaluated *(2,3,7,10,13,15,24)*. The generation of useful mechanistic data requires realization that the data obtained will not necessarily provide explanations for all manifestations of neurotoxicity seen in man and animals, including behavioral, cognitive, sensory, developmental, or age-related effects. Furthermore, standard protocols that include well-defined culture conditions and means to reduce potential for cell instability need to be followed to permit intralaboratory and interlaboratory validation of results *(2,3,7,10,13,15,22)*.

3. IN VITRO MODELING OF IN VIVO SYSTEMS: DOSE–RESPONSE CONSIDERATIONS

It is well recognized that risk assessment considers dose–response data for an adverse effect. Dose (concentration)–response studies can be done with relative efficiency using in vitro test systems, and test compounds can be applied directly without concern for the pharmacokinetic factors of absorption, distribution, metabolism, and excretion encountered in animals. Isolated test systems are often exposed to concentrations of chemicals that far exceed those achievable in tissues from exposed animals or humans. Interpretation of in vitro studies is aided dramatically by detailed knowledge concerning concentrations of the parent chemical or major metabolites in blood, brain, and other potential target tissues. In some cases (e.g., organophosphate insecticides, polychlorinated biphenyls, and ethanol) effects can occur in vitro at concentrations similar to those observed in vivo *(13,25)*. Effects occurring in vitro at lower concentrations than those achieved in vivo may indicate that the test chemical is metabolized in vivo to a less toxic form, the chemical or the active metabolites are excluded from the nervous system, or that compensatory or repair mechanisms occur that attenuate the toxicity of the chemical observed in vivo. Neurotoxic effects that require in vitro concentrations higher than blood concentrations of intoxicated animals may occur because concentrations in target tissues are higher than concentrations in blood. Concentration differences may also depend on the in vitro system used for testing (e.g., cells of neoplastic origin are notoriously resistant to chemical-induced cytotoxic effects). It is, therefore, important to consider the context in which the in vitro data are collected *(8,13,16,25)*.

A specific example of dosing considerations can be noted with exposure of neuronal cell lines of neoplastic origin to cholinesterase-inhibiting organophosphorus compounds. Inhibition of acetylcholinesterase, which is responsible for clinical signs seen in people and animals, occurs following minutes of exposure to physiological (nanomolar to micromolar) concentrations of these agents in neuroblastoma cells of mouse and human origin, yet cytotoxic and lethal effects require many hours and concentrations of these compounds in millimolar ranges *(25–28)*. Primary cell cultures (e.g., neurons isolated from chick dorsal root ganglia) exposed to these same test agents can demonstrate cytotoxic effects to organophosphorus compounds at micromolar concentrations (Massicotte and Ehrich, unpublished).

As noted in several reports, dose–response data obtained from in vitro studies do not generally consider pharmacokinetic differences between in vitro and in vivo systems, which can limit the potential for in vitro to in vivo extrapolations *(2,3,7,29)*. This, however, does not totally detract from their usefulness, for another application of in vitro test systems is to examine biological processes that may affect the pharmacokinetics of a chemical. For example, useful data concerning the transport of chemicals into the nervous system can be obtained from in vitro test systems. Studies using isolated primary rat neural cultures have demonstrated that the transferrin receptor plays a critical role in the uptake of aluminum, iron, and other metals *(30,31)*. Experiments conducted using isolated brain microvessels have demonstrated the role of amino acid carriers in the transport of mercury to the central nervous system *(32)*. Other investigators have used brain tissue slices, brain homogenates, and other in vitro test systems to examine the metabolism of *m*-dinitrobenzene *(33)*, 1-methyl-4-phenyl-1,2,3,6-tetrahydropyridine (MPTP) *(34,35)*, and other neurotoxicants. Predictive pharmacokinetic models that include in vitro metabolic data extrapolated to the whole animal are, however, still under development *(3,4,16,29)*.

A significant advantage of in vitro test systems is that concentration–response curves can be readily created and concentrations responsible for 50% effects (EC_{50} values) can be determined and compared *(4,13,16,19,25)*. These comparisons are very useful in considering structure–activity relationships among different chemicals. The best comparisons of EC_{50} values are made when concentration–response curves include several data points, when these curves are parallel, when the end point of interest is specific, and when all data are collected under the same conditions. EC_{50} values can also be used to examine whether tissue or species differences in response to a neurotoxicant occur *(3,19,25,36)*. Care, however, must be taken when EC_{50} values are used to compare sensitivity of different end points, especially when comparisons are between nonspecific end points (e.g., cytotoxicity) and specific targets of particular compounds (e.g., esterase inhibition caused by organophosphates), as mechanisms associated with expression of the end points may differ *(12,13,25)*. Considerable care must be taken when comparing in vitro data (e.g., EC_{50} values) and in vivo data (e.g., LD_{50} values, blood concentrations in intoxicated subjects, behavior of exposed subjects). The differences between in vivo and in vitro test systems are so great that correlation of EC_{50} values and LD_{50} values (or blood concentrations) may have little value. To date, the best correlations have occurred with very potent toxicants *(2,3,16,20,37)*.

4. RECOMMENDATIONS AND CONCLUSIONS

Inclusion of data collected during neurotoxicity testing using in vitro systems in risk assessment mandates that end points be relevant and that in vitro

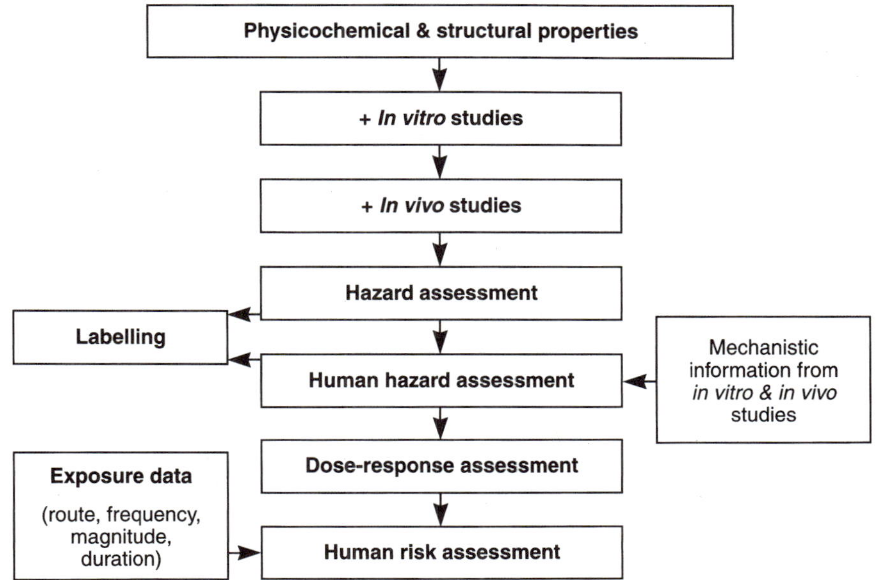

Fig. 3. Scheme for hazard and risk assessment. Reprinted from ref. *11* with permission of *ATLA*.

testing systems be validated. The validation needs to be at multiple test sites and include reproducibility, repeatability among various test sites, protocol standardization, chemical reference standardization, and quality assurance. In vivo methods with reasonably developed in vitro alternatives will be easiest to replace, although it must be recognized that statutory requirements must be met and acceptance may be slow *(2,4,10,11,13,15,16,21,22,25)*. In vitro systems could help classify test chemicals as to their likely mode of action, select chemicals from a larger group for further testing, and suggest which chemicals and which tests should be done in vivo *(8,11)*. In vitro and in vivo tests run in parallel may provide the most information about general toxicity and mechanisms of neurotoxicity, especially for new compounds. In this case, both types of data would be more likely to be included in the risk assessment process *(10,11,13,15)* (*see* Fig. 3).

REFERENCES

1. National Research Council (1983). *Risk Assessment in the Federal Government: Managing the Process*, National Academy Press, Washington, DC.
2. Costa, L. G. (1998a) Neurotoxicity testing: a discussion of *in vitro* alternatives. *Environ. Health Perspect.* **106S,** 505–510.

3. Harry, G. J., Billingsley, M., Bruinink, A., et al. (1998) In vitro techniques for the assessment of neurotoxicity. *Environ. Health Perspect.* **106S,** 131–158.

4. National Research Council Committee on Neurotoxicology and Models for Assessing Risk (1992) *Environmental Neurotoxicology*, National Academy Press, Washington, DC.

5. US Environmental Protection Agency (1991) *Pesticide Assessment Guidelines, Subdivision E. Hazard Evaluation: Human and Domestic Animals (Addendum 10: Neurotoxicity, series 81, 82, and 83)*, Office of Prevention, Pesticides and Toxic Substances, Washington, DC.

6. US Food and Drug Administration Center for Food Safety and Applied Nutrition. (1993) *Toxicological Principles for the Safety Assessment of Direct Food Additives and Color Additives Used in Food*, US Food and Drug Administration, Washington, D.C.

7. Ehrich, M. and Veronesi, B. (1999) *In vitro* neurotoxicology, in *Neurotoxicology* (Tilson, H. A. and Harry, G. J., eds.), Taylor & Francis, Philadelphia, pp. 37–51.

8. Flint, O. P. (1999) An introduction to the practical applications of new *in vitro* tests, in *Neurotoxicology in Vitro* (Pentreath, V. W., ed.), Taylor & Francis, Philadelphia, pp. 3–16.

9. Dorman, D. C. (2000). An integrative approach to neurotoxicology. *Toxicol. Pathol.* **28,** 37–42.

10. Campbell, I. C., Fletcher, L., Grant, P. A. A., and Abdulla, E. M. (1996) Validation of in vitro tests in neurotoxicology. *ATLA* **24,** 339–347.

11. Purchase, I. F. H. (1996) *In vitro* toxicology methods in risk assessment. *ATLA* **24,** 325–331.

12. Halks-Miller, M., Fedor, V., and Tyson, C. A. (1991) Overview of approaches to *in vitro* neurotoxicity testing. *J. Am. Coll. Toxicol.* **10,** 727–736.

13. Tiffany-Castiglioni, E., Ehrich, M., Dees, L., et al. (1999) Bridging the gap between *in vitro* and *in vivo* models for neurotoxicology. *Toxicol. Sci.* **51,** 178–183.

14. Veronesi, B., Ehrich, M., Blusztain, J. K., Oortgiesen, M., and Durham, H. (1997) Cell culture models of interspecies selectivity to organophosphorus insecticides. *Neurotoxicology* **18,** 283–298.

15. Atterwill, C. K., Bruinink, A., Drejer, J., et al. (1994) *In vitro* neurotoxicity tests, the report and recommendations of ECVAM workshop 3. *ATLA* **22,** 350–362.

16. Balls, M. and Walum, E. (1999) Towards the acceptance of *in vitro* neurotoxicity tests, in *Neurotoxicology in Vitro* (Pentreath, V. W., ed.), Taylor & Francis, Philadelphia, pp. 269–283.

17. Slikker, W. Jr., Crump, K. S., Anderson, M. E., and Bellinger, D. (1996) Biologically based, quantitative risk assessment of neurotoxicants. *Fundam. Appl. Toxicol.* **229,** 18–30.

18. Costa, L. G. (1998) Biochemical and molecular neurotoxicology: relevance to biomarker development, neurotoxicity testing and risk assessment. *Toxicol. Lett.* **102–103,** 417–421.

19. Forsby, A., Pilli, F., Bianchi V., and Walum. E. (1995) Determination of critical cellular neurotoxic concentrations in human neuroblastoma (SH-SY5Y) cell cultures. *ATLA* **23,** 800–811.
20. Clemedson, C., McFarlane-Abdulla, E., Andersson, M., et al. (1996) MEIC evaluation of acute systemic toxicity. Part II. *In vitro* results from 68 toxicity assays used to test the first 30 reference chemicals and a comparative cytotoxicity analysis. *ATLA* **24,** 273–311.
21. Walum, E., Forsby, A., Clemedson, C., and Ekwall, B. (1996) Dynamic qualities of validation and the evoluation of new *in vitro* toxicological tests. *ATLA* **24,** 333–338.
22. Ehrich, M. (1998) Human cells as *in vitro* alternatives for toxicological research and testing: neurotoxicity studies. *Comments Toxicol.* **6,** 189–198.
23. Dorman, D. C., Struve, M. F., and Morgan, K. T. (1993) In vitro neurotoxicity research at CIIT. *CIIT Activities* **13(11–12),** 1–8.
24. Ray, D. E. (1999) Toxic cell damage, in *Neurotoxicology in Vitro* (Pentreath, V. W., ed.), Taylor & Francis, Philadelphia, pp. 77–103.
25. Ehrich, M., Correll, L., and Veronesi, B. (1997) Acetylcholinesterase and neuropathy target esterase inhibitions in neuroblastoma cells to distinguish organophosphorus compounds causing acute and delayed neurotoxicity. *Fundam. Appl. Toxicol.* **38,** 55–63.
26. Veronesi, B. and Ehrich, M. (1993). Differential cytotoxic sensitivity in mouse and human cell lines exposed to organophosphate insecticides. *Toxicol. Appl. Pharmacol.* **120,** 240–246.
27. Ehrich, M. and Correll, L. (1998). Inhibition of carboxylesterases in SH-SY5Y human and NB41A3 mouse neuroblastoma cells by organophosphorus esters. *J. Toxicol. Environ. Health* **53A,** 385–399.
28. Carlson, K., Jortner, B. S., and Ehrich, M. (2000). Organophosphorus compound-induced apoptosis in SH-SY5Y human neuroblastoma cells. *Toxicol. Appl. Pharmacol.* 168, 102–113.
29. Barber, D., Correll, L., and Ehrich, M. (1999) Comparison of two *in vitro* activation systems for protoxicant organophosphorous esterase inhibitors. *Toxicol. Sci.* **47,** 6–22.
30. Golub, M. S., Han, B., and Keen, C. L. (1999). Aluminum uptake and effects on transferrin mediated iron uptake in primary cultures of rat neurons, astrocytes and oligodendrocytes. *Neurotoxicology* **20,** 961–970
31. Roberts, R., Sandra, A., Siek, G. C., Lucas, J. J., and Fine, R. E. (1992). Studies of the mechanism of iron transport across the blood–brain barrier. *Ann. Neurol.* **32 S,** 43–50.
32. Aschner, M. and Clarkson, T. W. (1989). Methyl mercury uptake across bovine brain capillary endothelial cells in vitro: the role of amino acids. *Pharmacol. Toxicol.* **64,** 293–297.

33. Hu, H. L., Bennett, N., Lamb, J. H., Ghersi-Egea, J.F., Schlosshauer, B., and Ray, D. E. (1997). Capacity of rat brain to metabolize m-dinitrobenzene: an *in vitro* study. *Neurotoxicology* **18,** 363–370.
34. Song, X. and Ehrich, M. (1998). Uptake and metabolism of MPTP and MPP$^+$ in SH-SY5Y human neuroblastoma cells. *In Vitro Mol. Toxicol.* **11,** 3–14.
35. Corsini, G. U., Pintus, S., Bocchetta, A., Piccardi, M. P., and Del Zompo, M. (1986). A reactive metabolite of 1-methyl-4-phenyl-1,2,3,6-tetrahydropyridine is formed in rat brain *in vitro* by type B monoamine oxidase. *J. Pharmacol. Exp. Ther.* **238,** 648–652.
36. Mortenson, S. R., Brimijoin, S., Hooper, M. J., and Padilla, S. (1998) Comparison of the in vitro sensitivity of rat acetylcholinesterase to chlorpyrifos-oxon: What do tissue IC50 values represent? *Toxicol. Appl. Pharmacol.* **148,** 46–59.
37. Clothier, R. H., Hulme, L. M., Smith, M., and Balls,M. (1987) Comparison of the in vitro cytotoxicities and acute in vivo toxicities of 59 chemicals. *Mol. Toxicol.* **1,** 571–577.

3

Exposure–Dose–Response Paradigm as It Relates to Toxicogenomics

William H. Hanneman, Melvin E. Andersen, Marie E. Legare, Christine T. French, Tami S. McMullin, Carolyn Broccardo, and Ruth E. Billings

1. INTRODUCTION

Over the past decades, the risk assessment of chemicals has frequently been considered a pseudoscientific process, primarily determined by public policy that masquerades as science, rather than representing a process well grounded in firm biological principles. Many toxicologists are uncomfortable when their work is linked to risk assessment or even when asked how their work will influence the risk assessment process. This chapter discusses the integration of toxicological data in risk assessment, emphasizing the applications of molecular toxicology (toxicogenomics) for improving the risk assessments of all chemical especially neurotoxicants. The chapter discusses the integration of toxicology information via an exposure–dose paradigm, provides a brief synopsis of the emerging consensus to increase the scientific basis of "neuroactive" chemical risk assessment, and notes the areas where molecular toxicology will likely contribute to refinements of the current risk assessment process.

2. EXPOSURE–DOSE–RESPONSE PARADIGM

Providing a risk assessment context for studying toxicological issues related to public health requires a more interdisciplinary approach than is available from the in-depth probing of a molecular mechanism by which a

From: *Methods in Pharmacology and Toxicology: In Vitro Neurotoxicology: Principles and Challenges*
Edited by: E. Tiffany-Castiglioni © Humana Press Inc., Totowa, NJ

chemical interacts with cellular constituents. In assessing real-world risks, the entire continuum, including exposure, absorption, distribution, cellular interactions, and, ultimately, impaired health, needs to be considered in context. This contextual basis for studying the health consequences of exposures to toxicants is referred to here as an exposure–dose–response paradigm (*see* Fig. 1). Frequently, the main issue that confronts a molecular toxicologist is the problem of how individual mechanistic studies fit into this larger perspective. The converse is the problem of the risk assessor in determining how in-depth mechanistic studies affect the larger problem of assessing public health consequences of exposures. Risk assessments have to consider the integration of all the steps in this exposure–dose–response continuum to make definitive statements of the risks at various levels of exposure. Risk assessment then requires the melding of various disciplines to arrive at a product that is generally larger than the contributions of the individual portions. What are the disciplines that contribute to a formal risk assessment? They include exposure assessment, toxicity testing, mechanistic and molecular toxicology, pathology, statistics, and mathematical modeling. The ongoing reassessment of the risks of exposure to 2,3,7,8-tetrachorodibenzo-*p*-dioxin (TCDD) by the US Environmental Protection Agency (US EPA) outlines the broad set of considerations that are necessary in arriving at estimates of human risk from toxicant exposures *(1–3)*.

To a large extent, the emphasis placed on an exposure–dose–response continuum for organizing toxicology data is directly related to the need to have the product of all the individual studies be useful for chemical risk assessment. The marriage of risk assessment methods and molecular toxicology requires close cooperation between risk assessment professionals and molecular toxicologists. The former will be challenged to keep abreast of the increase in the understanding of biological processes afforded by the new genomic and proteomic tools available for studying biological function and toxicological problems. This task is formidable even for experts in the area. For the molecular toxicologists, the challenge is to understand the exposure–dose–response paradigm and to articulate how individual pieces of their work link together to form the risk assessment process.

3. RISK ASSESSMENT:
AN HISTORICAL PROSPECTIVE

Risk assessment for chemical hazards in the workplace and in the general environment have become increasingly formalized over the past several decades. In early stages in the 1950s *(4)*, animal studies were used to determine no observed effect levels (NOELs). The US FDA derived acceptable

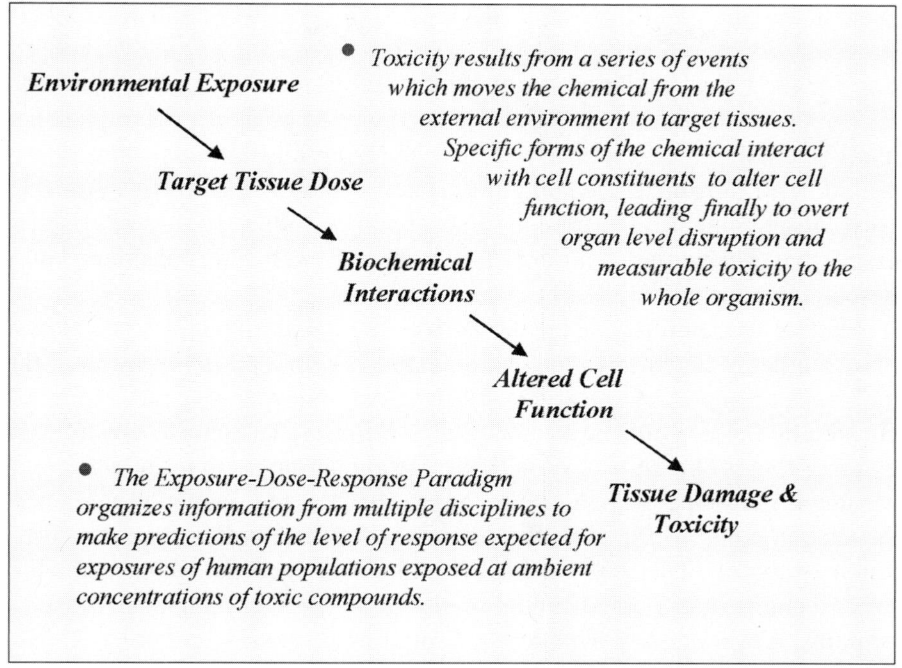

Fig. 1. Flowchart describing the continuum of the exposure–dose–response paradigm for organizing research in a manner useful for risk assessment applications. The major components to this continuum that need to be addressed include exposure, absorption, distribution, cellular interactions, and impaired health.

daily intakes (ADIs) by dividing animal NOELs by 100. The factor of 100 consisted of 2 safety factors of 10 each, intended in a general way to account for (1) differences in sensitivity of humans compared to animals and (2) variation in sensitivity of individuals in a heterogeneous human population compared to more homogeneous sensitivity in inbred animal stains. These ADIs were usually established based on organ- or organism-level responses that were clearly adverse to health. An underlying premise in this approach was the existence of a threshold dose (i.e., the belief that there were concentrations or exposure levels below which the risk of adverse health effects was zero).

In the 1970s, there was a refocusing of toxicological experimentation onto the biology of cancer and chemical carcinogenesis. The recognition of the role of mutagenesis as a requisite precursor to carcinogenesis brought attention to a variety of alternative test methods that could be used to assess mutagenesis in cells and simpler organisms. These alternative systems provided rapid screening of the mutagenic potential of many compounds. However, it was not clear how these data could be used to establish exposure standards. One obvious use for in vitro cell system data was in priority setting for long-term carcinogenicity studies in animals. If a compound had high exposures in human populations and showed evidence for mutagenicity, it would be a higher-priority compound for lifetime bioassay than a compound with similar exposure that lacked mutagenic activity. Another application is in product development. Compounds tested in short-term assays that proved mutagenic could be dropped from further consideration— in effect, a sieving process *(5)*.

Another contribution of the 1970s was the development of risk assessment methods for carcinogens. Animal studies provided information of the incidence of tumors at specific doses in test animals, usually rats and mice. How could these results be used to predict human risks at much lower doses by other routes of administration? Two extrapolations were introduced: One predicted the shape of the dose–response curve at low levels of incidence, the second adjusted the expected responses for different species. The low-dose extrapolation utilized a mathematical model of carcinogenesis, the linearized multistage (LMS) model. This model predicts some measure of response at every dose, no matter how small. Interspecies extrapolation, justified based on studies with various chemotherapeutic compounds, was calculated on a surface-area adjustment for dose. This extrapolation regards humans as more sensitive to toxic responses than are rodent species *(5)*.

Philosophically, however, this cancer risk assessment approach was quite distinct from that of other noncancer end points (i.e., neurotoxicity) *(6)*. Threshold approaches formed the basis for ADIs and carcinogens were treated as if they had no threshold. Although the cancer methods were primarily intended for carcinogens that interacted with DNA via mutational processes, these extrapolation tools were quickly applied to all chemical carcinogens. The LMS model and body surface-area dose adjustments were defined as defaults to be used for DNA-damaging carcinogens, but they came to be routine for all chemicals found to cause cancer. It bears emphasis that the understanding that multiple mechanisms contribute to chemical carcinogenesis was much less developed in the mid-1970s, when these initial cancer risk assessment paradigms were under development.

The concept of dose was also being refined by scientists who borrowed methods from the field of clinical pharmacokinetics (PK) to assess the relationship between exposure, sometimes called administered dose, and the concentrations of active chemical/metabolites at target tissues. The emphasis on compartmental pharmacokinetic models arose mainly as a result of the high doses used in many animal tests, doses at which capacity-limited processes (i.e., metabolism, renal tubular excretion in kidney, etc.) became saturated. Scientists in the chemical industry were the first to apply these PK methods to many commodity chemicals and to discuss the need to relate toxicity to target tissue dose rather than simple measures of dietary composition or concentration of inhaled chemical in the air. Work with vinyl chloride carcinogenesis showed a clear relationship between metabolized dose of this compound and carcinogenesis *(7)*.

The 1980s provided several important developments for toxicology. Among them were the increasing use of in vitro cell systems for assessing chemical interactions in living cells and the first applications of molecular techniques emerging from the new field of molecular biology. Another advance was the growing sophistication of techniques applied to assess how chemicals cause their effects (i.e., the mode of action of chemicals in biological systems). In addition, quantitative, mechanistic tools were increasingly being developed to assist in analysis of dose–response relationships. The earlier successes of compartmental PK models for unraveling dose–response curves continued in the development of physiologically based pharmacokinetic (PBPK) modeling to permit extrapolations across route, dose level, and species. At the same time, mechanistic models for carcinogenesis, primarily the Moolgavkar–Venzon–Knudson (MVK) model, provided a biological framework for considering the roles of mutation, cell birth and cell death, and cell differentiation within quantitative structures. This MVK model provided information on the role of promotion, defined as a growth advantage of preneoplastic versus normal cells, in giving rise to various shapes of dose–response curves. The MVK model for cancer was an early example of what is now referred to as biologically based dose–response (BBDR) models. These scientific contributions, coupled with the new quantitative tools in PBPK and BBDR modeling, provided pressure to apply this growing information to improve the scientific basis of chemical risk assessment *(7–9)*.

4. IN VITRO NEUROTOXICITY STUDIES: AN HISTORICAL PROSPECTIVE

In vitro studies involve the maintenance of primary cell cultures, established cell lines, cloned cells, reaggregate cultures, organotypic explants, and brain slices *(10,11)* in a state that is conducive to a variety of experimental techniques. They are traceable to investigations involving biochemistry, morphology, and electrophysiology. Additionally, molecular-biology techniques can be readily used to examine changes in gene and protein expression as a result of chemical treatment. In vitro studies are also used experimentally as screening tools to evaluate potential neurotoxicity of a chemical *(11)*. In vitro toxicity procedures are more simplistic and require less time and money than approaches through in vivo work. Additional advantages of in vitro toxicity testing include the creation of a uniform chemical and physical environment, strictly controlled continuous or intermittent exposure conditions, the use of only a small amount of chemical, bypassing systemic effects, and the availability of a large range of donor species and human materials *(10,11)*. Hence, the increasing attention to in vitro models in the past decade has, for the most part, contributed positively to the study of toxicology *(12)*.

The greatest potential for in vitro neurotoxicology work lies in the ability to examine the mechanism of action of toxicants. Prior to the 1990s, neurotoxicology studies generally lacked any mechanistic considerations. Yet, such mechanistic information is critical in assessing the potential toxicological impact of chemical compounds. Because in vitro systems permit the examination of mechanistic processes in isolated conditions, they facilitate characterization of the mode(s) of action in target tissues by elucidating information on cellular and molecular alterations caused by neurotoxicant exposure. Mechanistic understandings are also valuable in designing directed, hypothesis-driven, in vivo experiments *(12)* and aiding in the development of biomarkers of adverse effects. Such biomarkers can detect early biochemical modifications that may precede irreversible damage *(13)*. For example, in vitro studies aided in determining the underlying mechanism of organophosphorus toxicity, resulting in a renewed examination of interspecies sensitivity with regard to organophosphorus neurotoxicity *(14)*. Analyzing a toxicant's mechanism of action and evaluating the genetic contributions can elucidate potential varied responses within sensitive populations. Additionally, mechanistic in vitro studies, if conducted correctly, can help one construct and validate pharmacokinetic analyses and dose–response models, which play a critical role in the risk assessment of neuroactive compounds *(1,12)*.

Although in vitro methods play a crucial role in experimental research and provide valuable opportunities for more mechanistic risk assessments, they are associated with limitations and drawbacks, which must be considered when designing studies and extrapolating data to the dose–response paradigm. In vitro studies generally fail to account for the route of administration, distribution, and biotransformation of the toxicant within the body. Moreover, the detection of every neurotoxic end point from in vitro data extrapolation is virtually impossible. The in vitro conditions that cells are grown in are often a poor substitute for the intricate neuronal environment of the whole animal *(10)*. Other limitations include lack of integrated functions and the blood–brain barrier function, unknown target concentration, compensatory mechanisms cannot be determined, and single tests fail to cover every target and mechanism *(11)*. Because of these limitations, a variety of in vitro systems and a multitude of end points should be employed to parallel dose response in the intact animal. For example, end points should enable differentiation between cytotoxicants and neurotoxicants. Additionally, the experimental procedures of any in vitro neurotoxicity study should be standardized. Validation of any in vitro study is critical for consideration in risk assessment *(6)*.

5. NEW TOOLS FOR THE WAR ON NEUROTOXICANTS

With the advent of the "genomics revolution," creative new suites of methodologies for assessing molecular and cellular responses have increased exponentially. As the basic biological sciences provide new tools for research, these tools, in turn, become available for refining toxicological research. This theme recapitulates the other advances throughout the past 40 yr in the field of toxicology. However, from the risk assessment point of view, do these new tools automatically improve our ability to solve public health questions arising from chemicals in the environment? Without doubt, we are better able to assess molecular interactions at lower levels of exposure and to assess cellular level responses in vitro in a variety of organisms. Yet, it should be noted that research efforts utilizing these methods need to be placed in a risk perspective to provide useful data for assessing the public health consequences of exposures. Otherwise, the new field we now call "toxicogenomics" stands in jeopardy of creating a huge hazard identification database that will only serve to inflame public concerns about chemicals without providing the necessary exposure–dose–response perspective on the adversity of the observed alterations or a perspective on the linkage between these alterations and health consequences in target populations. Once again, from the point of view of risk assessment integration, there are a variety of disciplines that must contribute in addition to molecular genetics if the risk assessment is intended to have a strong basis in mechanistic biology *(see* Fig. 2). These disciplines can remain independent and Balkanized, as noted by the stark gridlines between them. In these cases, the integration process responsibility falls to the risk manager, who is unlikely to be trained in the disciplines of molecular and cellular biology. The jumble of information represents a formidable obstacle in creating the assessment.

A major problem in "handing these data off" for interpretation is that mechanistic data may fail to have a spokesperson arguing for their quantitative importance and noting how they might influence the risk assessment model. Molecular toxicology data collected and published, even in the most

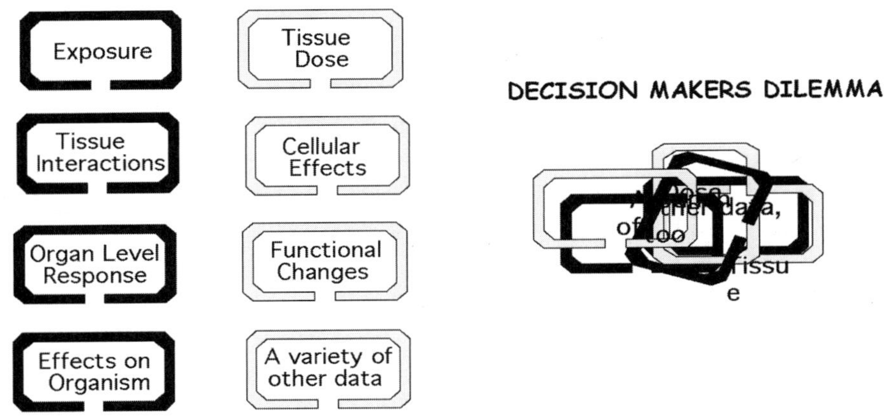

Hey buddy I've done my work... Somebody better use it!!

Fig. 2. An illustration of the dilemma faced by risk assessors on how to integrate and apply in-depth mechanistic data from seemingly independent disciplines into the exposure–dose–response paradigm. Commonly, research findings are passed on in the absence of interpretive context from the practicing scientist to the risk assessor who may not be knowledgeable about the applications of all the cutting edge science. This apparent jumble of information may represent a formidable task in creating the risk assessment.

prestigious journals, does not automatically convey information about how they fit into the exposure–dose–response paradigm. Basically, these data do not "speak for themselves." Scientists who collect the data need to serve as the spokesperson for their application and take responsibility for their inclusion in assessing risks of the chemicals in human populations. As noted earlier, the challenges with application of molecular-level data generally are twofold. The first question is in how these observations relate to portions of the exposure–dose–response continuum that are immediately upstream and immediately downstream. The second question with molecular-level observations is the relationship of precursor mechanistic end points to more obviously adverse responses at the organism level. The exposure–dose–response paradigm should be depicted by the more tightly integrated picture of a linked chain, connecting independent areas of research/testing to create a more seamless understanding of the responses of target organisms to toxic chemical exposures (*see* Fig. 3). Having provided the background on risk assessment methodologies, the remainder of the chapter discusses research strategies for improving risk assessment that introduce molecular methods within this exposure dose–response structure.

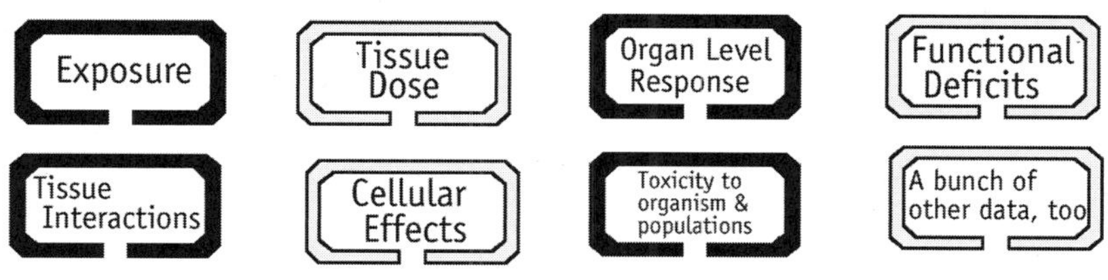

How do we plan the work so it will be used!!

Fig. 3. An illustration of a risk-assessment-oriented approach to integrating the various research disciplines. To achieve a cohesive set of data that can be linked to aid risk assessment, the contributions from individual disciplines need to be designed to fit into the exposure–dose–response continuum considering the adjacent disciplines and the relationship of all the steps to dose.

6. INTEGRATION OF TOXICOGENOMICS INTO THE EXPOSURE–DOSE–RESPONSE PARADIGM

In toxicology, the questions we ask are about how to reconstruct the normal circuitry and we examine the manner in which excesses of various exogenous and endogenous chemicals lead to physiological stress, alterations in gene batteries, and the resulting degradation of function. This manifesto for biology points to an integration of the multiple interacting cassettes that create normal cellular function and provide the main targets for assessing the actions of toxic compounds. An approach to studying these changes in batteries of coordinately controlled genes include observational assessment of the changes in gene/protein expression after dosing. This approach resembles studies in cancer in which the final aggressive transformed cell is compared with the initial normal cell to see the differences in characteristics between the two states. This strategy may place groups of compounds into categories in relation to their models of action while telling little about the cell alterations that move the cell from the initial to the final state. Uncovering the circuitry involved in these transitions may tell more about the molecular targets for the toxic responses and allow improved dose–response assessment of the toxic actions of the compounds.

Paramount to incorporation of molecular toxicological results in risk assessments would be a greater understanding of normal function of target macromolecules within the cell. The extent to which the normal function is understood both qualitatively and quantitatively would determine the extent to which the impact of the perturbation could be assessed at various doses and in various species. Although this idea may still be some distance off, it is no longer a fantasy. For example, although we still do not fully understand how the mammalian brain functions, there are documented learning deficits in toxicant-exposed human populations. In addition, recent gene targeting experiments suggest that the encoding process for learning and memory involve coordinated patterns of gene expression that result in stable changes in a discrete population of neuronal synapses, neurotransmitters, and brain enzymes *(14,15)*. Therefore, now more than ever, the science of toxicology, especially at the level of altered morbidity (i.e., learning and memory), is a study of perturbation of normal biological systems. In this case, the normal system is still somewhat of a "black box." However, there is light shining on virtually all of the critical processes. Instead of focusing on individual proteins or messenger RNA species, new genomic (microarray) and proteomic methods permit assessment of suites of genes and batteries of protein products that are coordinately regulated and allow a greater understanding of the manner in which toxicants alter their expression (*see* Fig. 4).

7. MECHANISTIC/COMPUTATIONAL CONCEPTS IN A MOLECULAR/CELLULAR CONTEXT

Despite the marvelous increase in sophistication of the methods available for studying cellular- and molecular-level responses, we are still faced with the same fundamental question in toxicology: What is the shape of the dose–response curve at low incidence levels for adverse effects? Moreover, will new technology answer these questions or will we simply continue to collect more and more information to form hazard identification without any insight for dose response in the intact animal?

Probably the most significant contribution that may arise from the combination of molecular toxicology coupled with a perturbation theory of toxicity is the ability to understand the molecular basis of dose–response

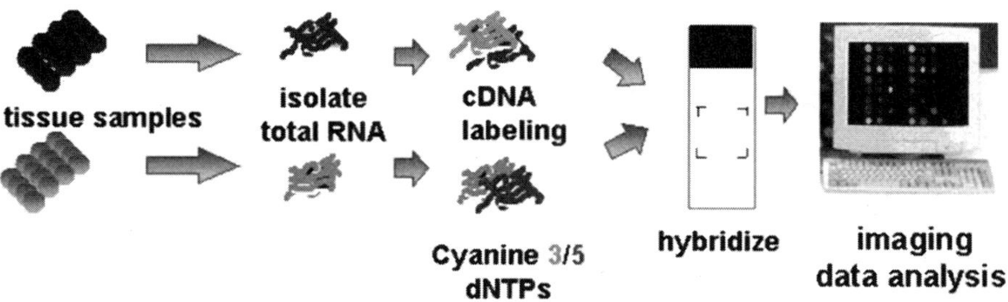

Fig. 4. Overview of cDNA microarray technology. This new genomic technique is increasingly being used to assess suites of genes that are coordinately regulated by toxicant treatment.

relationships for toxic compounds and provide biologically plausible methods for low-dose risk assessment. Dose–response assessment tools have largely been empirical or driven by defaults. A similar goal pervades the desire to create biological models of dose–response curves based on alterations in cell and tissue function (*see* Fig. 5). Whereas most dose–response assessment models have smooth continuous changes in response to dose, the real world of cells demonstrate a more complex variety of interacting circuits. Chemical processes can be described by statistical methods that average the behaviors of molecules, because the numbers of particles involved in most reactions and interactions are large. At the cellular level, behaviors are stochastic. For example, a cell either divides or it does not divide. A challenge in formulating the mathematical models of cellular functions is the requirement to grasp the manner in which continuous changes of chemical variables within the cell lead to dichotomous, discontinuous responses of the cell, such as apoptosis, proliferation, differentiation, or activation of global cellular circuitry by exposure to chemicals.

These stochastic, nonlinear models of cellular-level responses may provide the basis for developing tools that will predict threshold behaviors toward toxic exposures or predict dose regions where the proportionate response to increasing dose varies considerably from the dose–response structure at high doses of toxicants. Of course, some of the models applied for assessing cancer risks are stochastic models of cell division, cell death, and cell mutation. The MVK model represents a stochastic model of a biological process. As noted in perturbation approaches to biological–toxicological responses, the models have to be initially set to adequately describe tumor incidence in the control animals. In deriving the BBDR models, it is necessary to evaluate the effect of dose on intrinsic biological parameters of the model. The effects can be described empirically, as has been done, or

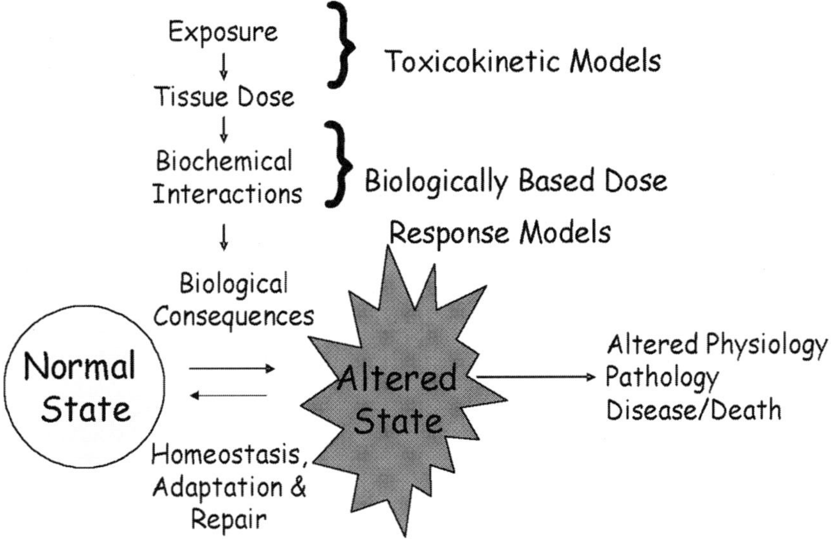

Fig. 5. Exposure–dose–response paradigm for toxic responses in relationship to perturbations of the normal control processes in the cell resulting from toxicant exposures. Mathematical, biologically based models are tools for describing and predicting these biological processes. Typically, toxicokinetic models are constructed to aid in linking exposure to tissue dose, whereas biologically based dose–response models aid in linking tissue dose to biological consequences at the cellular or physiological level.

mechanistically. Mechanistically, the relationship between dose and proliferation or dose and apoptosis are unlikely to be simple continuous functions. The control of biological circuitry and the transition between different states of the cellular circuitry in response to exogenous signaling molecules underlie the dose–response manifestations of the toxic responses.

Another area for interaction of dose–response modeling and molecular toxicology is the characterization of the relationship between molecular responses and ultimate toxic action. With 2,3,7,8-TCDD, the dose–response curves for simpler molecular responses tend to behave in a linear manner. For responses at the organ and organism level, the responses are less likely to be linear with apparent Hill-equation slope factors of greater than 1.0 *(8)*. Unraveling the control circuitry and the consequences of the molecular changes for the overall responses of the organism are important for providing the context to interpret many of the molecular changes that are measurable at much lower doses than are the overtly toxic responses. Therefore, the goal is to design molecular studies that make a difference. A good example

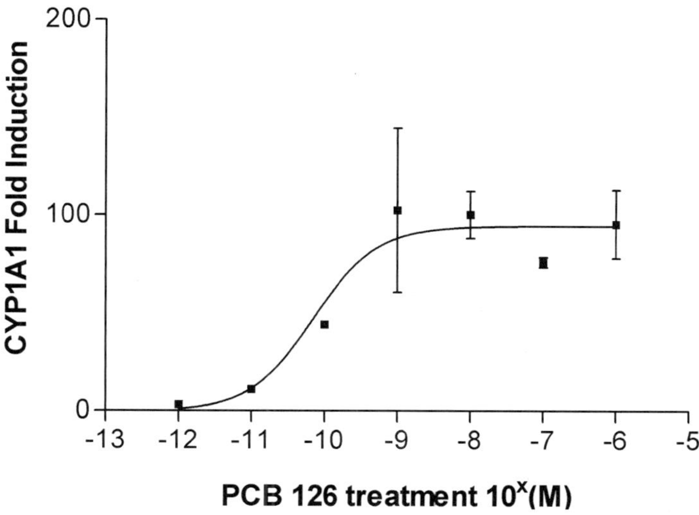

Fig. 6. The graph represents fold induction of CYP1A1 gene expression over a broad range of extremely low doses of PCB 126 (Hanneman Laboratory, unpublished data). CYP1A1 gene expression is quantified using "real-time" quantitative reverse transcription–polyacrylamide gel electrophoresis. This graph demonstrates the use of molecular techniques to quantify the lower end of the dose–response curve.

of this is an ongoing project in our laboratory that examines the nature of CYP1A1 induction within cells exposed to varying concentrations of PCB 126 (*see* Fig. 6). CYP1A1 mRNA induction is measured in these cells using "real-time" quantitative reverse transcription–polyacrylamide gel electrophoresis and, thus, affording us the opportunity to quantitatively examine the lower end of the dose–response curve in these cells.

8. OPPORTUNITIES AND CONCLUSIONS

It would seem that once every decade, new breakthroughs in biomedical technologies open up floodgates of new discoveries. These new findings are, in turn, followed by a fundamental shift in our basic understanding of biology. As toxicologists, we must try and position ourselves into research environments that will afford us the advantage of these new technologies and allow us to push the envelope of new discoveries in toxicology, thus creating more accurate assessments of risk of chemicals to humans. The traditional practice of one primary investigator studying one gene is fading fast and emerging in its wake are predictive screening strategies that the allow study of the complex interplay between hundreds to thousands of genes at both the in vitro and in vivo levels.

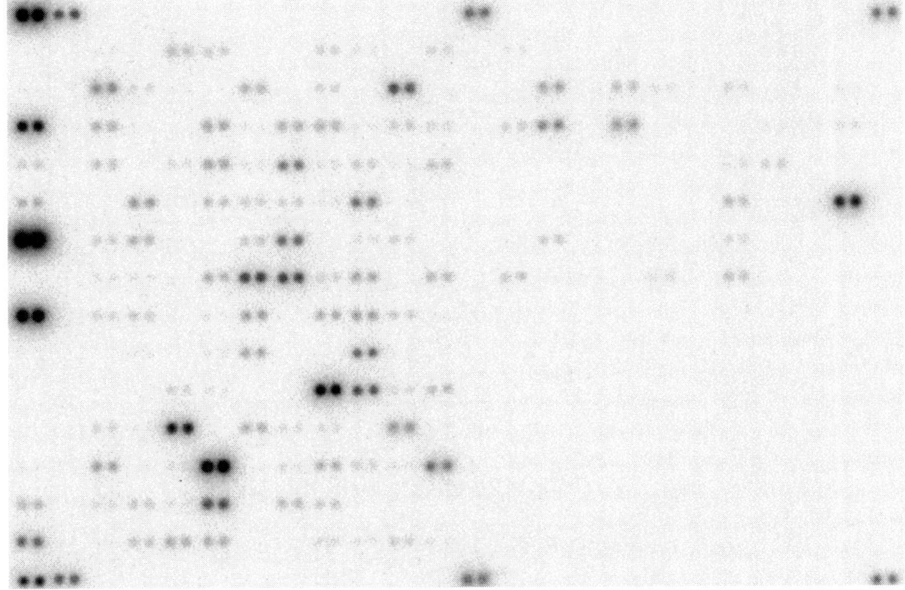

Fig. 7. An example of a selected area view of a cDNA microarray (Hanneman Laboratory) after hybridization of control and exposed cell samples. cDNA microarray technology is opening new avenues into investigating "large-scale" functional gene changes resulting from toxicant exposure.

Most certainly, our passing into a new millennium has marked the opening of a new floodgate during which we have seen major developments in widespread genome sequencing (human and mouse) and the development of technical platforms to support "large-scale" functional gene analysis. The availability of sequence information for thousands of genes (and, in most cases, the coding regions of these genes) has allowed investigators to construct large-scale gene microarrays (*see* Fig. 7) that enable semiquantitative measurement of the transcriptional activity of thousands of genes during chemical exposure *(16)*. As one can envision, these arrays can be either "broad spectrum" or custom designed to profile particular tissues (brain, liver, etc.) or specific toxicological pathways (aryl hydrocarbon receptor [AhR], poly-ADPribose polymerase [PARP], etc.) and may lead to a number of scientific windfalls (i.e., rapid fingerprints of chemical toxicity, a greater appreciation of molecular mechanisms of toxicity, and, finally an enhanced ability to extrapolate accurately between in vitro and in vivo approaches in the context of risk assessment. Clearly, the possibility of toxicogenomics giving us multiple data end points of adverse chemical effects (at low levels of exposure) is extremely exciting. It is reasonable to predict that accurate interpretation of expression changes will only be possible when the technologies of toxicogenomics are merged with classical experiments designed to understand toxicity at the physiological, pathological, and biochemical levels.

However, toxicogenomics also raises many questions in the context of interpreting gene expression changes with respect to hazard and risk assessment. Concerns are applicable with any new methodology brought to bear on issues related to the protection of public health from toxic compound exposures. Such questions arise as to the relationship of the concentrations used in cellular studies to doses that would be present in exposed persons. A second question that might arise is the relationship of the molecular markers to an adverse outcome (as described earlier). The answers to these latter questions all too often remain elusive. The converse is the opportunities provided by new technologies to make advances on primary issues that have resisted resolution with other tools. From the personal perspective of the authors of this chapter, the possibility of explaining the molecular basis of nonlinear dose–response curves with toxicants would be a significant contribution of molecular methods to public health in relation to toxic chemical exposures. Such insights would provide much more accurate risk assessments than estimates derived from arbitrary application of uncertainty factors and the proliferation of these factors for each new concern, such as the additional safety factor of 10 proposed for children in the Food Quality Protection Act of 1996 *(17)*.

In the final analysis, the primary challenge for linking molecular toxicology and/or toxicogenomics (especially the large-scale methods for assessing altered gene expression) with risk assessment is to avoid the collection of large bodies of data that serve only as hazard identification. Such uses of new methods tend to arouse public concern about potential risks of chemical exposures without providing any contextual analysis of the "actual risks" posed by exposures at low doses. Part of the solution to this is the design of careful studies that take advantage of the exposure–dose–response paradigm.

Interestingly, if one follows the ideas outlined in this chapter, one will find that his or her experiments will recapitulate the "essence" of the genomics revolution as stated so elegantly in an article entitled "Genomics: Journey to the Center of Biology" in which the authors note the overall goals of studies on genomics (see below) *(18)*:

> The long-term goal is to use this information to reconstruct the complex molecular circuitry that operates within the cell—to map out the network of interacting proteins that determines the underlying logic of various cellular biological functions including cell proliferation, responses to physiologic stresses, and acquisition and maintenance of tissue-specific differentiation

functions. A longer term goal, whose feasibility remains unclear, is to create mathematical models of these biological circuits and thereby predict these various types of cell biological behavior.

REFERENCES

1. Occapational Safety and Health Administration (OSHA) (1997) Occupational exposure to methylene chloride; final rule. *Fed. Reg.* **62(7),** 1493–1619.
2. US Environmenatal Protection Agency (2000) Toxicological review of vinyl chloride. EPA Report EPA/635R-00/004.
3. US EPA (2000) Exposure and human health reassessment of 2.3.7.8-tetrachlorodibenzo-*p*-dioxin (TCDD) and related compounds. Part II. Health assessment for 2.3.7.8-tetrachlorodibenzo-*p*-dioxin (TCDD) and related compounds. EPA Report NCEA-1-0835 (Science Advisory Board Review Draft).
4. Lehman, A. J. and Fitzhugh, O. G. (1954) 100-Fold margin of safety. *Assoc. Food Drug Off. U.S. Q. Bull.* **18,** 33–35.
5. Albert R. E., Train, R. E., and Anderson, E. (1977) Rationale developed by the Environment Protection Agency for the assessment of carcinogenic risks. *J. Natl. Cancer Inst.* **58,** 1537–1541.
6. Slikker, W., Crump, K. S., Andersen, M. E., and Bellinger, D. (1996) Biologically based, quantitative risk assessment of neurotoxicants. *Fundam. Appl. Toxicol.* **29,** 18–30.
7. Watanabe, P. G. and Gehring, P. J. (1976) Dose-dependent fate of vinyl chloride and its possible relationship to oncogenicity in rats. *Environ. Health Perspect.* **17,** 145–152.
8. Leung, H. W. (1991) Development and utilization of physiologically based pharmacokinetic models for toxicological applications. *J. Toxicol. Environ. Health* **32,** 247–267.
9. Moolgavkar, S. H. and Knudson, A. G., Jr. (1981) Mutation and cancer: a model for human carcinogenesis. *J. Natl. Cancer Inst.* **66,** 1037–1052.
10. Office of Research and Development, US Environmental Protection Agency 91998) Guidelines for neurotoxicity risk assessment. *Fed. Reg.* **63(93),** 26,926–26,954.
11. Costa, L. G. (1998) Neurotoxicity testing: a discussion of in vitro alternatives. *Environ. Health Perspect.* **106(Suppl. 2),** 505–510.
12. Tison, H. A. (2000) New horizons: future directions in neurotoxicology. *Environ. Health Perspect.* **108(Suppl. 3),** 439–441.
13. Costa, L. G. (1998) Biochemical and molecular neurotoxicology: relevance to biomarker development, neurotoxicity testing and risk assessment. *Toxicol. Lett.* **102–103,** 417–421.
14. Veronesi, B., Ehrich, M., Blusztajn, J. K., Oörtgiesen, M., and Durham, H. (1997) Cell culture models of interspecies selectivity to organophosphorous insecticides. *Neurotoxicology* **18(1),** 283–297.
15. Vohradsky, J. (2001) Neural network model of gene expression. *FASEB J.* **15,** 846–854.

16. Puga, A., Maire, A., and Medvedovic, P. (2000) Transcriptional signature of dioxin in human hepatoma HepG2 cells. *Biochem. Pharmacol.* **60,** 1129–1142.
17. The Food Quality and Protection Act (1996) Public Law 104-170.
18. Lander, E. S. and Weinberg, R. A. (2000) Genomics: journey to the center of biology. *Science* **287,** 1777–1782.

4

In Vitro Studies of Neurotoxicant Effects on Cellular Homeostasis

Gerald J. Audesirk and Ronald B. Tjalkens

1. INTRODUCTION

Homeostasis in neurons is regulated by interactions among many signaling pathways. We will loosely define the term "signaling pathways" to include any molecular mechanisms that transduce external environmental stimuli (e.g., neurotransmitters, hormones, or contact with other cells) and/ or intracellular metabolic conditions (e.g., intracellular free Ca^{2+} ion concentrations, redox status, or ATP demand) into cellular responses such as process growth, synthesis of neurotransmitters and/or their receptors, or changes in cellular respiration. This definition includes the interlinked pathways that lead to alterations in protein kinase or phosphatase activity and activation or repression of gene transcription and, perhaps less familiar mechanisms such as the stimulation of mitochondrial matrix enzymes by elevations in intramitochondrial Ca^{2+}.

Neurotoxicants can impact these pathways in many ways, but most effects fall into three categories. First, a neurotoxicant can block one or more steps in a pathway. A familiar example is the reduction of Ca^{2+} influx through a variety of voltage- or ligand- sensitive ion channels by extracellular heavy metals, which would reduce Ca^{2+} signaling in a number of different pathways. Second, a neurotoxicant can inappropriately stimulate signaling pathways. For example, a neurotoxicant can mimic an activating molecule, as inorganic Pb^{2+} can mimic Ca^{2+} in activation of calmodulin or protein kinase C. Third, a neurotoxicant can cause cellular effects that relatively nonspecifically stimulate or inhibit various pathways. One of these "non-

From: *Methods in Pharmacology and Toxicology: In Vitro Neurotoxicology: Principles and Challenges*
Edited by: E. Tiffany-Castiglioni © Humana Press Inc., Totowa, NJ

                                          Audesirk and Tjalkens

specific effects," which is receiving increasing attention as a possible factor in neurodegenerative disorders, is the production of and/or reduction in the clearance of reactive oxygen species (ROS) or reactive nitrogen species (RNS) by a variety of neurotoxicants. ROS or RNS affect many cellular processes, including damaging the mitochondrial respiratory chain, which increases ROS generation, stimulating apoptosis and/or necrosis, and oxidizing or nitrating many different lipids or proteins, including transmitter receptors and ion channels.

Evidence of mechanisms of action and/or toxic end points can be obtained following in vivo exposures, including changes in neurotransmitter turnover, receptor density, caspase activation, or oxidized lipids or proteins in brain samples. When used with caution, mice that overexpress specific genes or with knockout mutations in those same genes can be extraordinarily valuable in elucidating mechanisms of toxic action in vivo (and in vitro). However, detailed mechanistic studies, of both the basic biochemistry of signaling pathways and the effects of neurotoxicants, are most commonly carried out in vitro.

We will begin this chapter with a brief discussion of in vitro models, emphasizing the advantages and disadvantages of primary cultures and immortal cell lines. We will then discuss some of the known or suspected mechanisms whereby neurotoxicants can alter signaling pathways and, consequently, cellular homeostasis in neurons and glia, focusing on in vitro experiments. Despite a voluminous literature, the study of toxicant effects on cellular signaling is only in its infancy. Therefore, although we will discuss known toxicant effects on cell signaling, our emphasis will be to describe signaling pathways that are *likely* to be impacted by toxicants but that, in fact, have usually not been thoroughly investigated. Finally, where appropriate, we will discuss pitfalls in experimental design.

2. EVALUATING MODEL SYSTEMS

Although the extent of reduction varies, all in vitro experiments use model systems in which the complexity of in vivo metabolism and cell-to-cell interactions is significantly less than in living animals. Further, the culture conditions can never fully mimic in vivo conditions, and one must always consider the possibility that effects seen in vitro arise because of interactions between toxicant and culture conditions that would not occur in vivo. Probably the most common and serious of these possible interactions would be at least slightly impaired health of cultured cells and overstimulation or understimulation of various cellular processes by ingredients present in, or missing from, the culture media (e.g., hormones, neurotransmitters, or growth factors). Beyond these relatively unavoidable difficulties, there is also substantial debate over the merits of various in vitro systems, particularly primary cell cultures versus immortal cell lines.

Primary cultures of neurons or glia are those that are cultured directly from an animal and usually maintained in culture more than 1 d (acutely isolated cells are therefore not usually considered to be "cultured"). Neurons or glial cells can be cultured from defined brain regions, allowing the investigator to study the effects of neurotoxicants on neurons from, for example, both susceptible and resistant areas. In certain circumstances, relatively homogeneous neuronal cultures may be obtained, such as cerebellar granule neurons isolated from early postnatal rat or mice pups *(1)* [although granule neurons are not completely physiologically homogeneous, for example in their responses to stimulation of metabotropic glutamate receptors *(2)*]. Neurons or glia isolated from knockout or transgenic animals can be extremely useful for determining mechanisms of action. Newly developed, highly effective transfection methods for DNA, oligonucleotides, and proteins should also be utilized in mechanistic studies.

Although primary cultures consist of "normal" neurons or glia, their morphology and metabolic state may differ significantly from the same cell types in vivo. For example, cultured rat hippocampal neurons show enhanced dendritic growth when plated on polylysine as an attachment factor and enhanced axonal growth when plated on laminin *(3)*. Such differences can enhance neurotoxicology studies (e.g., by providing greater ease of studying certain phenomena, such as axonal elongation) or hinder interpretation of results if the in vitro mechanisms cannot readily be related to in vivo events.

Immortal cell lines are an alternative to primary cultures. Frequently used cell lines include neuroblastoma cells such as N1E-115 (mouse) or SH-SY5Y (human), pheochromocytoma (PC12) cells, and glioma cells such as C6. Immortal cell lines have certain advantages over primary cultures. First, because they multiply indefinitely in culture under the right conditions, they can simultaneously eliminate animal use and provide larger quantities of cells than are usually readily available in primary cultures. Second, many can be caused to differentiate in culture "on command," by the addition of appropriate differentiation factors such as nerve growth factor, retinoic acid, or dibutyryl cyclic AMP. Third, they can be relatively homogeneous compared to some types of primary culture. Fourth, there is an increasingly large catalog of well-characterized substrains of some cell lines, such as PC12 cells that are deficient in cyclic AMP-dependent protein kinase *(4)*, providing the equivalent of "knockout" cells in culture. Fifth, many cell lines, such as PC12, are easily transfected with foreign genes *(5)*. Finally, cultures of immortalized neurons are generally completely free of glial cells, which virtually always contaminate primary neuronal cultures to some extent. Glial cells often respond differently to many toxicants and can also protect neurons (e.g., by releasing glutathione or bilirubin into the medium). Therefore, it is often difficult to tease apart the response differences between neurons and glia in primary cultures.

Unfortunately, most immortal cell lines have significant drawbacks as well. Immortal cells differ significantly from "normal" neurons, perhaps most strikingly in their ability to multiply indefinitely under permissive culture conditions. Further, most immortal cell lines derived from tumors contain cells with widely differing numbers of chromosomes and, therefore, differing doses of genes. A recent development in cell lines is the use of the SV40 large T antigen, particularly a temperature-sensitive form, to immortalize cells. A transgenic mouse strain, called the Immortomouse (available from Charles River), carries a temperature-sensitive SV40 large T antigen and can be used to derive temperature-sensitive, immortal cell lines of many different cell types. Nevertheless, whether derived from tumors or transgenics, immortal cell lines may undergo evolution in culture. The cell lines can mutate and genetic drift or (usually unknown) selective pressures in culture can promote significant changes in phenotype; for example, PC12 cells from different laboratories can show different responses compared to the original line *(5)*. The "same" cell line could therefore differ significantly between laboratories or in the same laboratory over time. Finally, although individual molecules such as voltage-sensitive calcium channels might be functionally identical in primary neurons and immortal cell lines, the complex cascades of intracellular signaling could be somewhat different. Depending on the toxicant and cell line under study, these differences can lead to enhanced susceptibility, or enhanced resistance, in the immortal cells.

Therefore, there are both advantages and disadvantages to primary cultures and immortal cell lines. Each has some unique attributes that might be important for certain types of study. A thorough evaluation of the merits of alternative model systems is essential to ensure that the model chosen will provide appropriate data that can be extrapolated back to in vivo toxicology.

3. NEUROTOXICANTS AND CELL SIGNALING PATHWAYS

There are numerous cell signaling pathways in neurons and astrocytes, including the following: the classical pathways that activate serine/threonine protein kinases such as the protein kinase C family, cyclic AMP-dependent protein kinase, cyclic GMP-dependent protein kinase, and Ca^{2+}/calmodulin-dependent protein kinases; several MAP kinase pathways, including those that mediate activation of the extracellular signal regulated kinases (ERKs), p38 kinase, and JNK; and the caspase cascade, to name just a few. We will not attempt to provide an exhaustive catalog of neurotoxicant effects on all of these pathways. Rather, we will focus on a few selected pathways and toxicants and describe some important principles that will often apply, with some modification, to other pathways and other toxicants.

3.1. Ca^{2+} Homeostasis

Many signaling pathways are regulated to some extent by the intracellular free-Ca^{2+} ion concentration, $[Ca^{2+}]_i$, either globally within entire cells or more often locally near sites of Ca^{2+} entry through the plasma membrane or release from intracellular stores. Conversely, many signaling pathways also help to regulate Ca^{2+} concentrations, for example, by phosphorylation and dephosphorylation of Ca^{2+}-permeable membrane channels, thereby altering Ca^{2+} influx [e.g., voltage-sensitive Ca^{2+} channels *(6–12)*; NMDA receptor/channels *(13,14)*]. Toxicants may affect $[Ca^{2+}]_i$ in many ways, including altering Ca^{2+} influx or release, Ca^{2+} extrusion, or the many signaling pathways that affect $[Ca^{2+}]_i$. A few toxicants, particularly heavy metals, can also directly mimic or inhibit Ca^{2+}-sensitive processes.

3.1.1. Signaling Pathways and Ca^{2+} Homeostasis

We will begin with a brief description of the major cellular mechanisms controlling intracellular Ca^{2+} homeostasis, with some examples of important toxicant effects on these pathways (*see* Fig. 1). The free-Ca^{2+} concentration in the cytoplasm, $[Ca^{2+}]_i$, is normally in the range 50–200 nM. The extracellular Ca^{2+} concentration is about 2 mM, providing a very large gradient for Ca^{2+} influx through the plasma membrane and requiring constant extrusion of Ca^{2+} out of the cell. Intracellular free-Ca^{2+} concentrations are a dynamic balance among Ca^{2+} influx and extrusion through the plasma membrane, and Ca^{2+} sequestration and release from intracellular stores. These pathways for Ca^{2+} movement are composed of channels, exchange proteins, or pumps, which can be clustered in localized regions of a cell (e.g., postsynaptic membranes may have a high density of ligand-gated, Ca^{2+}-permeable receptor/channels). Further, because of many intracellular Ca^{2+}-binding molecules, the diffusion distance for Ca^{2+} in the cytoplasm is very small. Therefore, changes in intracellular Ca^{2+} usually begin as one or more "hot spots" near channels or channel clusters, where the intracellular free-Ca^{2+} concentration can reach tens of micromolar *(15)*. Increases in cytoplasmic Ca^{2+} can then spread throughout the cell, usually at much lower concentrations. Uptake of Ca^{2+} by intracellular organelles, especially endoplasmic reticulum or mitochondria, can limit such spread. Alternatively, Ca^{2+}-sensi-

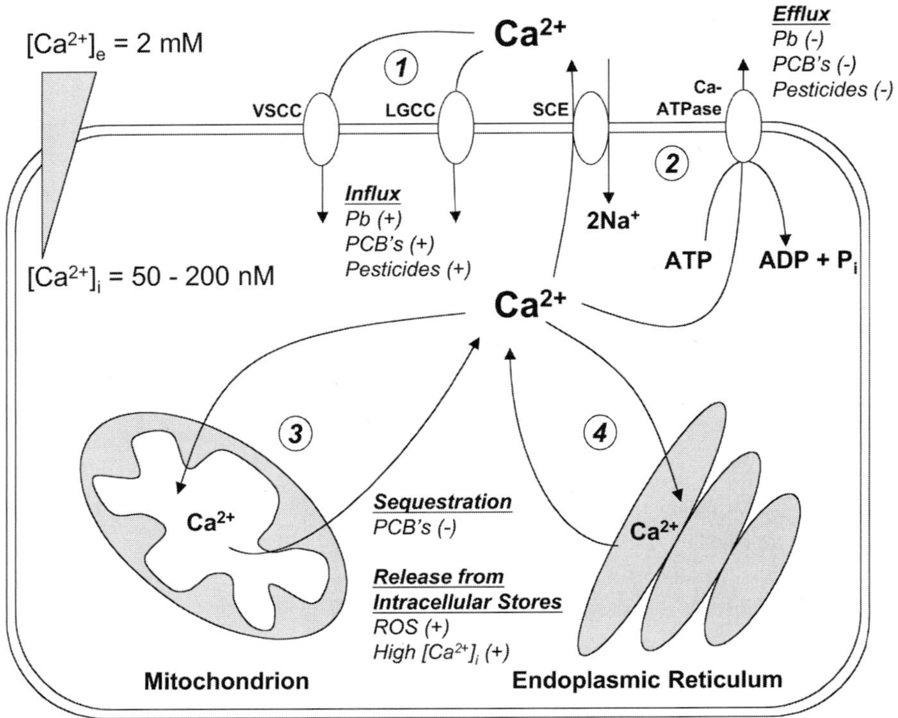

Fig. 1. Alteration of intracellular calcium regulation by neurotoxicants. The free-Ca^{2+} concentration in the cytoplasm, $[Ca^{2+}]_i$, is normally in the range 50–200 nM. The extracellular Ca^{2+} concentration is about 2 mM, providing a very large gradient for Ca^{2+} influx through the plasma membrane and requiring constant extrusion of Ca^{2+} out of the cell. (**1**) Calcium entry into the cell is tightly regulated and occurs primarily via voltage-sensitive calcium channels (VSCCs) and ligand-gated calcium channels (LGCC), such as the nicotinic acetylcholine receptors, NMDA receptor, and some AMPA/kainate types of glutamate receptor. VSCCs are sensitive to inhibition by various neurotoxic heavy metals including Pb^{2+}. (**2**) Calcium extrusion from the cell is achieved through the Na^+–Ca^{2+} exchanger (SCE) and the plasma membrane Ca^{2+} ATPase. The SCE can operate in reverse under certain conditions and actually contribute to increases in $[Ca^{2+}]_i$. (**3**) Ca^{2+} is sequestered by both mitochondria and endoplasmic reticulum. Mitochondria possess a low-affinity, high-capacity uptake channel that provides buffering of intracellular calcium levels during transient and oscillatory calcium signaling events. Mitochondria can also release large quantities of calcium during inner-membrane permeabilization from ROS and neurotoxicants. (**4**) The endoplasmic reticulum has a high- affinity Ca^{2+} ATPase uptake pump (SERCA pump) and can have at least two release channels: the ryanodine receptor (responsible for Ca^{2+}-induced Ca^{2+} release) and the IP_3 receptor (responsible for inositol trisphosphate-induced Ca^{2+} release). The ER calcium channels are sensitive to inhibition by ROS and several neurotoxicants including polychlorinated biphenyls.

tive release of Ca^{2+} from endoplasmic reticulum can lead to repetitive spikes or waves of elevated Ca^{2+}.

3.1.1.1. Ca^{2+} INFLUX

The principal pathways for Ca^{2+} influx are the following: voltage-sensitive calcium channels (VSCCs); ligand-gated channels, particularly some forms of nicotinic acetylcholine receptors and the NMDA and some AMPA/ kainate types of glutamate receptor; and, in some cell types, the "reverse operation" of the Na^+–Ca^{2+} exchanger. Many toxicants either directly or indirectly alter Ca^{2+}-entry $[Ca^{2+}]_i$ via these pathways. For example, it has been known for almost half a century that Pb^{2+} and many other heavy metals inhibit Ca^{2+} currents through VSCCs. It is much less clear whether most of these effects are toxicologically relevant, given the relatively high concentrations of metals required for significant block (usually micromolar to millimolar) and the low concentrations in blood or extracellular fluid (usually nanomolar to very low micromolar).

We hypothesize that intracellular actions of toxicants are, in many cases, more likely to be important in altering Ca^{2+} influx through these pathways. For example, picomolar concentrations of intracellular Pb^{2+} block Ca^{2+}-dependent inactivation of VSCCs in patch-clamped bovine chromaffin cells, causing increased Ca^{2+} influx *(16)*. Further, Ca^{2+} influx through most of these pathways is strongly regulated by intracellular signaling events, including binding of activated calmodulin and phosphorylation by any of several protein kinases. For example, calmodulin mediates Ca^{2+}-dependent inactivation in several types of VSCC *(17–19)* and in NMDA receptors *(20,21)*. Ca^{2+} entering through the channel binds to calmodulin, which, in turn, binds to an IQ-like motif near the intracellular mouth of the channel and reduces further Ca^{2+} influx (for reviews, see refs. *22* and *23*). Any toxicant that alters calmodulin concentrations or activity [as many heavy metals do; e.g., Pb^{2+} *(24–26)*] would be expected to alter Ca^{2+}-dependent inactivation. Whether this is the mechanism of the effects of Pb^{2+} on Ca^{2+}-dependent inactivation remains unknown.

The activity of many channels is altered by phosphorylation. Many serine–threonine protein kinases, including protein kinase C (PKC), cyclic AMP-dependent protein kinase (PKA), and Ca^{2+}/calmodulin-dependent protein kinase (CaM kinase), phosphorylate many types of VSCCs (e.g., refs. *6–12*), NMDA receptors *(13,14,27)*, AMPA receptors *(28–30)*, nicotinic receptors *(31–33)*, and the Na^+–Ca^{2+} exchange protein *(34)*, with variable effects on Ca^{2+} influx. Many toxicants alter the activity of these protein kinases in a variety of ways. For example, Pb^{2+} activates calmodulin *(24–26)*. Further, Pb^{2+} and Ca^{2+} are roughly additive in calmodulin activation *(26)*, so even very low concentrations of intracellular Pb^{2+} will probably impact calmodulin-stimulated enzymes, particularly at times when intracellular Ca^{2+} is increased. Thus, Pb^{2+} activates CaM kinase II, and combinations of low concentrations of Pb^{2+} and Ca^{2+} stimulate CaM kinase II more effectively than either cation alone (Wisniewski and Audesirk, unpublished results). Activation of calmodulin should also stimulate a host of other calmodulin-stimulated enzymes, thereby triggering numerous signaling cascades that should alter protein kinase activity. Thus, activation of calmodulin should stimulate isoforms I, III, and VIII of adenylate cyclase *(35)*, thereby increasing cyclic AMP concentrations and stimulating PKA. Alternatively, calmodulin activation also stimulates the PDE1 isoform of cyclic nucleotide phosphodiesterase *(35)*, which should reduce cyclic AMP concentrations. Which of these effects of Pb^{2+} would dominate in a cell will depend on the PDE and adenylate cyclase isoforms present in the cell and probably the relative concentrations of Pb^{2+} and Ca^{2+}. Pb^{2+} is also a partial agonist for Ca^{2+}-dependent isoforms of PKC, apparently as a partial Ca^{2+} mimic *(36,37)*. Because Ca^{2+} stimulates PKC more effectively than Pb^{2+} does, cellular PKC activity is likely to be a complex function of the concentrations of these two cations. Many other toxicants also alter protein kinase activity. For example, ortho-substituted polychlorinated biphenyl (PCB) congeners stimulate PKC activity in rat cerebellar granule cells by a Ca^{2+}–dependent mechanism *(38–40)*. In PC12 cells, a wide variety of pesticides, including endrin, chlordane, lindane, DDT, chlorpyrifos, and fenthion, stimulate PKC activity *(41)*. These toxicants would therefore also be expected to alter phosphorylation and activity of Ca^{2+}-permeable channels.

Total channel phosphorylation, of course, is determined by the activities of both kinases and phosphatases. Relatively little is known about toxicant effects on phosphatases. However, by activating calmodulin, picomolar concentrations of free Pb^{2+} stimulate calcineurin, a calmodulin-dependent phosphatase *(42)*. Higher Pb^{2+} concentrations reduce calcineurin activity. Several pyrethroid insecticides have been reported to inhibit calcineurin at extremely low concentrations *(43)* and are marketed commercially for that purpose, but these findings have been difficult to replicate *(44,45)*.

In summary, the influx of Ca^{2+} through the plasma membrane may be affected by toxicant actions both directly on the channels and via alteration of intracellular signaling. The impact of even a single toxicant on Ca^{2+} influx is likely to be the sum of a complex of interactions at multiple sites.

3.1.1.2. EXTRUSION OF Ca^{2+}

Ca^{2+} is transported out of cells by two principal mechanisms: Na^+–Ca^{2+} exchange proteins and Ca^{2+}ATPase pumps. The "normal" action of the exchange proteins uses the inward movement of Na^+ down its concentration gradient to transport Ca^{2+} out of the cytoplasm. However, under some circumstances, such as increased loading of the cytoplasm with Na^+ during intense neuronal activity, the exchanger can operate in reverse mode and actually transport Ca^{2+} into the cell. The affinity of the Na^+–Ca^{2+} exchange protein for Ca^{2+} is relatively low *(46)*; although Na^+–Ca^{2+} exchange may be important in clearing the cytoplasm of large, transient Ca^{2+} loads, this mechanism probably cannot reduce $[Ca^{2+}]_i$ significantly below 1 μM *(47,48)*. Therefore, this transport mechanism is unlikely to regulate the "resting" intracellular free-Ca^{2+} concentration. To our knowledge, there is nothing known about toxicant effects on Na^+–Ca^{2+} exchange. On the other hand, Na^+–Ca^{2+} exchange is regulated by phosphorylation by CaM kinase II *(34)*, making it likely that some toxicants might alter exchange activity through phosphorylation or dephosphorylation.

There are several isoforms of the plasma membrane Ca^{2+}ATPase pump (PMCA pump), with various affinities for Ca^{2+} and regulation by intracellular signaling pathways (see refs. *47–50*). Heavy metals can compete with Ca^{2+} for pumping action; Pb^{2+}, for example, can be pumped by the erythrocyte PMCA *(51,52)*. At least at high concentrations, Pb^{2+} might reduce the extrusion of Ca^{2+} *(53,54)*. The effects, if any, of likely intracellular metal concentrations on Ca^{2+} extrusion via the PMCA are largely unknown. The PMCA pumps are also stimulated by activated calmodulin; therefore, any toxicant that alters calmodulin activity should also alter Ca^{2+} extrusion by the PMCA. To our knowledge, appropriately designed experiments to test this possibility have not been reported.

3.1.1.3. STORAGE AND RELEASE OF Ca^{2+} FROM INTRACELLULAR ORGANELLES

Ca^{2+} is sequestered by both mitochondria and endoplasmic reticulum. Although it has long been considered that Ca^{2+} uptake into mitochondria is of low affinity *(55)*, probably too low to be important to cytoplasmic Ca^{2+} regulation, recent data show that mitochondria are important Ca^{2+} buffers. For example, mitochondria can be located close to sites of Ca^{2+} influx or release from endoplasmic reticulum. In these locations, mitochondria will be exposed to a high local Ca^{2+} concentration during periods of influx or release from stores and take up large amounts of Ca^{2+}, thereby strongly influencing cytoplasmic Ca^{2+} concentrations *(56–59)*. There is also at least one report that the affinity of mitochondrial Ca^{2+} uptake is much higher than commonly supposed *(60)*, allowing Ca^{2+} uptake from the "global" cytoplasmic Ca^{2+} pool as well as from "hot spots" near sites of influx or release. Mitochondria may then slowly release the accumulated Ca^{2+} over a relatively long period of time. Mitochondrial Ca^{2+} stores could also suffer catastrophic release during opening of the permeability transition pore, flooding the cytoplasm with a large Ca^{2+} load *(55,61,62)*. The permeability transition could occur as a result of a number of factors that may be affected by toxicants, particularly oxidative stress.

The endoplasmic reticulum has a high-affinity Ca^{2+}ATPase uptake pump (SERCA pump) and could have at least two release channels: the ryanodine receptor (responsible for Ca^{2+}-induced Ca^{2+} release) and the IP_3 receptor (responsible for inositol trisphosphate-induced Ca^{2+} release, for example, as a result of stimulation of the phospholipase C-coupled, class I metabotropic glutamate receptors). Unlike the PMCA pumps, the SERCA pumps are not calmodulin sensitive. Both release channels are modulated by Ca^{2+}/ calmodulin *(63,64)*, indicating that toxicants with effects on calmodulin activation should also modulate Ca^{2+} release from intracellular stores.

A variety of ortho-substituted PCBs inhibit Ca^{2+} sequestration by both microsomes (presumably endoplasmic reticulum) and mitochondria isolated from rat cerebellum *(65)*. Ortho-substituted PCBs also enhance Ca^{2+} release from rat cortical microsomes via ryanodine receptors *(66)*. These data indicate that these PCBs are likely to deplete Ca^{2+} stores in the endoplasmic reticulum by both blocking uptake and increasing release. Consequently, there will be at least a transient increase in cytoplasmic Ca^{2+}, as has indeed been shown in cerebellar granule cells *(67)*.

3.1.2. Measuring the Effects of Toxicants on Ca^{2+} Homeostasis

The introduction of fluorescent Ca^{2+}-sensitive dyes has transformed the study of intracellular Ca^{2+} homeostasis *(68)*. The ratiometric dyes fura-2 and indo-1 (and modified versions, especially of fura-2, with different Ca^{2+} affinities) can reliably report free Ca^{2+} over the normal intracellular concentration range, independent of variability in intracellular dye concentration, cell thickness, and excitation intensity. When suitable intracellular calibrations are performed, reasonably accurate true Ca^{2+} concentrations can be measured (although intracellular calibrations are not always trivial). There are many excellent descriptions of the use of these indicators and we will not describe the general methodology here. However, these dyes can interact with toxicants in ways that limit their usefulness or that require sophisticated and/ or tedious manipulations to achieve interpretable results. Even if there is no *a priori* reason to suspect that a toxicant directly interacts with Ca^{2+} indicators, it is wise to test for possible interference in cell-free assays. In the case of multivalent cation toxicants, interference is almost certain to occur.

3.1.2.1. METAL INTERFERENCE WITH Ca^{2+} INDICATORS

All Ca^{2+} indicators are based on Ca^{2+} chelators, with cation coordination patterns similar to EGTA or BAPTA *(68,69)*. Although most indicators have not be evaluated for their sensitivity to most other metals, virtually all toxicologically important metals, including Pb^{2+}, Al^{3+}, Cd^{2+}, Mn^{2+}, Zn^{2+}, Hg^{2+}, and Fe^{2+}, have a higher affinity for EGTA and 1,2-*bis*-(*o*-aminophenoxy)-ethane-*N,N,N',N'*-tetraacetic acid (BAPTA) than Ca^{2+} does, sometimes by several orders of magnitude. Therefore, one would expect that the metals would have a higher affinity for the Ca^{2+} indicators as well. Substantially higher affinity for fura-2, for example, has been shown for Fe^{2+}, Mn^{2+}, Zn^{2+} *(68)*, Cd^{2+} *(70)*, and Pb^{2+} *(36)*. Depending on the metal and indicator, metal binding can yield fluorescence changes that mimic increased or decreased Ca^{2+} concentrations.

Because of the large number of likely interactions between Pb^{2+} and Ca^{2+}, the effects of Pb^{2+} on Ca^{2+} indicators are probably the most intensively studied. Pb^{2+} is an almost perfect substitute for Ca^{2+} in its effects on fura-2 fluorescence (36); under normal imaging conditions, the fluorescence ratios caused by Pb^{2+} and Ca^{2+} binding are indistinguishable, although Pb^{2+} binds with much higher affinity *(36)*. In the cytoplasm of Pb^{2+}-exposed neurons, both Pb^{2+} and Ca^{2+} are present. In solutions containing any physiologically and toxicologically reasonable concentrations of Pb^{2+} and Ca^{2+}, Pb^{2+} increases the fura-2 ratio compared to the expected ratio caused by Ca^{2+} alone *(71)*. Therefore, if the fura-2 fluorescence ratio increases (which normally would indicate an increase in $[Ca^{2+}]_i$ concentration), one cannot tell if Ca^{2+}, Pb^{2+}, or both have increased or if Ca^{2+} might, in fact, have declined, but the effect of lower Ca^{2+} on the fura-2 ratio was overwhelmed by the effect of Pb^{2+}. However, if the fura-2 ratio decreases by any significant amount, this must mean that $[Ca^{2+}]_i$ has decreased. Using this method, Ferguson et al. *(71)* showed that exposure of hippocampal neurons to 100 n*M* Pb^{2+} for 2–48 h decreased $[Ca^{2+}]_i$.

Another commonly used (nonratiometric) Ca^{2+} indicator, fluo-3, also binds Pb^{2+} with high affinity, but Pb^{2+} causes almost no stimulation of fluorescence. In solutions containing both Pb^{2+} and Ca^{2+}, even quite low Pb^{2+} concentrations reduce fluo-3 fluorescence ("quench" fluorescence) compared to the fluorescence expected from Ca^{2+} binding alone (Kern and Audesirk, unpublished data). Therefore, a significant increase in fluo-3 fluorescence in Pb^{2+}-exposed cells should indicate that $[Ca^{2+}]_i$ increased. Unfortunately, the quenching effect of Pb^{2+} is very strong, so only quite large increases in $[Ca^{2+}]_i$ or more modest increases in $[Ca^{2+}]_i$ with extremely low intracellular free-Pb^{2+} concentrations can probably be detected.

An alternative method for using fluo-3 to detect changes in $[Ca^{2+}]_i$ in Pb^{2+}-exposed cells has been proposed by Dyatlov et al. *(72)* and He et al. *(73)*. In brief, cells are exposed to Pb^{2+} and fluo-3 fluorescence measured. Then, the intracellular heavy metal chelator, *N,N,N',N'*-tetrakis(2-pyridylmethyl)-

ethylenediamine (TPEN) *(74)*, is added to the bathing medium. After a short time, fluo-3 fluorescence is again measured. Ideally, TPEN chelates intracellular Pb^{2+}, leaving an "uncontaminated" Ca^{2+}/fluo-3 signal that measures the intracellular free Ca^{2+} that occurred during Pb^{2+} exposure. Unfortunately, there is nothing known about the relative rates of diffusion of TPEN into cells, chelation of Pb^{2+} by TPEN, and recovery of $[Ca^{2+}]_i$ to its "normal," unexposed state. Given the fact that Pb^{2+} activates many processes that might affect Ca^{2+} influx, extrusion, sequestration, or release from intracellular stores, it is likely that the fluo-3 signal after TPEN chelation does not accurately reflect the $[Ca^{2+}]_i$ that occurred during Pb^{2+} exposure and before TPEN application. In fact, the post-TPEN $[Ca^{2+}]_i$ concentration could be either higher or lower than $[Ca^{2+}]_i$ during Pb^{2+} exposure or, indeed, even before Pb^{2+} exposure, depending on the (largely unknown) effects, especially indirect effects, of Pb^{2+} on Ca^{2+} transport and sequestration.

3.2. Oxidative Stress

Oxidative stress in cells is most often the result of overproduction or inadequate detoxification of reactive oxygen species (ROS) or reactive nitrogen species (RNS). Reactive oxygen species are generated by several mitochondrial and cytoplasmic pathways (Fig. 2) (for reviews of ROS production, metabolism, and possible effects in cells and mitochondria, *see* refs. *75–79)*. Mitochondria use molecular oxygen as an electron receptor during respiration, with water as the principal product. However, about 1–4% of the O_2 consumed by mitochondria is converted to superoxide (O_2^-), much of it by the semiquinone form of coenzyme Q and by NADH dehydrogenase *(77,80)*. Superoxide dismutases (SODs), both the mitochondrial Mn-dependent and the cytosolic Cu/Zn-dependent forms, convert superoxide to H_2O_2. H_2O_2 may be converted to the highly reactive hydroxyl radical (OH·), usually through the Fenton reaction, catalyzed by iron *(75)*. H_2O_2 may also be metabolized to water by glutathione peroxidase (GPx), using reduced glutathione (GSH) in the process, or by catalase. There is some evidence that catalase may be more important than GPx in defense against peroxides *(81)*, particularly in neurons *(82)*. Superoxide may also react with nitric oxide (NO) to form peroxynitrite ($ONOO^-$), another highly reactive and potentially damaging species *(83,84)*.

In most cases, the primary generator of ROS (initially as superoxide) is mitochondrial respiration. ROS are generated both during "normal" respiration *(78,80,85)* and by inhibition of specific steps in the electron transport chain [e.g., complex I *(86)* *see also* refs. *78* and *87)*. Therefore, agents that either stimulate overall mitochondrial respiration and/or that inhibit these specific respiratory chain proteins increase ROS production.

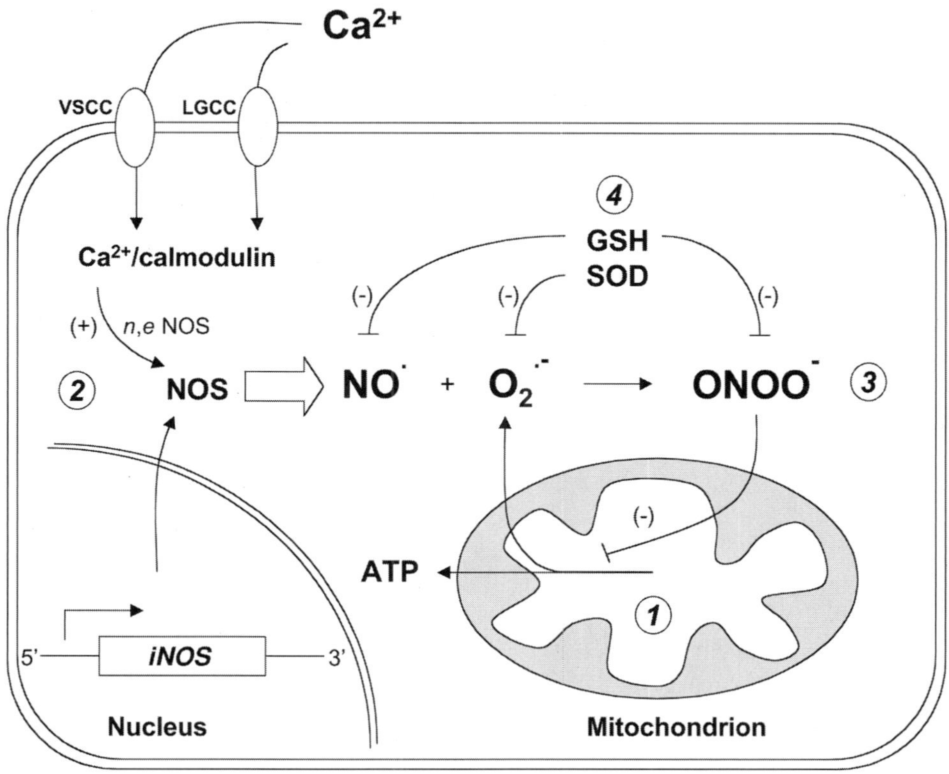

Fig. 2. Reactive oxygen and nitrogen species in neurotoxicity. (**1**) Mitochondrial respiration is the principal source of reactive oxygen in the cell, where 1–4% of the oxygen consumed is converted to superoxide by via reaction with partially reduced electron carriers such as coenzyme Q semiquinone. High mitochondrial calcium concentrations stimulate respiratory activity but also may dramatically increase levels of ROS. (**2**) Nitric oxide (NO) is produced by nitric oxide synthase (NOS) following activation of constitutively expressed isoforms (neuronal [nNOS] and endothelial [eNOS]) or by increased expression of the inducible isoform (iNOS; expressed primarily in glia). Elevated $[Ca^{2+}]_i$ from voltage-sensitive or ligand-gated calcium channels can increase NO synthesis by stimulating calmodulin-mediated activation of nNOS or eNOS. (**3**) During periods of oxidative stress, NO reacts with $O_2^{\cdot-}$ to form peroxynitrite ($ONOO^-$), which inhibits mitochondrial respiration at multiple sites, initiates peroxidation of mitochondrial membrane lipids, and can result in mitochondrial membrane permeabilization (MMP) via activation of the mitochondrial permeability transition pore. MMP results in release of pro-apoptic factors from the mitochondrial intermembrane space such as cytochrome-*c* and apoptosis-inducing factor (AIF) that trigger apoptotic demise of the neuron. (**4**) Cellular antioxidant defenses reduce levels of ROS/RNS by converting them to less reactive species through enzyme-catalyzed (SOD) or spontaneous (GSH) reactions.

One of the most important regulators of respiratory rate is the Ca^{2+} concentration in the mitochondrial matrix *(55,57)*. Low to moderate Ca^{2+} loads increase respiration [e.g., by stimulating several matrix dehydrogenases, which therefore provide more reducing substrates to the electron transport chain *(88)*]. Presumably, this is adaptive in that ATP synthesis is increased, providing energy for Ca^{2+} extrusion and/or sequestration *(55)*. Perhaps by a combination of overall respiratory stimulation and other, poorly understood mechanisms *(77,78)*, Ca^{2+} loading increases the production of ROS *(89–92)*, including superoxide *(89)*. Higher mitochondrial Ca^{2+} causes increased ROS generation, which can, by several pathways, ultimately kill the cell; indeed, some authors attribute glutamate excitotoxicity at least partly to high superoxide synthesis (e.g., ref. *93*). Very high Ca^{2+} loads can trigger opening of the mitochondrial permeability transition pore, causing catastrophic mitochondrial depolarization and release of pro-apoptotic factors such as cytochrome-*c (55,61,62)*.

Nitric oxide and peroxynitrite are the principal RNS in cells. NO has both protective and deleterious effects in neurons, probably depending on the NO concentration [very high levels are usually harmful, but lower concentrations may be protective *(83,94)*]. At low to moderate concentrations, NO may reduce oxidative stress and/or cellular damage by several mechanisms, including directly reacting with some ROS *(83,95)*, by reacting with GSH to form *S*-nitrosoglutathione, which is 100 times more potent an antioxidant than GSH itself *(95)*, by S-nitrosylation of some NMDA receptor subunits, which reduces Ca^{2+} influx through the receptor/channel *(96)*, and by S-nitrosylation of caspases *(96a)*. Although peroxynitrite is probably mostly harmful, there is some debate even about that *(83)*. One well-characterized harmful effect of NO is inhibition of mitochondrial respiration (e.g., refs. *80*, *97*, and *98*) and, consequently, ATP synthesis *(99)*. NO production can be varied by upregulation of nitric oxide synthase (NOS) enzyme levels and by regulation of NOS enzyme activity. Neurons contain mostly the "constitutive" NOS isoforms, neuronal NOS (nNOS), and, in some cases, endothelial NOS (eNOS), which are both stimulated by Ca^{2+}/calmodulin. Glial cells may contain both constitutive NOS *(100)* and inducible NOS (iNOS; e.g., ref. *101*); iNOS contains "permanently" bound calmodulin and is not Ca^{2+} dependent, but enzyme concentrations are strongly upregulated by a variety of stimuli. The constitutive NOS isoforms can also be upregulated in some cell types; for example, eNOS is upregulated in endothelial cells by estradiol *(102)*. In neurons, increased activity, leading to elevated intracellular Ca^{2+}, increases synthesis of both NO and superoxide and therefore increases peroxynitrite formation. NOS activity is also be regulated by phosphorylation by several protein kinases, including Ca^{2+}/calmodulin-dependent protein kinase, PKA, and PKC *(103–106)*

Glial-derived reactive nitrogen species can also result in neurotoxicity. Following stimulation by cytokines, chemokines, prostaglandins, or ROS during physiologic and pathophysiologic conditions, astrocytes can dramatically increase production of NO with resultant injury to neuronal mitochondrial respiration. Increased inducible expression of iNOS within glia and subsequent overproduction of NO causes neuronal injury in several experimental models. Neuronal cell death induced by the peptide S100beta, which is overexpressed in Alzheimer's disease, requires the presence of astrocytes and is dependent on induction of iNOS; cell death correlates with the levels of NO and is blocked by inhibiting iNOS *(107)*. Cytokine-stimulated astrocytes incubated with neurons produce NO that leads to inhibition of respiratory complexes II, III, and IV in neuronal mitochondria *(108)*. Inhibition of neuronal respiratory complex activity becomes irreversible after 24–48 h of coincubation with astrocytes and neuronal death ensues. Similarly, cytokine-mediated iNOS induction in mixed glial–neuronal cultures results in neuronal cell death after 24–48 h that is attenuated by inhibition of iNOS with 100 μ*M N*-methylarginine *(109)*. Astroglial-derived NO is implicated in the neurotoxicity of glutamate *(110)*, NMDA *(111)*, dopamine *(112)*, ceramide *(113)*, and ischemia–reperfusion injury *(114)*. Collectively, these studies indicate that astroglial-derived NO causes lethal damage to associated neurons principally via inhibition of neuronal respiration.

3.2.1. Cellular Defenses Against Oxidative Stress: Oxidant-Metabolizing Enzymes and Intracellular Antioxidants

Cells synthesize a variety of molecules that help to reduce oxidative stress and/or the damage caused by ROS/RNS: SOD, catalase, GSH, and GPx, mentioned earlier, are examples found in most cells. SOD might or might not be protective against ROS, depending on the relative concentrations of SOD and catalase/GPx and the type of oxidative stress. By metabolizing superoxide to H_2O_2, SOD can help to reduce oxidative stress if the levels of catalase and GPx/GSH are high enough to handle the H_2O_2. If not, then SOD may actually contribute to stress *(115)*. On the other hand, SOD action keeps superoxide from reacting with NO to form peroxynitrite and, therefore, is protective against peroxynitrite-mediated damage *(115)*. Catalase and GPx/GSH are at least superficially interchangeable in metabolizing H_2O_2 to H_2O *(116)*

Reduced glutathione and its associated enzymes are important in intracellular defense against oxidative stress, binding to and/or assisting in the metabolism of such diverse species as H_2O_2, NO, and peroxynitrite. There appear to be substantial differences between neurons and astrocytes in GSH-based defenses. For example, astrocytes contain much more GSH than neurons do *(117–119)*, although this may not necessarily confer superior resistance to oxidative stress [e.g., the metabolism of H_2O_2 might not differ between cultured neurons and astrocytes, because of higher neuronal catalase activity *(82,116)*]. Nevertheless, it is thought that GSH protects astrocytes against some stresses, such as peroxynitrite damage to mitochondria *(120)*. It is also significant that GSH levels can be maintained in mitochondria, even though GSH is severely depleted in the cytosol *(121)*.

3.2.2. Toxicant Effects on ROS/RNS Production and Clearance

Toxicants can interact with most, if not all, of these processes. For example, Pb^{2+} alters mitochondrial respiration, with reports of both increases *(122,123)* and decreases *(124–126)*. Most of these experiments used high doses of Pb^{2+} either in vivo (often causing encephalopathy) or in vitro (often >1 μM in isolated mitochondria or >50 μM in intact cells). The effects of more realistic Pb exposures are unknown. If intramitochondrial free-Pb^{2+} substitutes for Ca^{2+} in stimulating respiration, superoxide production should increase. Further, probably depending on the Pb^{2+} exposure level and cell type, Pb^{2+} can increase intracellular free-Ca^{2+} ion concentrations *(127)*, which can increase mitochondrial Ca^{2+} loading and also stimulate respiration and superoxide production. As with Ca^{2+}, it is also possible that high Pb^{2+} loading would cause catastrophic effects, including collapse of the mitochondrial potential, opening of the permeability transition pore, and release of pro-apoptotic factors. Exposing rat rods to high Pb concentrations (1 μM free Pb^{2+}) causes apoptosis by opening the mitochondrial permeability transition pore *(73)*, presumably by overloading the matrix with Ca^{2+} or Pb^{2+} (or both).

In cell-free assays, Pb^{2+} stimulates iron-catalyzed lipid peroxidation *(128)* and ROS production *(129)*, although the concentrations used were very high. If similar effects occur at the much lower Pb^{2+} concentrations within cells, hydroxyl radical concentrations would probably increase via the Fenton reaction. Pb^{2+} also enhances glutamate-stimulated ROS formation in both GT1-7 hypothalamic cells and SH-SY5Y neuroblastoma cells *(130,131)*; however, the Pb^{2+} concentrations in these experiments were extremely high (1 mM), casting doubt on whether this effect is of toxicological relevance. Using partially purified enzymes, Ariza et al. *(132)* reported that Pb^{2+} does not affect the activities of catalase or GPx, but stimulates the activity of Cu/Zn-SOD. In contrast, Mylroie et al. *(133)* found no effect of in vitro Pb^{2+} on bovine blood SOD. The PCB mixture Aroclor 1242 and the PCB congener 2,2'4,4'-tetrachlorobiphenyl inhibit SOD in leukocytes and in cell-free assays *(134)*.

Many toxicants alter GSH production or utilization. For example, methylmercury upregulates glutathione synthesis in cultured rat CNS cells *(135)*, whereas aluminum decreases GSH content in glioma cells but not neuroblastoma cells *(136)*. Ethanol increases GPx activity, but decreases GSH content in cultured astrocytes *(137)*. In vivo Pb^{2+} exposure decreases GSH levels in rat brain *(138,139)* and human erthrocytes *(140)*. GPx levels have been reported to decrease *(139)* or increase *(141)* in rat brain after in vivo exposure. The activities of other enzymes involved in ROS metabolism [glutathione reductase, SOD, and catalase *(133,138,139,142)*] are also usually reduced. Note that these reports did not separately analyze neurons and glial cells, and many involved very high Pb^{2+} exposures and/or cell types that take up a great deal of Pb^{2+} (e.g., erythrocytes). In cultured rat astrocytes, 0.1–1 μM extracellular Pb^{2+} initially decreases GSH levels, but after 48 h, GSH levels exceed normal *(143)*.

Remarkably little is known about the effects of neurotoxicants on nitric oxide synthase expression or activity. Constitutive NOS (nNOS and eNOS) is Ca^{2+}/calmodulin dependent, so any toxicant that alters Ca^{2+} homeostasis and/or activates calmodulin would be expected to alter NOS activity. NOS activity is also modulated by phosphorylation, which also provides numerous pathways for toxicant effects on NO production. Direct effects on the NOS enzyme itself are also possible. Finally, toxicants can alter NOS activity by multiple pathways, with possible differences depending on toxicant concentration. Not surprisingly, the literature on toxicant effects on NO production is unclear. For example, Pb^{2+} has been reported to stimulate *(144,145)* or inhibit *(146,147)* constitutive NOS activity. Methylmercury inhibits nNOS in cell- free assays, but upregulates nNOS content in vivo *(148)*.

Nitric oxide synthase enzyme concentrations may be impacted by toxicant exposure. For example, inducible NOS (iNOS) activity is stimulated in pancreatic β cells by a combination of Pb^{2+} (as low as 100 nM) and suboptimal amounts of interleukin (IL)-1β, probably by upregulation of iNOS expression *(149)*, but iNOS activity is decreased in macrophages *(150)*. In a rat β-cell line, Pb^{2+} upregulates and Hg^{2+} downregulates iNOS gene expression *(149)*. Some pesticides, including *p,p'*-DDT and endosulfan, upregulate iNOS synthesis in rat liver *(151)*. Constitutive NOS expression can also be altered by toxicant exposure; for example, methylmercury increases nNOS content of both the cerebrum and cerebellum *(148,152,153)*.

3.3. Stress Proteins

In many cells, a variety of stresses induce the rapid synthesis of several proteins collectively called stress proteins. Common stress proteins include HSP (heat shock protein) 90, HSP 70, HSP 27, GRP (glucose regulated protein) 94, GRP 78, and heme oxygenase-1 (also called HSP32) *(154–156)*. Although their cellular functions have not been completely characterized, many stress proteins, including HSP25, HSP70, and HSP90 act as "molecular chaperones" that assist in protein folding and/or targeting proteins to specific cellular locations *(155,157,158)*. In this review, we will focus on heme oxygenase and GRP78.

Heme oxygenase is a family of enzymes that break down heme, producing carbon monoxide, iron, and biliverdin as products (for reviews, see refs. *159–161*). Biliverdin is usually rapidly converted to bilirubin by biliverdin reductase. There are three isoforms of heme oxygenase. Heme oxygenase-1 is normally found in very low levels in many cells, but is upregulated several-fold in response to a great variety of stresses, including oxidative stress, ischemia, NO, metals, heat, and heme, which can activate HO-1 gene transcription via several different regulatory elements in its promoter region, including AP-1, AP-2, C/EPB, Sp1, heat shock factor, metal responsive element, antioxidant response element, and necrosis factor (NF)-κB (e.g., refs. *160–164*). HO-1 is absent, or nearly so, in most (unstressed) neurons, although a few do contain HO-1 *(165)*. It appears that a much smaller set of stresses induce HO-1 in neurons than in astrocytes. For example, in cerebellum, kainate injection induces HO-1 in Bergmann glia but not in Purkinje neurons, despite a high concentration of kainate receptors on Purkinje neurons *(166)*. Kainate also induces HO-1 protein almost exclusively in astrocytes and microglia in the hippocampus, although HO-1 mRNA is also induced in some neurons *(167)*. However, under some circumstances, HO-1 is induced in neurons. For example, HO-1 is induced in Purkinje neurons following hyperthermia *(168)* and in cultured cortical and hippocampal neurons by thapsigargin, which causes release of Ca^{2+} from intracellular stores *(169,170)*. HO-2 is constitutively present in many neurons, with prominent expression in hippocampal pyramidal cells *(160)*; its concentration usually does not change greatly in response to stresses *(163,171,172)*. HO-3 is a poor heme catalyst *(159,173)*, and will not be discussed further.

Heme oxygenase activity (usually HO-1) protects a variety of tissues against many different cellular stresses, including β-amyloid *(174)*, H_2O_2 *(174,175)*, peroxynitrite *(176)*, hyperoxia *(177–179)*, depletion of GSH *(180)*, and hemoglobin *(181,182)*. Further, it appears that HO-1 levels must be "just right" for optimal protection; although low or moderate induction of HO-1 is usually protective, excessive HO-1 expression can actually increase susceptibility to insults *(161,177,179)*. Overall, the literature suggests that because most stresses induce HO-1 effectively in glia, including astrocytes, but poorly in neurons, neurons can be more susceptible to a variety of insults *(175,182)*. Transfecting cells with HO-1 provides some protection against ischemia *(183)* and H_2O_2 *(184)*. Transgenic mice overexpressing HO-1 under the neuron-specific enolase promoter are resistant to ischemia *(185)*. Cerebellar granule neurons from these mice resist glutamate and H_2O_2 cytotoxicity *(186)*. These cells also produce much less ROS in response to glutamate *(186)*. Fibroblasts from mice with a defective HO-1 gene show increased cytotoxicity to H_2O_2 and hemin, but not paraquat, a superoxide generator *(187)*.

The cellular effects of HO activity are complex. CO may act as a diffusible messenger, stimulating guanylate cyclase, with multiple effects. Iron may be prooxidant, accelerating the conversion of H_2O_2 to hydroxyl radical. However, iron released by heme oxygenase often upregulates ferritin *(161,188)*, which binds iron and results in lower intracellular free iron concentrations. HO-1 may also enhance iron efflux from cells *(189)*. Less iron will usually mean less conversion of H_2O_2 to the more damaging hydroxyl radical. Bilirubin usually acts as an antioxidant *(161,190,191)*, particularly for hydroxyl radicals *(192)*, and has been reported to be more potent against hydroxyl radicals than ascorbate or Trolox *(192)*. In cultured hippocampal neurons, exogenously applied bilirubin mimics the protective effect of HO-2 activity against H_2O_2 *(193)*. Although there is little direct evidence for or against the proposition that bilirubin provides significant *intracellular* protection against oxidants *(161)*, Dore et al. *(193)* found that stimulating HO-2 activity with phorbol esters (to enhance PKC-mediated phosphorylation of HO-2) increased intracellular bilirubin and increased protection against H_2O_2.

The glucose-related protein 78 (GRP78) is a protein located in the endoplasmic reticulum, where it aids in glycoprotein processing (for reviews, see refs. *194* and *195*). GRP78 is induced by a wide variety of stresses, including hypoxia, hypoglycemia, and calcium ionophores *(194)*; focal cerebral ischemia and kainate *(196)*; release of Ca^{2+} from the endoplasmic reticulum *(197,198)* and/or the concomitant increase in cytoplasmic free Ca^{2+} *(199)*; and glutamate, oxidative stress (Fe^{2+}), and β-amyloid *(200,201)*. GRP78 may provide protection against stresses by multiple mechanisms, including maintaining Ca^{2+} homeostasis, reducing oxidative stress, and maintaining mitochondrial membrane potential *(201)*.

3.3.1. Toxicant Interactions with Stress Proteins

Many toxicants induce stress protein synthesis. For example, Pb^{2+} induces synthesis of several stress proteins in cultured neonatal rat cerebral cortical astrocytes *(202,203)* and hippocampal astrocytes *(204)*, including HO-1. Pb^{2+} also induces GRP78 synthesis in C6 rat glioma cells *(205)* and recombinant HepG2 cells *(206)*. It is not known whether either of these stress proteins defends against Pb^{2+} toxicity. However, Pb^{2+} induces oxidative stress in cell-free assays *(128,129)* and in several cell types *(130,131,207)*, and both HO-1 and GRP78 provide some protection against oxidative stress (see earlier discussion). GRP78 also binds Pb^{2+} with high affinity *(205)*, which can reduce free Pb^{2+} concentrations within the cell or specifically in the endoplasmic reticulum. GRP78 is also induced in several cell types by other metals [e.g., cadmium *(206,208)*] and by ethanol *(209,210)*.

How might stress proteins defend against such a wide variety of toxicants? One possibility is that each stress protein might have several actions. This is probably at least part of the explanation for the benefit of GRP78 induction, which can defend against some insults (e.g., Fe^{2+}) through reducing oxidative stress, some (e.g., glutamate and kainate) both by reducing oxidative stress and regulating intracellular Ca^{2+}, and some (e.g., Pb^{2+}) by directly binding the offending cation. HO-1 also clearly has multiple mechanisms for reducing oxidative stress. Another, possibly simultaneous, mechanism might be that many stressors generate one or several common metabolic defects (e.g., alteration of Ca^{2+} homeostasis or generation of ROS). In this case, any stress protein that reduces any of these defects will provide at least some protection against toxicants with similar mechanisms of action. Pb^{2+}, for example, probably simultaneously impairs Ca^{2+} homeostasis, increases oxidative stress, alters protein phosphorylation and dephosphorylation, and induces or represses synthesis of many proteins. Some of these actions could also depend on one another. Increased ROS, for example, could cause increased cytosolic Ca^{2+} concentrations; induction of protein synthesis could be stimulated by phosphorylation of transcription factors.

Induction of stress proteins by toxicants and how stress proteins defend against toxicant actions promises to be an important avenue of research in neurotoxicology. Different cell types (e.g., neurons vs glia) and different brain regions (e.g., substantia nigra vs cerebellum) might display markedly different susceptibilities to toxicants. In many cases, these cell types or brain regions might also show very different stress protein responses. Differential susceptibility to toxicant insult might be caused by different magnitudes of toxicant effects (e.g., nigral dopaminergic neurons are particularly susceptible to oxidative stress because of high iron concentrations and generation of H_2O_2 by dopamine metabolism) or by different cellular defense capabilities. Differing abilities to induce stress protein synthesis can be an important source of variability in defensive capacity and, hence, in susceptibility to neurotoxicants.

4. FUTURE DIRECTIONS

In this chapter, we have provided a few examples of the multiple effects of neurotoxicants on cell signaling pathways, with emphasis on Ca^{2+}

homeostasis, generation and response to ROS, and stress proteins. Most of these effects have been investigated both in vivo and in vitro. In general, we feel that elucidating mechanisms of action and detailed pathways from toxicant exposure to cellular damage can be most effectively done in in vitro preparations.

Cells derived from transgenic and mutant animals, and newly developed, more efficient transfection techniques (for DNA, oligonucleotides, and protein) should allow methodical dissection of the sites in cellular signaling pathways at which toxicants exert their effects. In the past, toxicants were often assumed to have a single primary molecular target. Over the past decade, multiple toxicant actions have been found to be very common, perhaps most strikingly for inorganic lead and ethanol. Investigating effects in cellular signaling pathways that are "downstream" from the primary targets can be important for understanding the ensemble of toxicant actions in individual cells and for understanding differential susceptibility of certain cell populations. Finally, it should be kept in mind that "downstream" interventions might be reasonably effective in treating toxicant damage, even if damage to the "primary" target cannot be prevented or reversed.

REFERENCES

1. Trenkner, E. (1991) Cerebellar cells in culture, in *Culturing Nerve Cells* (Banker, G. and Goslin, K., eds.), MIT Press, Cambridge, MA, pp. 283–307.
2. Milani, D., Candeo, P., Favaron, M., Blackstone, C. D., and Manev, H. (1993) A subpopulation of cerebellar granule neurons in culture expresses a functional mGluR1 metabotropic glutamate receptor: effect of depolarizing growing conditions. *Receptors Channels* **1,** 243–250.
3. Wheeler, B. C. and Brewer, G. J. (1994) Selective hippocampal neuritogenesis: axon growth on laminin or pleiotrophin, dendrite growth on poly-D-lysine. *Soc. Neurosci. Abstract.* **20,** 1292.
4. Glowacka, D. and Wagner, J. A. (1990) Role of the cAMP-dependent protein kinase and protein kinase C in regulating the morphological differentiation of PC12 cells. *J. Neurosci. Res.* **25,** 453–462.
5. Greene, L. A., Sobeih, M. M., and Teng, K. K. (1991) Methodologies for the culture and experimental use of the PC12 rat pheochromocytoma cell line, in *Culturing Nerve Cells* (Banker, G. and Goslin, K., eds.), MIT Press, Cambridge, MA, pp. 208–226.
6. Armstrong, D. and Eckert, R. (1987) Voltage-activated calcium channels that must be phosphorylated to respond to membrane depolarization. *Proc. Natl. Acad. Sci. USA* **84,** 2518–2522.
7. Kavalali, E. T., Hwang, K. S., and Plummer, M. R. (1997) cAMP-dependent enhancement of dihydropyridine-sensitive calcium channel availability in hippocampal neurons. *J. Neurosci.* **17,** 5334–5348.

8. McCarron, J. G., McGeown, J. G., Reardon, S., Ikebe, M., Fay, F. S., and Walsh, J. V., Jr. (1992) Calcium-dependent enhancement of calcium current in smooth muscle by calmodulin-dependent protein kinase II. *Nature* **357,** 74–77.

9. Schuhmann, K., Romanin, C., Baumgartner, W., and Groschner, K. (1997) Intracellular Ca^{2+} inhibits smooth muscle L-type Ca^{2+} channels by activation of protein phosphatase 2B and by direct interaction with the channel. *J. Gen. Physiol.* **110,** 503–513.

10. Stea, A., Soong, T. W., and Snutch, T. P. (1995) Determinants of PKC-dependent modulation of a family of neuronal calcium channels. *Neuron* **15,** 929–940.

11. Yuan W. and Bers, D. M. (1994) Ca-dependent facilitation of cardiac Ca current is due to Ca-calmodulin-dependent protein kinase. *Am. J. Physiol.* **267,** H982–H993.

12. Zhu, Y. and Ikeda, S. R. (1994) Modulation of Ca^{2+}-channel currents by protein kinase C in adult rat sympathetic neurons. *J. Neurophysiol.* **72,** 1549–1560.

13. Lieberman, D. N. and Mody, I. (1994) Regulation of NMDA channel function by endogenous Ca^{2+}-dependent phosphatase. *Nature* **369,** 235–239.

14. Raman, I. M., Tong, G., and Jahr, C. E. (1996) β-adrenergic regulation of synaptic NMDA receptors by cAMP-dependent protein kinase. *Neuron* **16,** 415–421.

15. Spigelman, I., Tymianski, M., Wallace, C. M., Carlen, P. L., and Velumian, A. A. (1996) Modulation of hippocampal synaptic transmission by low concentrations of cell- permeant Ca^{2+} chelators: effects of Ca^{2+} affinity, chelator structure and binding kinetics. *Neuroscience* **75,** 559–572.

16. Sun, L. R. and Suszkiw, J. B. (1995) Extracellular inhibition and intracellular enhancement of Ca^{2+} currents by Pb^{2+} in bovine adrenal chromaffin cells. *J. Neurophysiol.* **74,** 574–581.

17. Lee, A., Wong, S. T., Gallagher, D., et al. (1999) Ca^{2+}/calmodulin binds to and modulates P/Q-type calcium channels. *Nature* **399,** 155–159.

18. Qin, N., Olcese, R., Bransby, M., Lin, T., and Birnbaumer, L. (1999) Ca^{2+}-induced inhibition of the cardiac Ca^{2+} channel depends on calmodulin. *Proc. Natl. Acad. Sci. USA* **96,** 2435–2438.

19. Zuhlke, R. D., Pitt, G. S., Deisseroth, K., Tsien, R. W., and Reuter, H. (1999) Calmodulin supports both inactivation and facilitation of L-type calcium channels. *Nature* **399,** 159–162.

20. Ehlers, M. D., Zhang, S., Bernhardt, J. P., and Huganir, R. L. (1996) Inactivation of NMDA receptors by direct interaction of calmodulin with the NR1 subunit. *Cell* **84,** 745–755.

21. Zhang, S., Ehlers, M. D., Bernhardt, J. P., Su, C.-T., and Huganir, R. L. (1998) Calmodulin mediates calcium-dependent inactivation of *N*-methyl-D-aspartate receptors. *Neuron* **21,** 443–453.

22. Ehlers, M. D. and Augustine, G. J. (1999) Calmodulin at the channel gate. *Nature* **399,** 105–108.

23. Levitan, I. B. (1999) It is calmodulin after all! Mediator of the calcium modulation of multiple ion channels. *Neuron* **22,** 645–648.

24. Goldstein, G. W. and Ar, D. (1983) Lead activates calmodulin sensitive processes. *Life Sci.* **33,** 1001–1006.
25. Habermann, E., Crowell, K., and Janicki, P. (1983) Lead and other metals can substitute for Ca^{2+} in calmodulin. *Arch. Toxicol.* **54,** 61–70.
26. Kern, M., Wisniewski, M., Cabell, L., and Audesirk, G. (2000) Inorganic lead and calcium interact positively in activation of calmodulin. *NeuroToxicology* **21,** 353–364.
27. Omkumar, R. V., Kiely, M. J., Rosenstein, A. J., Min, K.-T., and Kennedy, M. B. (1996) Identification of a phosphorylation site for calcium/calmodulin-dependent protein kinase II in the NR2B subunit of the *N*-methyl-D-aspartate receptor. *J. Biol. Chem.* **271,** 31,670–31,678.
28. Barria, A., Derkach, V., and Soderling, T. (1997) Identification of the Ca^{2+}/calmodulin-dependent protein kinase II regulatory phosphorylation site in the α-amino-3-hydroxyl-5-methyl-4-isoxazole-propionate-type glutamate receptor. *J. Biol. Chem.* **272,** 32,727–32,730.
29. Derkach, V., Barria, A., and Soderling, T. R. (1999) Ca^{2+}/calmodulin-kinase II enhances channel conductance of α-amino-3-hydroxy-5-methyl-4-isoxazolepropionate type glutamate receptors. *Proc. Natl. Acad. Sci. USA* **96,** 3269–3274.
30. Roche, K. W., O'Brien, R. J., Mammen, A. L., Bernhardt, J., and Huganir, R. L. (1996) Characterization of multiple phosphorylation sites on the AMPA receptor GluR1 subunit. *Neuron* **16,** 1179–1186.
31. Fenster, C. P., Beckman, M. L., Parker, J. C., et al. (1999) Regulation of α4β2 nicotinic receptor desensitization by calcium and protein kinase C. *Mol. Pharmacol.* **55,** 432–443.
32. Voitenko, S. V., Bobryshev, A. Y., and Skok, V. I. (2000) Intracellular regulation of neuronal nicotinic cholinoreceptors. *Neurosci. Behav. Physiol.* **30,** 19–25.
33. Wecker, L., Guo, X., Rycerz, A. M., and Edwards, S. C. (2001) Cyclic AMP-dependent protein kinase A (PKA) and protein kinase C phosphorylate sites in the amino acid sequence corresponding to the M3/M4 cytoplasmic domain of α4 neuronal nicotinic receptor subunits. *J. Neurochem.* **76,** 711–720.
34. Isosaki, M., Minami, N., and Nakashima, T. (1994) Pharmacological evidence for regulation of Na^+–Ca^{2+} exchange by Ca^{2+}/calmodulin-dependent protein kinase in isolated bovine adrenal medullary cells. *J. Pharmacol. Exp. Ther.* **270,** 104–110.
35. Sonnenburg, W. K., Wayman, G. A., Storm, D. R., and Beavo, J. A. (1998) Cyclic nucleotide regulation by calmodulin, in *Calmodulin and Signal Transduction* (Van Eldik, L. J. and Watterson, D. M., eds.), Academic, San Diego, CA, pp. 237–286.
36. Tomsig, J. L. and Suszkiw, J. B. (1995) Multisite interactions between Pb^{2+} and protein kinase C and its role in norepinephrine release from bovine adrenal chromaffin cells. *J. Neurochem.* **64,** 2667–2673.

37. Long, G. J., Rosen, J. F., and Schanne, F. A. X. (1994) Lead activation of protein kinase C from rat brain. Determination of free calcium, lead, and zinc by ^{19}F NMR. *J. Biol. Chem.* **269,** 834–837.

38. Kodavanti, P. R. S., Shafer, T. J., Ward, T. R., et al. (1994) Differential effects of polychlorinated biphenyl congeners on phosphoinositide hydrolysis and protein kinase C translocation in rat cerebellar granule cells. *Brain Res.* **662,** 75–82.

39. Kodavanti, P. R. S., Ward, T. R., McKinney, J. D., and Tilson, H. A. (1995) Increased [^{3}H]phorbol ester binding in rat cerebellar granule cells by polychlorinated biphenyl mixtures and congeners: structure-activity relationships. *Toxicol. Appl. Pharmacol.* **130,** 140–148.

40. Kodavanti, P. R. S. and Ward, T. R. (1998) Interactive effects of environmentally relevant polychlorinated biphenyls and dioxins on [^{3}H]phorbol ester binding in rat cerebellar granule cells. *Environ. Health Perspect.* **106,** 479–486.

41. Bagchi, D., Bagchi, M., Tang, L., and Stohs, S. J. (1997) Comparative in vitro and in vivo protein kinase C activation by selected pesticides and transition metal salts. *Toxicol. Lett.* **91,** 31–37.

42. Kern, M. and Audesirk, G. (2000a) Stimulatory and inhibitory effects of inorganic lead on calcineurin. *Toxicology* **150,**173–180.

43. Enan, E. and Matsumura, F. (1992) Specific inhibition of calcineurin by type II synthetic pyrethroid insecticides. *Biochem. Pharmacol.* **43,** 1777–1784.

44. Enz, A. and Pombo-Villar, E. (1997) Class II pyrethroids: noninhibitors calcineurin. *Biochem. Pharmacol.* **54,** 321–323.

45. Fakata, K. L., Swanson, S. A., Vorce, R. L., and Stemmer, P. M. (1998) Pyrethroid insecticides as phosphatase inhibitors. *Biochem. Pharmacol.* **55,** 2017–2022.

46. Matsuda, T., Takuma, K., and Baba, A. (1997) Na$^+$–Ca^{2+} exchanger: physiology and pharmacology. *Jpn. J. Pharmacol.* **74,** 1–20.

47. Racay, P., Kaplan, P., and Lehotsky, J. (1996) Control of Ca^{2+} homeostasis in neuronal cells. *Gen. Physiol. Biophys.* **15,** 193–210.

48. Brandt, P. C. and Vanaman, T. C. (1998) Calmodulin and ion flux regulation, in *Calmodulin and Signal Transduction* (Van Eldik, L. J. and Watterson, D.M., eds.), Academic, San Diego, CA, pp. 397–471.

49. Carafoli, E. (1991) Calcium pump of the plasma membrane. *Physiol. Rev.* **71,** 129–153.

50. Miller, R. J. (1991) The control of neuronal Ca^{2+} homeostasis. *Prog. Neurobiol.* **37,** 255–285.

51. Simons, T. J. B. (1984) Active transpot of lead by human red blood cells. *FEBS Lett.* **172,** 250–254.

52. Simons, T. J. B. (1988) Active transport of lead by the calcium pump in human red blood cells. *J. Physiol.* **405,** 105–113.

53. Calderon-Salinas, J. V., Quintanar-Escorza, M. A., Hernandez-Luna, C. E., and Gonzalez-Martinez, M. T. (1999) Effect of lead on the calcium transport in human erythrocyte. *Hum. Exp. Toxicol.* **18,** 146–153.

54. Mas-Oliva, J. (1989) Effect of lead on the erythrocyte (Ca^{2+}, Mg^{2+})-ATPase activity. Calmodulin involvement. *Mol. Cell. Biochem.* **89,** 87–93.

55. Duchen, M. R. (1999) Contributions of mitochondria to animal physiology: from homeostatic sensor to calcium signalling and cell death. *J. Physiol.* **516,** 1–17.

56. Rizzuto, R., Pinton, P., Brini, M., Chiesa, A., Filippin, L., and Pozzan, T. (1999) Mitochondria as biosensors of calcium microdomains. *Cell Calcium* **26,** 193–199.

57. Rutter, G. A. and Rizzuto, R. (2000) Regulation of mitochondrial metabolism by ER Ca^{2+} release: an intimate connection. *Trends Biochem. Sci.* **25,** 215–221.

58. Wang, G. J. and Thayer, S. A. (1996) Sequestration of glutamate-induced Ca^{2+} loads by mitochondria in cultured rat hippocampal neurons. *J. Neurophysiol.* **76,** 1611– 1621.

59. Werth, J. L. and Thayer, S. A. (1994) Mitochondria buffer physiological calcium loads in cultured rat dorsal root ganglion neurons. *J. Neurosci.* **14,** 348–356.

60. Colegrove, S. L., Albrecht, M. A., and Friel, D. D. (2000) Dissection of mitochondrial Ca^{2+} uptake and release fluxes in situ after depolarization-evoked $[Ca^{2+}]_i$ elevations in sympathetic neurons. *J. Gen. Physiol.* **115,** 351–369.

61. Liu, X., Kim, C. N., Yang, J., Jemmerson, R., and Wang, X. (1996) Induction of apoptotic program in cell-free extracts: requirements for dATP and cytochrome c. *Cell* **86,** 147–157.

62. Smaili, S.S., Hus, Y.-T., Youle, R. J., and Russell, J. T. (2000) Mitochondria in Ca^{2+} signaling and apoptosis. *J. Bioenerg. Biomembr.* **32,** 35–46.

63. Buratti, R., Prestipino, G., Menegazzi, P., Treves, S., and Zorzato, F. (1995) Calcium dependent activation of skeletal muscle Ca^{2+} release channel (ryanodine receptor) by calmodulin. *Biochem. Biophys. Res. Commun.* **213,** 1082–1090.

64. Missiaen, L., Parys, J. B., Weidema, A. F., et al. (1999) The bell-shaped Ca^{2+} dependence of the inositol 1,4,5-trisphosphate-induced Ca^{2+} release is modulated by Ca^{2+}/calmodulin. *J. Biol. Chem.* **274,** 13,748–13,751.

65. Kodavanti, P. R. S., Ward, T. R., McKinney, J. D., and Tilson, H. A. (1996) Inhibition of microsomal and mitochondrial Ca^{2+} sequestration in rat cerebellum by polychlorinated biphenyl mixtures and congeners: structure-activity relationships. *Arch. Toxicol.* **70,** 150–157.

66. Wong, P. W., Brackney, W. R., and Pessah, I. N. (1997) Ortho-substituted polychlorinated biphenyls alter microsomal calcium transport by direct interaction with ryanodine receptors of mammalian brain. *J. Biol. Chem.* **272,** 15,145–15,153.

67. Kodavanti, P. R. S., Shin, D., Tilson, H. A., and Harry, G. J. (1993) Comparative effects of two polychlorinated biphenyl congeners on calcium homeostasis in rat cerebellar granule cells. *Toxicol. Appl. Pharmacol.* **123,** 97–106.

68. Grynkiewicz, G., Poenie, M., and Tsien, R. Y. (1985) A new generation of Ca^{2+} indicators with greatly improved fluorescence properties. *J. Biol. Chem.* **260,** 3440–3450.

69. Minta, A., Kao, J. P. Y., and Tsien, R. Y. (1989) Fluorescent indicators for cytosolic calcium based on rhodamine and fluorscein chromophores. *J. Biol. Chem.* **264,** 8171–8178.
70. Hinkle, P. M., Shanshala, E. D., and Nelson, E. J. (1992) Measurement of intracellular cadmium with fluorescent dyes. Further evidence for the role of calcium channels in cadmium uptake. *J. Biol. Chem.* **267,** 25,553–25,559.
71. Ferguson, C., Kern, M., and Audesirk, G. (2000) Nanomolar concentrations of inorganic lead increase Ca^{2+} efflux and decrease intracellular free Ca^{2+} ion concentrations in cultured rat hippocampal neurons by a calmodulin-dependent mechanism. *NeuroToxicology* **21,** 365–378.
72. Dyatlov, V. A., Dyatlova, O. M., Parsons, P. J., Lawrence, D. A., and Carpenter, D. O. (1998) Lipopolysaccharide and interleukin-6 enhance lead entry into cerebellar neurons: application of a new and sensitive flow cytometric technique to measure intracellular lead and calcium concentrations. *NeuroToxicology* **19,** 293–302.
73. He, L., Poblenz, A. T., Medrano, C. J., and Fox, D. A. (2000) Lead and calcium produce rod photoreceptor cell apoptosis by opening the mitochondrial permeability transition pore. *J. Biol. Chem.* **275,** 12175–12184.
74. Arslan, P., DiVirgilio, F., Beltrame, M., Tsien, R. Y., and Pozzan, T. (1985) Cytosolic Ca^{2+} homeostasis in Ehrlich and Yoshida carcinomas. A new, membrane- permeant chelator of heavy metals reveals that these ascites tumor cell lines have normal cytosolic free Ca^{2+}. *J. Biol. Chem.* **260,** 2719–2727.
75. Halliwell, B. (1992) Reactive oxygen species and the central nervous system. *J. Neurochem.* **59,** 1609–1623.
76. Kelly, S. A., Havrilla, C. M., Brady, T. C., Abramo, K. H., and Levin, E. D. (1998) Oxidative stress in toxicology: established mammalian and emerging piscine model systems. *Environ. Health. Perspect.* **106,** 375–384.
77. Kowaltowski, A. J. and Vercesi, A. E. (1999) Mitochondrial damage induced by conditions of oxidative stress. *Free Radical. Biol. Med.* **26,** 463–471.
78. Nicholls, D. G. and Budd, S. L. (2000) Mitochondria and neuronal survival. *Physiol. Rev.* **80,** 315–360.
79. Olanow, C. W. (1993) A radical hypothesis for neurodegeneration. *Trends Neurosci.* **16,** 439–444.
80. Sastre, J., Pallardo, F. V., Garcia de al Asuncion, J., and Vina, J. (2000) Mitochondria, oxidative stress and aging. *Free Radical Res.* **32,** 189–198.
81. Johnson, R. M., Goyette, G., Jr., Ravindranath, Y., and Ho, Y.-S. (2000) Red cells from glutathione peroxidase-1-deficient mice have nearly normal defenses against endogenous peroxides. *Blood* **96,** 1985–1988.
82. Dringen, R., Kussmaul, L., Gutterer, J. M., Hirrlinger, J., and Hamprecht, B. (1999) The glutathione system of peroxide detoxification is less efficient in neurons than in astroglial cells. *J. Neurochem.* **72,** 2523–2530.
83. Halliwell, B., Zhao, K., and Whiteman, M. (1999) Nitric oxide and peroxynitrite. The ugly, the uglier and the not so good. *Free Radical Res.* **31,** 651–669.

84. Murphy, M. P., Packer, M. A., Scarlett, J. L., and Martin, S. W. (1998) Peroxynitrite: a biologically significant oxidant. *Gen. Pharmacol.* **31,** 179–186.

85. Di Donato, S. (2000) Disorders related to mitochondrial membranes: pathology of the respiratory chain and neurodegeneration. *J. Inherit. Metab. Dis.* **23,** 247–263.

86. Pitkanen, S. and Robinson, B. H. (1996) Mitochondrial complex I deficiency leads to increased production of superoxide radicals and induction of superoxide dismutase. *J. Clin. Invest.* **98,** 345–351.

87. Capaldi, R. A. (2000) The changing face of mitochondrial research. *Trends Biochem. Sci.* **25,** 212–214.

88. Murphy, A. N., Fiskum, G, and Beal, M. F. (1999) Mitochondria in neurodegeneration: bioenergetic function in cell life and death. *J. Cerebral Blood Flow Metab.* **19,** 231–245.

89. Bindokas, V. P., Jordan J., Lee, C. C., and Miller, R. J. (1996) Superoxide production in rat hippocampal neurons: sensitive imaging with ethidine. *J. Neurosci.* **16,** 1324–1336.

90. Dugan, L. L., Sensi, S. L., Canzoniero, L. M. T., et al. (1995) Mitochondrial production of reactive oxygen species in cortical neurons following exposure to *N*-methyl-D-aspartate. *J. Neurosci.* **15,** 6377–6388.

91. Nicholls, D. G. and Ward, M. W. (2000) Mitochondrial membrane potential and neuronal glutamate excitotoxicity: mortality and millivolts. *Trends Neurosci.* **23,** 166–174.

92. Reynolds, I. J. and Hastings, T. G. (1995) Glutamate induces the production of reactive oxygen species in cultured forebrain neurons following NMDA receptor activation. *J. Neurosci.* **15,** 3318–3327.

93. Patel, M., Day, B. J., Crapo, J. D., Fridovich, I., and McNamara, J. O. (1996) Requirement for superoxide in excitotoxic cell death. *Neuron* **16,** 345–355.

94. Lipton, S. A. (1999) Neuronal protection and destruction by NO. *Cell Death Differ.* **6,** 943–951.

95. Chiueh, C. C. and Rauhala, P. (1999) The redox pathway of *S*-nitrosoglutathione, glutathione and nitric oxide in cell to neuron communications. *Free Radical Res.* **31,** 641–650.

96. Choi, Y.-B., Tenneti, L., Le, D. A., et al. (2000) Molecular basis of NMDA receptor-coupled ion channel modulation by S- nitrosylation. *Nature Neurosci.* **3,** 15–21.

96a. Liu, L. and Stamler, J. S. (1999) NO: an inhibitor of cell death. *Cell Death Differ.* **6,** 937–942.

97. Beltran, B., Orsi, A., Clementi, E., and Moncada, S. (2000) Oxidative stress and S- nitrosylation of proteins in cells. *Br. J. Pharmacol.* **129,** 953–960.

98. Heales, S. J. R., Bolanos, J. P., Stewart, V. C., Brookes, P. S., Land, J. M., and Clark, J. B. (1999) Nitric oxide, mitochondria and neurological disease. *Biochim. Biophys. Acta* **1410,** 215–228.

99. Brookes, P. S., Bolanos, J. P., and Heales, S. J. R. (1999) The assumption that nitric oxide inhibits mitochondrial ATP synthesis is correct. *FEBS Lett.* **446,** 261–263.

100. Tolias, C. M., McNeil, C. J., Kazlauskaite, J., and Hillhouse, E. W. (1999) Superoxide generation from constitutive nitric oxide synthase in astrocytes in vitro regulates extracellular nitric oxide availability. *Free Radical Biol. Med.* **26,** 99–106.

101. Kitamura, Y., Matsuoka, Y., Nomura, Y., and Taniguchi, T. (1998) Induction of inducible nitric oxide synthase and heme oxygenase-1 in rat glial cells. *Life Sci.* **62,** 1717–1721.

102. MacRitchie, A. N., Jun, S. S., Chen, Z., et al. (1997) Estrogen upregulates endothelial nitric oxide synthase gene expression in fetal pulmonary artery endothelium. *Circ. Res.* **81,** 355–362.

103. Bredt, D. S., Ferris, C. D., and Snyder, S. H. (1992) Nitric oxide synthase regulatory sites. Phosphorylation by cyclic AMP-dependent protein kinase, protein kinase C, and calcium/calmodulin protein kinase: identification of flavin and calmodulin binding sites. *J. Biol. Chem.* **267,** 10,976–10,981.

104. Brune, B. and Lapetina, E. G. (1991) Phosphorylation of nitric oxide synthase by protein kinase A. *Biochem. Biophys. Res. Commun.* **181,** 921–926.

105. Dinerman, J. L., Steiner, J. P., Dawson, T. M., Dawson, V., and Snyder, S. H. (1994) Cyclic nucleotide dependent phosphorylation of neuronal nitric oxide synthase inhibits catalytic activity. *Neuropharmacology* **33,** 1245–1251.

106. Nakane, M., Mitchell, J., Forstermann, U., and Murad, F. (1991) Phosphorylation by calcium calmodulin-dependent protein kinase II and protein kinase C modulates the activity of nitric oxide synthase. *Biochem. Biophys. Res. Commum.* **180,** 1396–1402.

107. Hu, J., Ferreira, A., and Van Eldik, L. J. (1997) S100beta induces neuronal cell death through nitric oxide release from astrocytes. *J. Neurochem.* **69,** 2294–2301.

108. Stewart, V. C., Sharpe, M. A., Clark, J. B., and Heales, S. J. (2000). Astrocyte- derived nitric oxide causes both reversible and irreversible damage to the neuronal mitochondrial respiratory chain. *J. Neurochem.* **75,** 694–700.

109. Dawson, V. L., Brahmbhatt, H. P., Mong, J. A., and Dawson, T. M. (1994) Expression of inducible nitric oxide synthase causes delayed neurotoxicity in primary mixed neuronal–glial cortical cultures. *Neuropharmacology* **33,** 1425–1430.

110. Cardenas, A., Moro, M. A., Hurtado, O., et al. (2000). Implication of glutamate in the expression of inducible nitric oxide synthase after oxygen and glucose deprivation in rat forebrain slices. *J. Neurochem.* **74,** 2041–2048.

111. Lecanu, L., Verrecchia, C., Margaill, I., Boulu, R. G., and Plotkine, M. (1998). iNOS contribution to the NMDA-induced excitotoxic lesion in the rat striatum. *Br. J. Pharmacol.* **125,** 584–590.

112. Weingarten, P., Bermak, J., and Zhou, Q. Y. (2001). Evidence for non-oxidative dopamine cytotoxicity: potent activation of NF-kappa B and lack of protection by antioxidants. *J. Neurochem.* **76,** 1794–1804.

113. Hunot, S., Brugg, B., Ricard, D., et al. (1997). Nuclear translocation of NF-kappaB is increased in dopaminergic neurons of patients with parkinson disease. *Proc. Natl. Acad. Sci. USA* **94,** 7531–7536.

114. Seegers, H., Grillon, E., Trioullier, Y., Vath, A., Verna, J. M., and Blum, D. (2000). Nuclear factor-kappa B activation in permanent intraluminal focal cerebral ischemia in the rat. *Neurosci. Lett.* **288,** 241–245.

115. Ying, W., Anderson, C. M., Chen, Y., et al. (2000) Differing effects of copper, zinc superoxide dismutase overexpression on neurotoxicity elicited by nitric oxide, reactive oxygen species, and excitotoxins. *J. Cereb. Blood Flow Metab.* **20,** 359–368.

116. Dringen, R. and Hamprecht, B. (1997) Involvement of glutathione peroxidase and catalase in the disposal of exogenous hydrogen peroxide by cultured astroglial cells. *Brain Res.* **759,** 67–75.

117. Bolanos J. P., Heales, S. J. R., Land, J. M., and Clark, J. B. (1995) Effect of peroxynitrite on the mitochondrial respiratory chain: differential susceptibility of neurones and astrocytes in primary cultures. *J. Neurochem.* **64,** 1965–1972.

118. Huang, J. and Philbert, M. A. (1995) Distribution of glutathione-related enzyme systems in mitochondria and cytosol of cultured cerebellar astrocytes and granule cells. *Brain Res.* **680,** 16–22.

119. Philbert, M. A., Beiswanger, C. M., Manson, M. M., et al. (1995) Glutathione *S*-transferases and γ-glutamyl transpeptidase in the rat nervous system: a basis for differential susceptibility to neurotoxicants. *NeuroToxicology* **16,** 349–362.

120. Barker, J. E., Bolanos, J. P., Land, J. M., Clark, J. B., and Heales, S. J. R. (1996) Glutathione protects astrocytes from peroxynitrite-mediated mitochondrial damage: implications for neuronal/astrocytic trafficking and neurodegeneration. *Dev. Neurosci.* **18,** 391–396.

121. Wüllner, U., Seyfried, J., Groscurth, P., et al. (1999) Glutathione depletion and neuronal cell death: the role of reactive oxygen intermediates and mitochondrial function. *Brain Res.* **826,** 53–62.

122. Holtzman, D., Shen Hsu, J., and Mortell, P. (1978) In vitro effects of inorganic lead on isolated rat brain mitochondrial respiration. *Neurochem. Res.* **3,** 195–206.

123. Wielgus-Serafinska, E., Zawadzka A., and Falkus, B. (1980) The effect of lead acetate on rat liver mitochondria. *Acta Physiol. Pol.* **31,** 659–668.

124. Holtzman, D., DeVries, C., Nguyen, H., Olson, J., and Bensch, K. (1984) Maturation of resistance to lead encephalopathy: cellular and subcellular mechanisms. *NeuroToxicology* **5,** 97–124.

125. Holtzman, D., Olson, J. E., DeVries, C., and Bensch, K. (1987) Lead toxicity in primary cultured cerebral astrocytes and cerebellar granule neurons. *Toxicol. Appl. Pharmacol.* **89,** 211–225.

126. Medrano, C. J., Shulman, L. M., and Fox, D. A. (1993) Lead-induced alterations in retinal energy metabolism. *Toxicologist* **13,** 166.

127. Van Rossum, G. D., Kapoor, S. C., and Rabinowitz, M. S. (1985) Effects of inorganic lead in vitro on ion exchanges and respiratory metabolism of rat kidney cortex. *Arch. Toxicol.* **56,** 175–181.

128. Schanne, F. A. X., Moskal, J. R., and Gupta, R. K. (1989) Effect of lead on intracellular free calcium ion concentration in a presynaptic neuronal model: ^{19}F-NMR study of NG108-15 cells. *Brain Res.* **503,** 308–311.

129. Quinlan, G. J., Halliwell, B., Moorhouse, C. P., and Gutteridge, J. M. (1988) Action of lead(II) and aluminum(III) ions on iron-stimulated lipid peroxidation in liposomes, erythrocytes and rat liver microsomal fractions. *Biochim. Biophys. Acta* **962,** 196–200.

130. Bondy, S. C. and Guo, S. X. (1996) Lead potentiates iron-induced formation of reactive oxygen species. *Toxicol. Lett.* **87,** 109–112.

131. Naarala, J. T., Loikkanen, J. J., Ruotsalainen, M. H., and Savolainen, K. M. (1995) Lead amplifies glutamate-induced oxidative stress. *Free Radical Biol. Med.* **19,** 689–693.

132. Loikkanen, J. J., Naarala, J. T., and Savolainen, K. M. (1998) Modification of glutamate-induced oxidative stress by lead: the role of extracellular calcium. *Free Radical Biol. Med.* **24,** 377–384.

133. Ariza, M. E., Bijur, G. N., and Williams, M. V. (1998) Lead and mercury mutagenesis: role of H_2O_2, superoxide dismutase, and xanthine oxidase. *Environ. Mol. Mutagen.* **31,** 352–361.

134. Mylroie, A. A., Collins, H., Umbles, C., and Kyle, J. (1986) Erythrocyte superoxide dismutase activity and other parameters of copper status in rats ingesting lead acetate. *Toxicol. Appl. Pharmacol.* **82,** 512–520.

135. Narayanan, P. K., Carter, W. O., Ganey, P. E., Roth, R. A., Voytik-Harbin, S. L., and Robinson, J. P. (1998) Impairment of human neutrophil oxidative burst by polychlorinated biphenyls: inhibition of superoxide dismutase activity. *J. Leukocyte Biol.* **63,** 216–224.

136. Ou, Y. C., White, C. C., Krejsa, C. M., Ponce, R. A., Kavanagh, T. J., and Faustman, E. M. (1999) The role of intracellular glutathione in methylmercury-induced toxicity in embryonic neuronal cells. *NeuroToxicology* **20,** 793–804.

137. Campbell, A., Prasad, K. N., and Bondy, S. C. (1999) Aluminum-induced oxidative events in cell lines: glioma are more responsive than neuroblastoma. *Free Radical Biol. Med.* **26,** 1166–1171.

138. Eysseric, H., Gonthier, B., Soubeyran, A., Richard, M. J., Daveloose, D., and Barret, L. (2000) Effects of chronic ethanol exposure on acetaldehyde and free radical production by astrocytes in culture. *Alcohol* **21,** 117–125.

139. Jindal, V. and Gill, K. D. (1999) Ethanol potentiates lead-induced inhibition of rat brain antioxidant defense systems. *Pharmacol. Toxicol.* **85,** 16–21.

140. Sandhir, R., Julka, D., and Gill, K. D. (1994) Lipoperoxidative damage on lead exposure in rat brain and its implications on membrane bound enzymes. *Pharmacol. Toxicol.* **74,** 66–71.

141. Sugawara, E., Nakamura, K., Miyake, T., Fukumura, A., and Seki, Y. (1991) Lipid peroxidation and concentration of glutathione in erythrocytes from workers exposed to lead. *Br. J. Ind. Med.* **48,** 239–242.

142. Adonaylo, V. N. and Oteiza, P. I. (1999) Lead intoxication: antioxidant defenses and oxidative damage in rat brain. *Toxicology* **135,** 77–85.

143. Correa, M., Miquel, M., Sanchis-Segura, C., and Aragon, C. M. (1999) Effects of chronic lead administration on ethanol-induced locomotor and brain catalase activity. *Alcohol* **19,** 43–49.

144. Legare, M. E., Barhoumi, R., Burghardt, R. C., and Tiffany-Castiglioni, E. (1993) Low-level lead exposure in cultured astroglia: identification of cellular targets with vital fluorescent probes. *Neurotoxicology* **14,** 267–272.
145. Gonick, H. C., Ding, Y., Bondy, S. C., Ni, Z., and Vaziri, N. D. (1997) Lead-induced hypertension: interplay of nitric oxide and reactive oxygen species. *Hypertension* **30,** 1487–1492.
146. Swanson, S. P. and Angle, C. R. (1995) Lead stimulates nitric oxide synthase of cultured cerebellar granule cells: another toxic manifestation due to activation of protein kinase C? *Toxicologist* **15,** 9.
147. Mittal, C. K., Harrell, W. B., and Mehta, C. S. (1995) Interaction of heavy metal toxicants with brain constitutive nitric oxide synthase. *Mol. Cell. Biochem.* **149/150,** 263–265.
148. Quinn, M. R. and Harris, C. L. (1995) Lead inhibits Ca^{2+}-stimulated nitric oxide activity from rat cerebellum. *Neurosci. Lett.* **196,** 65–68.
149. Shinyashiki, M., Kumagai, Y., Nakajima, H., et al. (1998) Differential changes in rat brain nitric oxide synthase in vivo and in vitro by methylmercury. *Brain Res.* **798,** 147–155.
150. Eckhardt, W., Bellmann, K., and Kolb, H. (1999) Regulation of inducible nitric oxide synthase expression in β cells by environmental factors: heavy metals. *Biochem. J.* **338,** 695–700.
151. Tian, L. and Lawrence, D. A. (1996) Metal-induced modulation of nitric oxide production in vitro by murine macrophages: lead, nickel and cobalt utilize different mechanisms. *Toxicol. Appl. Pharmacol.* **141,** 540–547.
152. Dhouib, M. and Lugnier, A. (1996) Induction of nitric oxide synthase by chlorinated pesticides (p,p'-DDT, chlordane, endosulfan) in rat liver. *Cent. Eur. J. Public Health* **4(Suppl.),** 48.
153. Craig, E. A., Weissman, J. S., and Horwich, A. L. (1994) Heat shock proteins and molecular chaperones: mediators of protein conformation and turnover in the cell. *Cell* **78,** 365–372.
154. Ikeda, M., Komachi, H., Sato, I., Himi, T., Yuasa, T., Murota, S. (1999) Induction of neuronal nitric oxide synthase by methylmercury in the cerebellum. *J. Neurosci. Res.* **55,** 352–356.
155. De Maio, A. (1999) Heat shock proteins: facts, thoughts and dreams. *Shock* **11,** 1–12.
156. Welch, W. J. (1992) Mammalian stress response: cell physiology, structure/function of stress proteins, and implications for medicine and disease. *Physiol. Rev.* **72,** 1063–1081.
157. Welch, W. J. (1993) Heat shock proteins functioning as molecular chaperones: their roles in normal and stressed cells. *Phil. Trans. R. Soc. Lond. B* **339,** 327–333.
158. Ang, D., Liberek, K., Skowyra, D., Zylicz, M., and Georgopoulos, C. (1991) Biological role and regulation of the universally conserved heat shock proteins. *J. Biol. Chem.* **266,** 24,233–24,236.

159. Galbraith, R. (1999) Heme oxygenase: who needs it? *Proc. Soc. Exp. Biol. Med.* **222,** 299–305.
160. Maines, M. D. (1997) The heme oxygenase system: a regulator of second messenger gases. *Annu. Rev. Pharmacol. Toxicol.* **37,** 517–554.
161. Ryter, S. W. and Tyrrell, R. M. (2000) The heme synthesis and degradation pathways: role in oxidant sensitivity. *Free Radical Biol. Med.* **28,** 289–309.
162. Alam, J. (1994) Multiple elements within the 5' distal enhancer of the mouse heme oxygenase-1 gene mediate induction by heavy metals. *J. Biol. Chem.* **269,** 25,049–25,056.
163. Elbirt, K. K. and Bonkovsky, H. L. (1999) Heme oxygenase: recent advances in understanding its regulation and role. *Proc. Assoc. Am. Physicians* **111,** 438–447.
164. Lavrovsky, Y., Schwartzman, M. L., Levere, R. D., Kappas, A., and Abraham, N. G. (1994) Identification of binding sites for transcription factors NF-B and AP-2 in the promoter region of the human heme oxygenase 1 gene. *Proc. Natl. Acad. Sci. USA* **91,** 5987–5991.
165. Vincent, S. R., Das, S., and Maines, M. D. (1994) Brain heme oxygenase isoenzymes and nitric oxide synthase are co-localized in select neurons. *Neuroscience* **63,** 223–231.
166. Nakaso, K., Kitayama, M., Fukuda, H., et al. (2000) Oxidative stress-related proteins A170 and heme oxygenase-1 are differently induced in the rat cerebellum under kainate-mediated excitotoxicity. *Neurosci. Lett.* **282,** 57–60.
167. Nakaso, K., Kitayama, M., Fukuda, H., et al. (1999) Induction of heme oxygenase-1 in the rat brain by kainic acid-mediated excitotoxicity: the dissociation of mRNA and protein expression in the hippocampus. *Biochem. Biophys. Res. Comm.* **259,** 91–96.
168. Ewing, J. F., Haber, S. N., and Maines, M. D. (1992) Normal and heat-induced patterns of expression of heme oxygenase-1 (HSP32) in rat brain: hyperthermia causes rapid induction of mRNA and protein. *J. Neurochem.* **58,** 1140–1149.
169. Gissel, C., Doutheil, J., and Paschen, W. (1997) Activation of heme oxygenase-1 expression by disturbance of endoplasmic reticulum calcium homeostasis in rat neuronal culture. *Neurosci. Lett.* **231,** 75–78.
170. Linden, T., Doutheil, J., and Paschen, W. (1998) Role of calcium in the activation of erp72 and heme oxygenase-1 expression on depletion of endoplasmic reticulum calcium stores in rat neuronal cell culture. *Neurosci. Lett.* **247,** 103–106.
171. Dwyer, B. E., Nishimura, R. N., Lu, S.-Y., and Alcaraz, A. (1996) Transient induction of heme oxygenase after cortical stab wound injury. *Mol. Brain Res.* **38,** 251–259.
172. Ewing, J. F. and Maines, M. D. (1991) Rapid induction of heme oxygenase mRNA and protein by hyperthermia in rat brain: Heme oxygenase 2 is not a heat shock protein. *Proc. Natl. Acad. Sci. USA* **88,** 5364–5368.

173. McCoubrey, W. K., Huang, T. J., and Maines, M. D. (1997) Isolation and characterization of a cDNA from the rat brain the encodes hemoprotein heme oxygenase-3. *Eur. J. Biochem.* **247,** 725–732.

174. Le, W.-D., Xie, W.-J., and Appel, S. H. (1999) Protective role of heme oxygenase- 1 in oxidative stress-induced neuronal injury. *J. Neurosci. Res.* **56,** 652–658.

175. Dwyer, B. E., Nishimura, R. N., and Lu, S.-Y. (1995) Differential expression of heme oxygenase-1 in cultured neurons and astrocytes determined by the aid of a new heme oxygenase antibody. Response to oxidative stress. *Mol. Brain Res.* **30,** 37–47.

176. Foresti, R., Sarathchandra, P., Clark, J. E., Green, C. J., and Motterlini, R. (1999) Peroxynitrite induces haem oxygenase-1 in vascular endothelial cells: a link to apoptosis. *Biochem. J.* **339,** 729–736.

177. Dennery, P. A., Sridhar, K. J., Lee, C. S., et al. (1997) Heme oxygenase-mediated resistance to oxygen toxicity in hamster fibroblasts. *J. Biol. Chem.* **272,** 14,937–14,942.

178. Otterbein, L. E., Kolls, J. K., Mantell, L. L., Cook, J. L., Alam, J., and Choi, A. M. K. (1999) Exogenous administration of heme oxygenase-1 by gene transfer provides protection against hyperoxia-induced lung injury. *J. Clin. Invest.* **103,** 1047–1054.

179. Suttner, D. M. and Dennery, P. A. (1999) Reversal of HO-1 related cytoprotection with increased expression is due to reactive iron. *FASEB J.* **13,** 1800–1809.

180. Ewing, J. F. and Maines, M. D. (1993) Glutathione depletion induces heme oxygenase-1 (HSP32) mRNA and protein in rat brain. *J. Neurochem.* **60,** 1512–1519.

181. Abraham, N. G., Lavrovsky, Y., Schwartzman, M. L., et al. (1995) Transfection of the human heme oxygenase gene into rabbit coronary microvessel endothelial cells: protective effect against heme and hemoglobin toxicity. *Proc. Natl. Acad. Sci. USA* **92,** 6798–6802.

182. Regan, R. F., Guo, Y., and Kumar, N. (2000) Heme oxygenase-1 induction protects murine cortical astrocytes from hemoglobin toxicity. *Neurosci. Lett.* **282,** 1–4.

183. Hegazy, K. A., Dunn, M. W., and Sharma, S. C. (2000) Functional human heme oxygenase has a neuroprotective effect on adult rat ganglion cells after pressure- induced ischemia. *NeuroReport* **11,** 1185–1189.

184. Takeda, A., Perry, G., Abraham, N. G., et al. (2000) Overexpression of heme oxygenase in neuronal cells, the possible interaction with tau. *J. Biol. Chem.* **275,** 5395–5399.

185. Panahian, N., Yoshiura, M., and Maines, M. D. (1999) Overexpression of heme oxygenase-1 is neuroprotective in a model of permanent middle cerebral artery occlusion in transgenic mice. *J. Neurochem.* **72,** 1187–1203.

186. Chen, K., Gunter, K., and Maines, M. D. (2000a) Neurons overexpressing heme oxygenase-1 resist oxidative stress-mediated cell death. *J. Neurochem.* **75,** 304–313.
187. Poss, K. D. and Tonegawa, S. (1997b) Reduced stress defense in heme oxygenase 1-deficient cells. *Proc. Natl. Acad. Sci. USA* **94,** 10,925–10,930.
188. Eisenstein, R. S., Garcia, M. D., Pettingell, W., and Munro, H. N. (1991) Regulation of ferritin and heme oxygenase synthesis in rat fibroblasts by different forms of iron. *Proc. Natl. Acad. Sci. USA* **88,** 688–692.
189. Ferris, C. D., Jaffrey, S. R., Sawa, A., et al. (1999) Haem oxygenase-1 prevents cell death by regulating cellular iron. *Nature Cell Biol.* **1,** 152–157.
190. Minetti, M., Mallozzi, C., DiStasi, A. M. M., and Pietraforte, D. (1998) Bilirubin is an effective antioxidant of peroxynitrite-mediated protein oxidation in human blood plasma. *Arch. Biochem. Biophys.* **352,** 165–174.
191. Stocker, R., Yamamoto Y., McDonagh, A. F., Glazer, A. N., and Ames, B. N. (1987) Bilirubin is an antioxidant of possible physiological importance. *Science* **235,** 1043–1046.
192. Neuzil J., and Stocker, R. (1993) Bilirubin attenuates radical-mediated damage to serum albumin. *FEBS Lett.* **331,** 281–284.
193. Dore, S., Takahashi, M., Ferris, C. D., Hester, L. D., Guastella, D., and Snyder, S. H. (1999) Bilirubin, formed by activation of heme oxygenase-2, protects neurons against oxidative stress injury. *Proc. Natl. Acad. Sci. USA* **96,** 2445–2450.
194. Lee, A. S. (1987) Coordinated regulation of a set of genes by glucose and calcium ionophores in mammalian cells. *Trends Biochem. Sci.* **12,** 20–23.
195. Lee, A. S. (1992) Mammalian stress response: induction of the glucose-regulated protein family. *Curr. Opin. Cell Biol.* **4,** 267–273.
196. Wang, S., Longo, F. M., Chen, J., et al. (1993) Induction of glucose regulated protein (grp78) and inducible heat shock protein (hsp70) mRNAs in rat brain after kainic acid seizures and focal ischemia. *Neurochem. Int.* **23,** 575–582.
197. Li, W. W., Alexandre, S., Cao, X., and Lee, A. S. (1993) Transactivation of the grp78 promoter by Ca^{2+} depletion: a comparative analysis with A23187 and the endoplasmic reticulum Ca^{2+}-ATPase inhibitor thapsigargin. *J. Biol. Chem.* **268,** 12,003–12,009.
198. Stevens, J. L., Liu, H., Halleck, M., Bowes, R. C., Chen, Q. M., and van de Water, B. (2000) Linking gene expression to mechanisms of toxicity. *Toxicol. Lett.* **112-113,** 479–486.
199. Chen, L. Y., Chiang, A. S., Hung, J. J., Hung., H. I., and Lai, Y. K. (2000) Thapsigargin-induced grp78 expression is mediated by the increase of cytosolic free calcium in 9L rat brain tumor cells. *J. Cell. Biochem.* **78,** 404–416.
200. Yang, Y., Turner, R. S., and Gaut, J. R. (1998) The chaperone BiP/GRP78 binds to amyloid precursor protein and decreases Aβ40 and Aβ42 secretion. *J. Biol. Chem.* **273,** 25,552–25,555.
201. Yu, Z., Luo, H., Fu, W., and Mattson, M. P. (1999) The endoplasmic reticulum stress-responsive protein GRP78 protects neurons against excitotoxicity and apoptosis: suppression of oxidative stress and stabilization of calcium homeostasis. *Exp. Neurol.* **155,** 302–314.

202. Opanashuk, L. A. and Finkelstein, J. N. (1995) Induction of newly synthesized proteins in astroglial cells exposed to lead. *Toxicol. Appl. Pharmacol.* **131,** 21–30.

203. Opanashuk, L. A., and Finkelstein, J. N. (1995) Relationship of lead-induced proteins to stress response proteins in astroglial cells. *J. Neurosci. Res.* **42,** 623–632.

204. Audesirk, G., Ferguson, C. A., Kern, M., and Cabell, L. (1997) Cultured rat hippocampal neurons and astrocytes differ greatly in the induction of protein synthesis by inorganic lead. *Soc. Neurosci. Abstracts* **23,** 2209.

205. Qian, Y., Harris, E. D., Zheng, Y., and Tiffany-Castiglioni, E. (2000) Lead targets GRP78, a molecular chaperone, in C6 rat glioma cells. *Toxicol. Appl. Pharmacol.* **163,** 260–266.

206. Tully, D. B., Collins, B. J., Overstreet, J. D., et al. (2000) Effects of arsenic, cadmium, chromium, and lead on gene expression regulated by a battery of 13 different promoters in recombinant HepG2 cells. *Toxicol. Appl. Pharmacol.* **168,** 79–90.

207. Ferguson, C., Kern, M., and Audesirk, G. (2000) Nanomolar concentrations of inorganic lead increase Ca2+ efflux and decrease intracellular free Ca2+ ion concentrations in cultured rat hippocampal neurons by a calmodulin-dependent mechanism. *NeuroToxicology* **21,** 365–378.

208. Timblin, C. R., Janssen, Y. M., Goldberg, J. L., and Mossman, B. T. (1998) GRP78, HSP72/73, and cJun stress protein levels in lung epithelial cells exposed to asbestos, cadmium, or H_2O_2. *Free Radical Biol. Med.* **24,** 632–642.

209. Miles, M. F., Wilke, N., Elliot, M., Tanner, W., and Shah, S. (1994) Ethanol-reponsive genes in neural cells include the 78-kilodalton glucose-regulated protein (GRP78) and the 94-kilodalton glucose-regulated protein (GRP94) molecular chaperones. *Mol. Pharmacol.* **46,** 873–879.

210. Tunici, P., Schiaffonati, L., Rabellotti, E., Tiberio, L., Perin, A., and Sessa, A. (1999) In vivo modulation of 73 kDa heat shock cognate and 78 kDa glucose-regulating protein gene expression in rat liver and brain by ethanol. *Alcohol Clin. Exp. Res.* **23,** 1861–1867.

5

Role of Apoptosis in Neurotoxicology

**Lori D. White, Sid Hunter, Michael W. Miller,
Marion Ehrich, and Stanley Barone, Jr.**

1. INTRODUCTION

The role of apoptosis in development and neurodegeneration has become
increasingly apparent in the past 10 yr. Normal apoptosis occurs in the central nervous system (CNS) from the embryonic stage through senescence,
with different cells in each region of the nervous system having characteristic temporal patterns of programmed cell death. Several different stimuli
trigger the apoptotic cascade, initiating diverse intracellular signaling pathways. These include mitochondrial calcium overload, generation of reactive
oxygen species, and alterations in neurotrophic factor signaling. Neurotrophic factor-mediated signaling is achieved though the interaction of
p75NTR and Trk receptors to modulate apoptotic cell death in developing
and adult neural tissues. Both in vivo and in vitro experiments have suggested that exposure to a number of neurotoxicants results in apoptosis. For
example, exposure of organogenesis-stage mouse embryos to a wide variety
of xenobiotics, including ethanol, arsenic, hydroxyurea, chemotheraputic
drugs, or haloacetic acids, results in increased apoptosis during neurulation.
Ethanol, a widely used neurotoxicant, has been shown to affect apoptosis, as
well as proliferation and migration, in developing animals. Exposure to
heavy metal contaminants has been implicated in apoptotic cell death. This
has been demonstrated with methylmercury with in vivo exposure producing apoptosis in the cerebellum and in vitro studies in PC12 cells implicat-
ing a neurotrophic factor dependent mechanism for this effect. Also,
exposure to some organophosphates targets mitochondrial function by alter-

From: *Methods in Pharmacology and Toxicology: In Vitro Neurotoxicology: Principles and Challenges*
Edited by: E. Tiffany-Castiglioni © Humana Press Inc., Totowa, NJ

ing membrane potential and substrate adhesion, resulting in apoptosis. Thus, a variety of neurotoxicants modulate or produce apoptosis through alterations in developmental processes or alterations in cellular and subcellular homeostasis. This chapter presents current research in this area and illustrates how alterations in apoptosis result in morphological or functional deficits in the nervous system. Our aim is to address the distinction between apoptosis and programmed cell death, to discuss methodologies for detection/measurement of apoptosis, to describe the developmental time-course of programmed cell death, to illustrate the relevance of this process in neurotoxicology, and to demonstrate how both in vitro and in vivo methods can be used to study this process of cell death.

2. APOPTOSIS AND PROGRAMMED CELL DEATH

Apoptosis and programmed cell death are terms often used synonymously, but there are, in fact, distinctions. Apoptosis was originally described by Kerr et al. in 1972 *(1)* as a set of morphological changes in a degenerating cell, including cell shrinkage, membrane blebbing, chromatin condensation, nuclear fragmentation, and, finally, the formation of apoptotic bodies. On the other hand, programmed cell death refers to the temporally and spatially reproducible loss of cells during the development of an organism, which is a genetically defined process that leads to the morphological characteristics of apoptosis.

A recent review of apoptosis in development *(2)* stated,

> During ontogeny of many organs, cells are over-produced only to be etched or whittled away to generate the rococo structures of functional tissue. Early distaste among biologists for the "wastefulness" of such a process has given away to the recognition that the ability to ablate cells is as essential a constructive process in animal ontogeny as are the abilities to replicate and differentiate them.

There are two major kinds of cell death, apoptosis and necrosis, which have been likened to suicide and accidental death, respectively *(3)*. Actually, apoptosis and necrosis are not mutually exclusive, but are, instead, at two ends of the spectrum of cell death. Of great importance to the nervous system is the fact that cells undergoing apoptosis do not create an inflammatory response. Furthermore, apoptosis is a highly regulated event, whereas necrosis is a generalized breakdown of the cell membrane, with the contents spilling into the surrounding area where macrophages and microglia then phagocytose the dead cells. Cell death can further be classified by how the corpses of cells are cleared from the site *(4)*. Early in apoptosis, there are changes in the cellular volume and ion composition of the cells. Then, proteins start to be cleaved, the nucleus begins to degrade, and the chromatin condenses along the periphery of the nucleus. Finally, the cell breaks into apoptotic bodies, which are dealt with by local phagocytic cells (reviewed in ref. *5*).

3. PROGRAMMED CELL DEATH DURING NERVOUS SYSTEM DEVELOPMENT

The process of programmed cell death in conjunction with cell proliferation is critical in pattern formation. Together, these processes help shape a flat sheet of cells into a neural tube. This is mediated by genetic and epigenetic signaling and leads to the diverse and segmented structures of the nervous system. One specific example where this genetic regulation of pattern formation is clearly linked to apototic cell death is in the rhombomeres of the hind brain of the mouse *(6)*.

Although apoptosis has been studied intensively for the past decade, significant information gaps still exist in the regional and temporal characterization of normally occurring apoptosis in nervous system development. The magnitude of cell death that occurs during neural development is unknown, but it is thought that approximately half of all neurons produced during development die *(7)*, some during the fetal period in mainly proliferative zones and some during a second wave of programmed cell death in postmitotic cells *(8)*.

The proliferative capacity of most regions of the nervous system is limited to finite periods of time during development, but apoptosis can occur less synchronously and over a more protracted period of time depending on environmental stimuli or insults. Thus, both neural proliferation and apoptosis determine the cell number of a specified neural structure. Therefore, to have an understanding of the apoptosis that may be induced by neurotoxicant exposure, we have quantitatively and qualitatively characterized this time-course in an attempt to establish a baseline for further neurotoxicological studies *(9)*.

Postnatally, brainstem, neocortex, and hippocampus (*see* Fig. 1A) had similar patterns of apoptosis as determined by cell death enzyme-linked immunosorbent assay (ELISA). Fragmented DNA was at high levels at postnatal day (PD) 1 followed by a reduction during the first postnatal week to a basal plateau by PD90. The brainstem levels reached a plateau more gradually than neocortex or hippocampus. Apoptosis in the hippocampus peaked at PD1, but its level was less than half of that occurring in the neocortex and brainstem at PD1.

Patterns of cerebellar apoptosis were unique compared to other regions in that a peak in DNA fragmentation was observed at PD10 followed by a

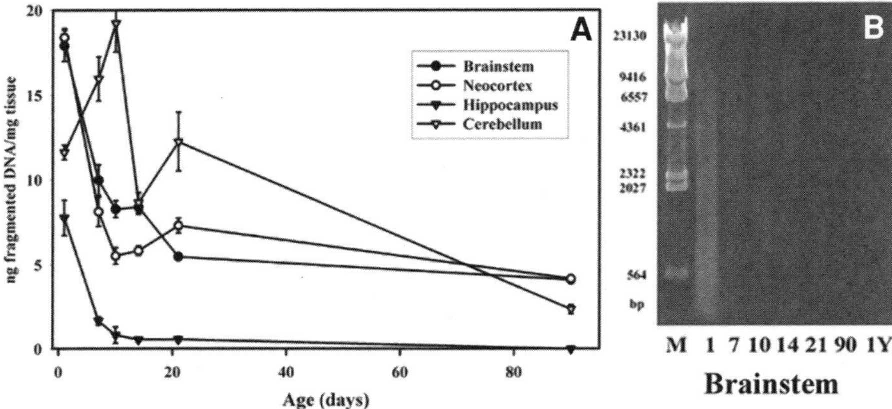

Fig.1. Developmental time-course of apoptosis. (**A**) Apoptosis detected with an ELISA for quantitation of levels of cytosolic fragmentation of nucleosomal DNA from the neocortex, hippocampus, brainstem, and cerebellum during the postnatal period (PD1–90), (**B**) Apoptosis in brainstem detected by agarose gel electrophoresis to demonstrate DNA fragmentation.

smaller increase at PD21 *(9)*. Adult levels of apoptosis were also low in the cerebellum. An important point is that the brainstem is ontogenically the oldest region of the brain where apoptosis is highest on the first postnatal day of the rat. Conversely, the cerebellum develops mostly postnatally and has a peak of apoptosis at PD10 and a smaller peak at PD21. In all brain regions, there was good correlation between data gathered from ELISA and agarose gels for measurement of DNA fragmentation, although the gel results of in vivo samples did not display discrete banding patterns (*see* Fig. 1B), as is often seen in gels of DNA from apoptotic cultured cells. However, the fragmented DNA was the correct size for oligonucleosomal fragments. Others have observed similar "smeared" results with DNA isolated from tissue containing apoptotic cells *(10)* or have been unable to demonstrate "ladders" in cultured cells that are undergoing apoptosis. Another technical consideration of agarose gel data is the sensitivity to the small percentage of cells undergoing apoptosis at a given time in the tissue. Even at PD1 in the neocortex, the dying cells are at differing degrees of cell death, demonstrating the early 50- to 300-kb fragments, multiples of the 180- to 200-base oligonucleosomes, and further degraded pieces of nucleic acids.

Terminal transferase-mediated dUTP nick-end-labeling (TUNEL) histochemistry also provides an index of apoptosis, wherein presumptive apoptotic cells are darkly stained and other cells are lightly counterstained with methyl green. The TUNEL data corroborated ELISA and DNA gel results. TUNEL immunoreactivity is depicted in this collage of camera lucida drawings of the ontogeny from gestational day 18 (GD18) to 2-yr-old rats with each dot representing an apoptotic cell (*see* Fig. 2). The neocortex, brainstem, and hippocampus, the regions quantified by ELISA, have the most dense populations of apoptotic cells at PD1. High levels of apoptosis were also noted on PD1 in the thalamus, hypothalamus, and striatum. To summarize this ontogenetic study of programmed cell death during rat brain development, (1) brain regions have unique spatiotemporal patterns of apoptosis qualitatively and quantitatively during prenatal and postnatal development, (2) in the brainstem, neocortex, and hippocampus, levels are highest at PD1 and decrease to lower levels in adulthood, and (3) cerebellar apoptosis peaks at PD10 with low levels in adulthood. These data provide a temporal and regional baseline for further studies of the effects of perturbations of cell death during neural development.

4. CLINICAL RELEVANCE OF APOPTOSIS IN THE NERVOUS SYSTEM

Disturbances in the tightly controlled spatiotemporal pattern of proliferation, migration, differentiation, and apoptosis can occur in a number of developmental disorders. In addition to nonrandomly occurring programmed cell death occurring during development, apoptosis is relevant in a number of human neurological diseases. Perturbations of programed cell death, with the end result being either too few or too many cells, are associated both with learning disabilities and neurodegenerative disorders (reviewed in ref. *11*). For example, in Down syndrome, there is a decreased brain cell number as a result of increased apoptosis in early development. In early adulthood, Down's syndrome individuals usually develop an Alzheimer's-like dementia *(12)*. In schizophrenia, alterations in cell number, mainly in cortical regions [e.g., an increase in neuronal density in dorsolateral prefrontal cortex *(13)* and a decrease in Bcl-2 levels *(14)*, volume, and neuron number *(15)* in temporal regions] implicate alterations in proliferation and/or apoptosis. In addition, the striatum of schizophrenics has been shown to have increased cell numbers *(16)*, whereas the corpus callosum demonstrated a reduced cross-sectional area compared to controls *(17)*. Macrocephaly appears to occur in many autistic individuals *(18,19)*. This increase in the size of the autistic brain has been demonstrated *in situ* with magnetic resonance imaging with an increase in volume of the caudate nucleus of the basal ganglia *(20)*, whereas anterior subregions of the corpus callosum were found to be smaller than in age-matched controls *(21)* and altered asymmetry of the frontal lobes was observed *(22)*. Changes in cell number or cell density

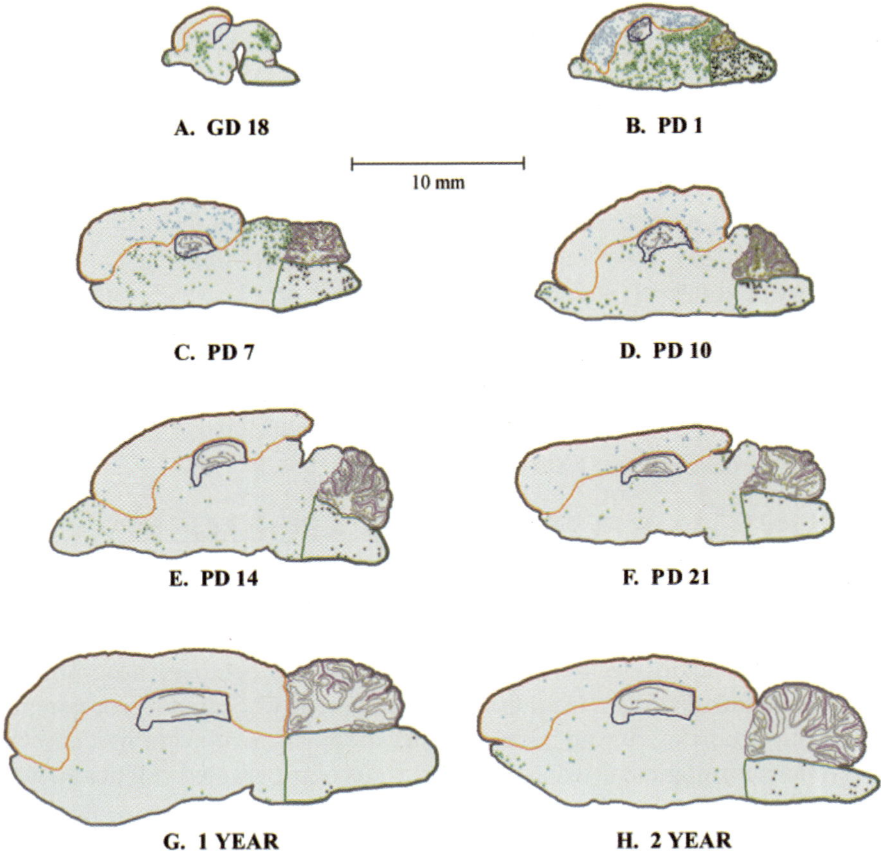

Fig. 2. Camera lucida drawings of TUNEL-stained presumptive apoptotic cells during developmental of rat brain from GD18, PD1, PD7, PD10, PD14, PD21, 1-yr, and 2-yr-olds. Brains were cut sagitally at 12 μm and stained according to kit protocols (Intergen). Tissue is counterstained with methyl green.

appear to be region dependent, with increases in the cerebral cortex and decreases in Purkinje cells of the posterior cerebellum and inferior olivary nucleus *(23)*. Although apoptosis is not conclusively involved in all of these regional differences, disruption of regulation of this process could explain why, in some regions, there is an increase in cell number and a decrease in cell number in others.

5. REGULATORS OF APOPTOSIS

Genes and proteins regulating apoptosis were first characterized in the nematode *Caenorhabditis elegans* (reviewed in ref. *24*). The adult worm is comprised of 959 cells subsequent to the programmed cell death of 131 of the original 1090 somatic cells. The genes and their protein products controlling this process have been highly conserved throughout evolution.

The genetic regulation of apoptosis was further characterized in the fruit fly *Drosophila melanogaster* (reviewed in ref. *25*). In mammals, the apoptotic machinery is even more complex, although there is basic homology with the invertebrates. Two families of proteins are involved in the control of apoptosis, the caspase family (also known as interleukin-converting enzymes [ICEs]) and the Bcl (for B-cell lymphoma) family. Caspases (reviewed in ref. *26*), which are intracellular cysteine proteases, are important in the initiation and execution of cell death. There are currently about 14 known caspases, some of which are involved in immune responses and others involved with apoptosis. The caspases involved in apoptosis are either "upstream" initiator caspases (e.g., caspase-8 and caspase-9) or "downstream" effector caspases. Initiator caspases have either death-effector domains (DEDs) or caspase activation and recruitment domains (CARDs), which are prodomains that fold into similar structures to allow protein–protein interactions and the creation of apoptosomes (reviewed in ref. *27*).

The effector caspases lack these prodomains and are instead activated by upstream caspases. Their role is to implement apoptosis by cleavage of structural proteins and metabolic and repair enzymes, the substrates which, when cleaved, allow the orderly death of the cell. Caspases are typically present in cells constitutively as inactive zymogens and are then cleaved to yield a p20 and a p10 subunit. Two of each subunit combine to form the active protein.

The other protein family involved in the regulation of apoptosis is the Bcl family. Members, including Bcl-2 *(28,29)* and Bcl-X_L *(30)* are antiapoptotic, are localized to the outer surface of mitochondria and endoplasmic reticulum, and have C-terminal hydrophobic tails with the bulk of the protein in the cytosol. Bax *(31)* and Bak *(32)* are proapoptotic with a similar structure. In developing rats, the balanced expression of bcl-2 and bax transiently changes at times that are concurrent with naturally occurring neuronal death *(33,34)*.

6. THE APOPTOTIC CASCADES

There are three major pathways of apoptosis in mammalian cells (reviewed in ref. *2*). The first pathway, which does not appear to have a counterpart in insect and nematode apoptosis, utilizes a family of death receptors, which include the tumor necrosis factor (TNF) receptor, the CD95 receptor *(35)*, and the p75 receptor *(36)* (*see* Fig. 3). Binding of TNF, Fas ligand, or nerve growth factor (NGF), respectively, initiates a cascade of events ulti-

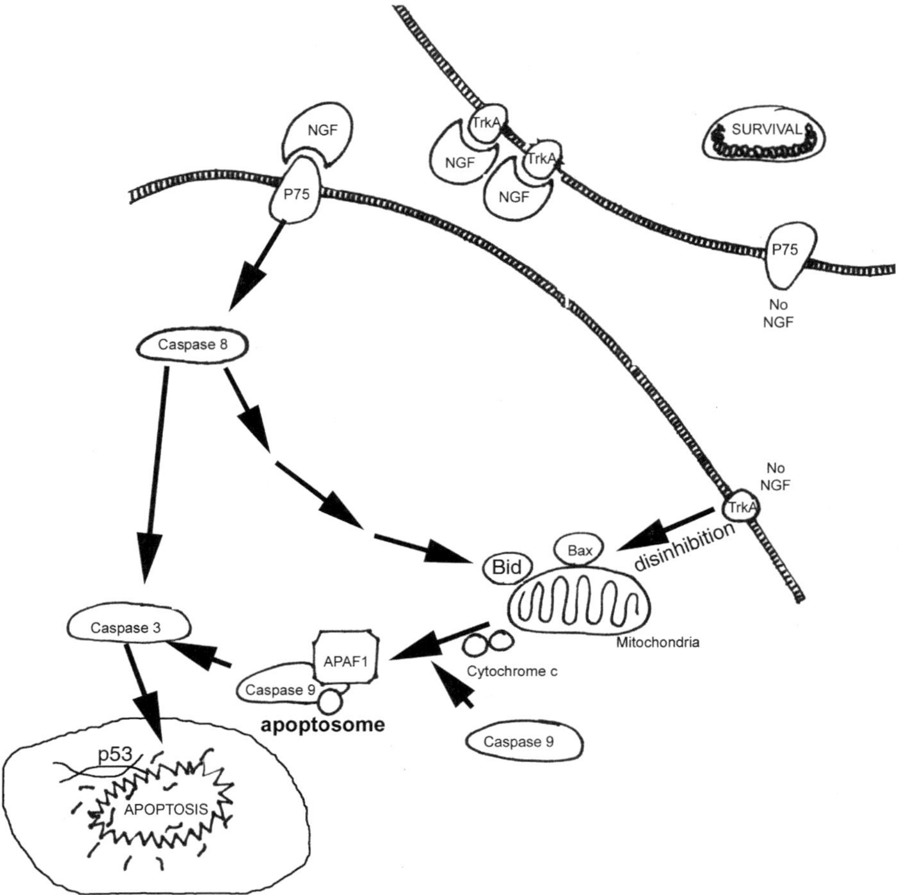

Fig. 3. Apoptosis cascade demonstrating the p75-mediated pathway and the trkA-mediated pathway and the various caspases involved in neuronal apoptosis. There is a balance between trophic support through trk activation and trophic factor regulation of survival through p75. This balance is shifted with trophic factor withdrawal (e.g., NGF) leading to increases in activity through both legs of the caspase cascade (caspase-8 and caspase-9), leading to increased apoptotic activity.

mately ending in apoptosis of the cell, unless the cascade is stopped by antiapoptotic components within the cell. The context in which these death receptors are present is also a determinant of their role in apoptosis. For example, p75 receptors, in the presence of trkA receptors, enhance the antiapoptotic role of trkA/NGF binding (reviewed in ref. *37*).

Receptor-mediated apoptosis is initiated by recruitment of a number of procaspase-8 zymogens using the adaptor protein fas-associated death domain (FADD). The procaspase-8 molecules are mutually cleaved, presumably because of their proximity, and become active caspase-8, which can subsequently cleave downstream caspases. A second pathway, involving serine proteases called granzymes, is involved in immune cell apoptosis, but, as yet, does not appear particularly relevant to the nervous system. A third pathway in mammals involves mitochondria, wherein release of proapoptotic molecules, including cytochrome-*c*, initiates apoptosis by binding to procaspase-9 and a protein cofactor, Apaf-1. Cytochrome-*c* complexes with Apaf-1, and this oligomer recruits procaspase-9 into an apoptosome complex. Procaspase-9 is activated by means of a conformational change, through its protein–protein interactions with cytochrome-*c* and Apaf-1. Release of cytochrome-*c* is regulated by members of the Bcl family, which are thought to control channel formation in the mitochondrial outer membrane, membrane potential, and/or membrane permeability. Caspase-8 can also cleave Bid *(38)*, a proapoptotic Bcl family member, which then mediates release of cytochrome-*c* from mitochondria *(39,40)*, thus creating amplification of the death receptor pathway by the mitochondrial pathway.

In addition to the use of death receptors, mammalian apoptosis differs from the invertebrates in another important way: Many apoptosis-inducing cell stressors have the effect of inducing openings in the mitochondrial membrane to initiate the mitochondrial pathway described earlier. DNA damage from genotoxic insults (reviewed in ref. *41*) activates the proapoptotic signal p53, the transcription factor E2F-1, and the proto-oncogene c-Abl. These same basic pathways of apoptosis are common to most cell types; however, specificity is achieved though the interactions of the Bcell family members, the caspase family members, and the presence or absence of death receptors. Different types of neuron and neurons at different developmental stages, express myriad combinations of Bcl-2 and caspase family members. This multiplicity is necessary to provide the tightly controlled regulation of cell death in the developing nervous system. Perturbations in this balance can underlie neurotoxicant-induced vulnerability of the developing nervous system.

7. APOPTOSIS METHODOLOGIES

The accurate detection and quantification of apoptosis are important in studies of the role of cell death in neurotoxicology. Presented here are a number of methodologies utilized by the authors in their studies of this process.

7.1. Lysotracker Staining/Whole-Mount Techniques

Apoptosis in organogenesis-stage mouse embryos can be studied by use of confocal laser scanning microscopy and a vital stain *(42)*. Mouse embryos

are harvested on gestational day (GD) 8 or 9, stained with the vital lysoso-
mal dye LysoTracker Red, fixed with paraformaldehyde, and then dehy-
drated and cleared. The stained embryo is then optically sectioned with the
use of confocal microscopy and the dye visualized in three-dimensional
reconstructions.

7.2. Terminal Transferase-Mediated dUTP Nick End Labeling

Terminal transferase-mediated dUTP nick end labeling (TUNEL) can be
used both quantitatively and qualitatively to assay apoptosis *in situ*. This
method enzymatically labels the myriad free 3' OH ends generated by DNA
fragmentation. Cells undergoing apoptosis stain darkly and thus allow both
for quantification and qualitative information about cellular localization and
anatomical detail. False positives can occur with this method *(43)*, so it is
important to use it in conjunction with other detection methods.

7.3. Flow Cytometry

Flow cytometry can be used to distinguish apoptotic cells from live or
necrotic cells. This method measures changes in scattered and fluoresced
light of dissociated cells pumped through an optical system. The fluorescence parameters that can be detected in apoptotic cells are uptake of
Hoechst 33258 dye, DNA strand breaks labeled by the TUNEL method (*see*
Subheading 7.2.), changes in plasma membrane asymmetry visualized with
annexin V labeling (*see* Subheading 7.11.), and nuclear condensation.

7.4. Cell Death ELISA

Quantification of fragmented DNA in apoptotic cells can be done with a
cell death ELISA. This method uses an antihistone capture antibody and an
anti-DNA detection antibody in a sandwich ELISA format to detect the
DNA/histone mononucleosomes and oligonucleosomes generated by nu-
clease cleavage of nuclear DNA *(9)*.

7.5. Gel Electrophoresis

Agarose gel electrophoresis of fragmented DNA, which is sometimes
considered the hallmark assay of apoptosis, illustrates cleavage into
oligonucleosomal fragments, or ladders, in multiples of 180–200 bp, from
the initial cleavage into fragments of 50–300 kbp. DNA is extracted from
cells with phenol/choroform/isoamyl alcohol, followed by ethanol precipitation. The DNA is then electrophoresed in a 1% agarose gel to separate
fragments of DNA by size, with the creation of the typical "apoptotic lad-
der" in only some cell types (*see* Subheading 3.).

7.6. *Immunohistochemistry for Apoptosis-Related Proteins*

A number of proteins are implicated in apoptosis, including p53, p38, members of the caspase and Bcl-2 families, Jun, and Alzheimer's-specific protein. Polyclonal or monoclonal antibodies to these proteins can be used to identify cells undergoing or about to undergo apoptosis. As such, they are only markers, not expressed in all cell types, and thus immunopositive reactions only suggest apoptosis. Additionally, antibodies to caspases can specifically recognize either the inactive proenzyme or the cleaved active enzyme.

7.7. *Caspase-3 Assays*

Caspase-3 activation is measured by adding phycoerythrin-conjugated antiactive caspase-3 antibodies to cultured cells after harvest. Harvested cells are fixed, permeabilized, and washed with a Cytofix/Cytoperm Kit (Pharmagen, San Diego, CA). Antiactive caspase-3 antibodies (1 : 1000) are then added and allowed to incubate overnight at 4°C. Flow cytometry is utilized to examine 5000–8000 gated cell samples (excitation 488 nm, emission 575 nm). Mean fluorescence intensity of the x channel in the gated field of treated cultures is compared to values of control cultures, with activation expressed as percent of control.

Pretreatment (8 h) with 25 μM caspase inhibitors (Ac-DEVD-CHO for caspase-3 and Ac-IETD-CHO for caspase-8 [Pharmagen]) or with a serine–protease inhibitor (phenylmethylsulfonyl fluoride [PMSF], 1 mM) can be used to verify that caspase activation is occurring. Cyclosporin A pretreatment (500 nM, 8 h) also decreases caspase activation and serves as a positive control for enzyme inhibition *(44)*.

7.8. *Fluorescent Microscopy of Nuclear Morphology/Hoechst Staining*

Cells grown in four- and eight-well multichamber slides are treated with test compounds or with 50–500 nM staurosporine (positive control). At various times after compound addition, cells are centrifuged on a Hettich cytospin (Tuttlingen, Germany) for 5 min at 32–89g and then fixed in acetone/ethanol (1 : 1 v/v). The slides are then air-dried and stained with the DNA-specific fluorochrome Hoechst 33342 (10 µg/mL) for 15 min before they are examined on a Nikon Diaphot-TMD inverted microscope equipped with a 40× fluorescence objective and an ultraviolet (UV) filter cube. The percentage of apoptotic nuclei can be determined from photographs, with comparisons made between controls and treated cells *(44)*.

7.9. Transmembrane Potential

Transmembrane potential can be evaluated *(45)* by utilizing the mitochondrial-specific, cationic fluorescent dye rhodamine 123 (Molecular Probes, Eugene, OR). Following 3–4 d growth in standard media in microtiter wells, cells are changed to a medium supplemented with 5 µg/mL rhodamine 123 and incubated for 8–12 h before the addition of test compounds. At various times after test compound exposure, fluorescence is measured with a Cytofluor II multiwell fluorescence spectrophotometer, with excitation at 530 nm and emission at 590 nm. Comparisons are made between treated and control cells.

7.10. Mitochondrial Transition Pore

The integrity of the mitochondrial transition pore can be evaluated with the Focht Live-Cell Chamber System [FCS2, Bioptechs, PA *(46)*] Control and toxicant-treated cell cultures are incubated with medium containing 500 nM of tetramethylrhodamine methyl ester (TMRM) for 15 min, followed by TMRM plus 1 µM acetoxymethyl ester of calcein (calcein-AM) for 15 min at a controlled temperature of 37°C. Effects on the mitochondrial transition pore are monitored by laser scanning confocal microscopy. Red fluorescence of TMRM associated with intact mitochondria passes through a 590-nm (long-pass) filter and green fluorescence of calcein passes through a 515-nm (25-nm bandpass) barrier filter to a variable-pinhole photodetector. Images can be transferred to a computer where they are analyzed for regions where the dyes are colocalized (where the mitochondrial-specific dye has leaked into the cytosol). Increases in colocalization of the dyes from that seen in control cells indicate treatment-induced damage to the mitochondrial transition pore.

7.11. Annexin Cell Membrane Assays

Alterations in cell membrane phospholipids, resulting in membrane asymmetry, also occur as an early event in cells undergoing apoptosis. Phosphatidylserine (PS), which is usually located on the inner membrane, translocates to the outer membrane during apoptosis. This characteristic can be exploited to identify those cells undergoing apoptosis (reviewed in ref. *47*). A calcium-dependent phospholipids-binding protein, annexin V, which has a high and specific affinity for PS, is labeled with either biotin or a fluorophor and allowed to bind to and identify apoptotic cells by flow cytometry or light microscopy.

8. RESULTS OF STUDIES EXAMINING NEUROTOXICANT-INDUCED APOPTOSIS

8.1. Early Effects of Xenobiotics on Apoptosis During Organogenesis and Neurulation

Neurulation is one of the earliest morphogenetic events in brain development. Development of the neural tube includes the closure of the neural plate and an epithelio-mesenchymal transformation of the lateral cells of the neuroectoderm to form the migratory neural crest (NC) cells. Apoptosis is a normal event in the development of the neuroepithelium and neural crest cells. In chick embryos, blockage of caspase activity induces neural tube defects, suggesting that apoptosis is a requirement for closure of the tube. Thus, prevention of cell death leading to insufficient apoptosis by xenobiotics might be a cause of anencephaly/exencephaly. Xenobiotic-induced excess cell death in neuroepithelial and NC cells has been associated with neural tube and craniofacial defects. Day 8 (plug day = 0) early-somite-staged (four to six pairs of somites) CD-1 mouse conceptuses in whole-embryo culture exposed to the haloacetic acids (HAs) dichloroacetate, bromochloroacetate, or dibromoacetate exhibit craniofacial dysmorphogenesis after a 24-h culture period (*see* Fig. 4) *(48)*. These effects include a lack of neural tube closure as well as prosencephalic and pharyngeal arch hypoplasia. Based on the morphology, both NC cells and neural tube closure appear susceptible to HA-induced toxicity. To characterize the pathogenic effects produced by HAs, vital staining was used to evaluate cell death and flow cytometry was used to determine the distribution of cells in the cell cycle. Lysotracker staining and whole-mount evaluation indicated that cell death was present in the neuroepithelium, but was especially widespread in the pharyngeal arches following a 24-h exposure to HAs. No changes in the distribution of nuclei in the cell cycle were detected. The colocalization of anatomical defects and cell death, especially in the first pharyngeal arch, suggests that these may be causally related. Based on studies in adult tissues, our working hypothesis is that HA-induced dysmorphogenesis arises from altered signal transduction. Embryos exposed to staurosporine, a broad-spectrum kinase inhibitor, Bisindolmaleimide 1, a PKC inhibitor, or PD98059, a MAP kinase inhibitor exhibit dysmorphology *(49)*. These studies confirm the susceptibility of the neurulation-staged embryo to xenobiotic perturbation of signal transduction pathways. High levels of embryonic cell death were induced by staurosporine

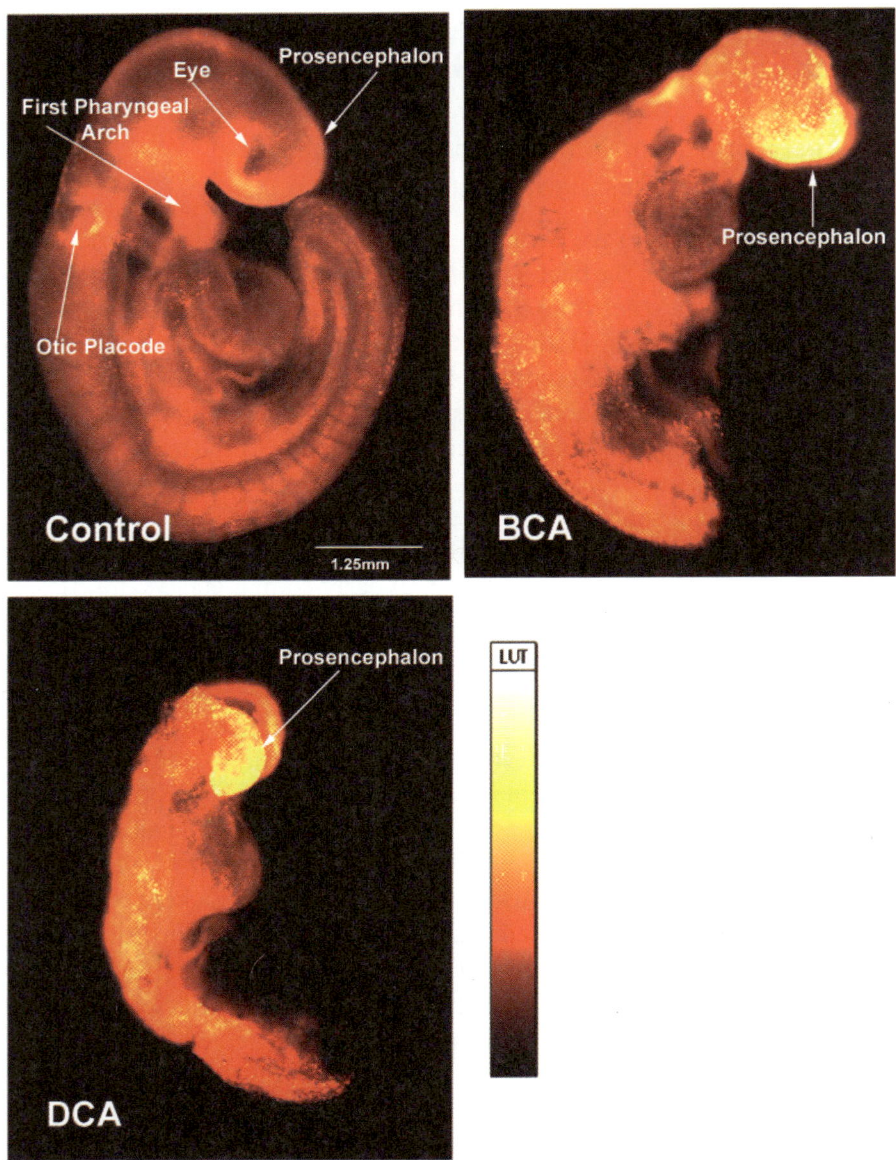

Fig. 4. Pseudocolor images of mouse embryos stained with Lysotracker Red after a 24-h exposure to control medium, 11 m*M* dichloroacetic acid (DCA) or 300 µ*M* bromochloroacetic acid (BCA). The look-up table (LUT) from lowest to highest fluorescence is included. Regions of cell death in the control embryo occur in the prosencephalon, base of the first arch and otic pit. Extensive cell death in observed in the prosencephalon of embryos exposed to BCA or DCA. Scale bar = 1.25 mm.

and PD98059, but not by Bis1, indicating that regulation of cell death by signal transduction pathways, especially MAP kinase, are active at this stage of development. The types of malformation and distribution of cell death in staurosporine and PD98059-exposed embryos also indicate that the neural crest are very susceptible to kinase inhibitors. Staurosporine perturbed NC cell development and induced high levels of cell death in primary NC cell culture. Cell death was also observed following exposure to the HAs in primary NC culture (*see* Fig. 5) (unpublished observation). The adverse effects of staurosporine on the embryo and NC cells are consistent with our hypothesis that altered signal transduction pathways might be responsible for HA-induced defects; however, the critical pathway(s) for alterations in neurulation remains to be determined *(50)*.

8.2. Methylmercury Studies

Nerve growth factor (NGF) has long been recognized as essential for survival of PC12 cells that have been primed to differentiate following repeated exposure to this neurotrophic factor. In the presence of NGF, PC12 cells decrease their rate of proliferation and begin to differentiate by extending neurites at a much faster rate than cells not exposed to NGF (reviewed in ref. *51*). The effect of NGF on this cell line provided for a model system that can be used to test early effects on proliferating cells and later effects on differentiating cells. Withdrawal of NGF from differentiated PC12 cells induced apoptosis in a dose-dependent fashion with a rescue from apoptosis seen at 5 ng/mL NGF (*see* Fig. 6).

The effects of methylmercury on apoptosis in PC12 cells, both differentiated and undifferentiated, have recently been characterized *(52)*. Differentiated PC12 cells exposed to methylmercury, with or without NGF, clearly show increased apoptosis with NGF withdrawal. A dose-dependent increase in apoptosis was noted with methylmercury exposure (data not shown).

The TUNEL assays of differentiated or undifferentiated PC12 cells treated with methylmercury, either with or without NGF, were done to further characterize the effects on apoptosis. Results show a concentration-dependent increase in apoptosis with methylmercury in both differentiated and undifferentiated cells, with the differentiated cells showing overall greater levels of apoptotic cells (*see* Fig. 7). ELISA data for cytoplasmic oligonucleosomal fragments from similar exposure paradigms demonstrated a clear dose response at low ($< 3\ \mu M$) methylmercury levels. At higher doses of methylmercury ($> 3\ \mu M$), the cells exhibited signs of necrosis, with many of them detaching from the substrate *(52)*.

The rat has been utilized as an in vivo model for studies of the neuropathology of mercury exposure. Nagashima *(53)* reviewed these data, which

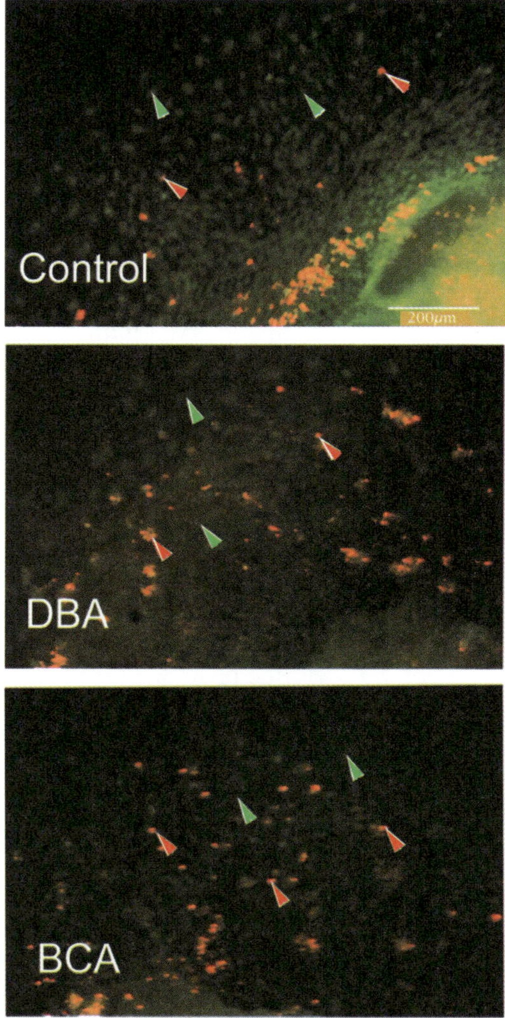

Fig. 5. Live/Dead Staining (Molecular Probes) of primary cultures of NC cells after a 24-h exposure to control medium, 300 μM dibromoacetic acid (DBA) or 300 μM bromochloroacetic acid (BCA). Green fluorescence shows living cells with intact membranes and red fluorescence indicates dead cells. Few dead cells are observed in control cultures, but cell death is observed throughout the cells exposed to DBA or BCA. Scale bar = 200 μm.

demonstrated degeneration of cerebellar granule cells, posterior funiculus of the spinal cord, sensory root nerve, and peripheral nerve. In these studies, the cell death in cerebellar granule cells was shown to be apoptotic and functionally the rats displayed ataxic behavior.

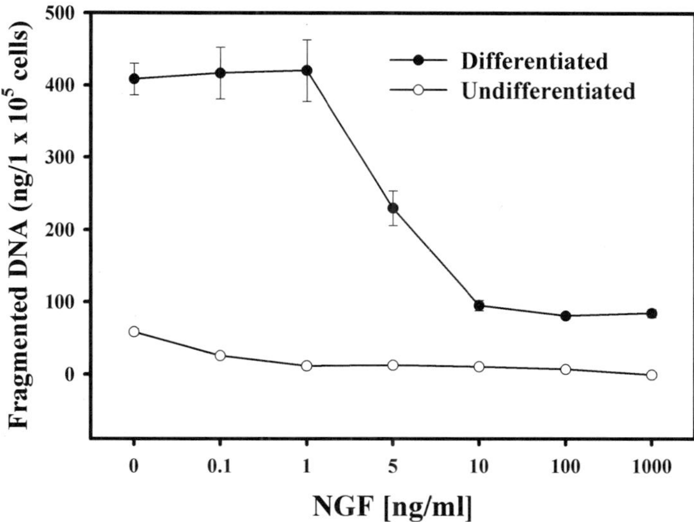

Fig. 6. Dose–response curve showing the concentration-dependent effect of NGF on DNA fragmentation in both differentiated and undifferentiated PC12 cells. Cell death ELISA recognizes cytoplasmic oligonucleaosomal DNA. Number (n=6) per dose and means are expressed with S.E. bars.

8.3. Ethanol Studies

8.3.1. In Vitro Studies of Ethanol-Induced Death Among Cultured Cortical Neurons

In vitro studies provide insight into the mechanism underlying the effects of ethanol on cell survival. The effect of ethanol on neuronal survival has been determined by use of primary cultured neurons from cerebral cortex *(54)*. Over a 3-d period, 25% of the cells are lost, which we equate to naturally occurring neuronal death. Following the addition of ethanol, an additional 25% of the cells are lost. This decrease is associated with a significant increase in TUNEL staining among the cultured cortical neurons *(55)*. Unfortunately, TUNEL, as mentioned earlier, is not a definitive method and it often leads to false-positive results by labeling some necrotic cells.

The results of the TUNEL study were verified by examining, the effects of ethanol on caspase-3 expression. The expression of caspase-3 parallels the pattern of TUNEL positivity; hence, three pieces of evidence (cell counting, TUNEL and caspase-3) show that ethanol kills primary cultured neurons.

8.3.2. Nerve Growth Factor Is a Key Survival Factor

The effects of three neurotrophins on the survival of cultured cortical neurons have been examined *(54,56)*. These neurotrophins include NGF,

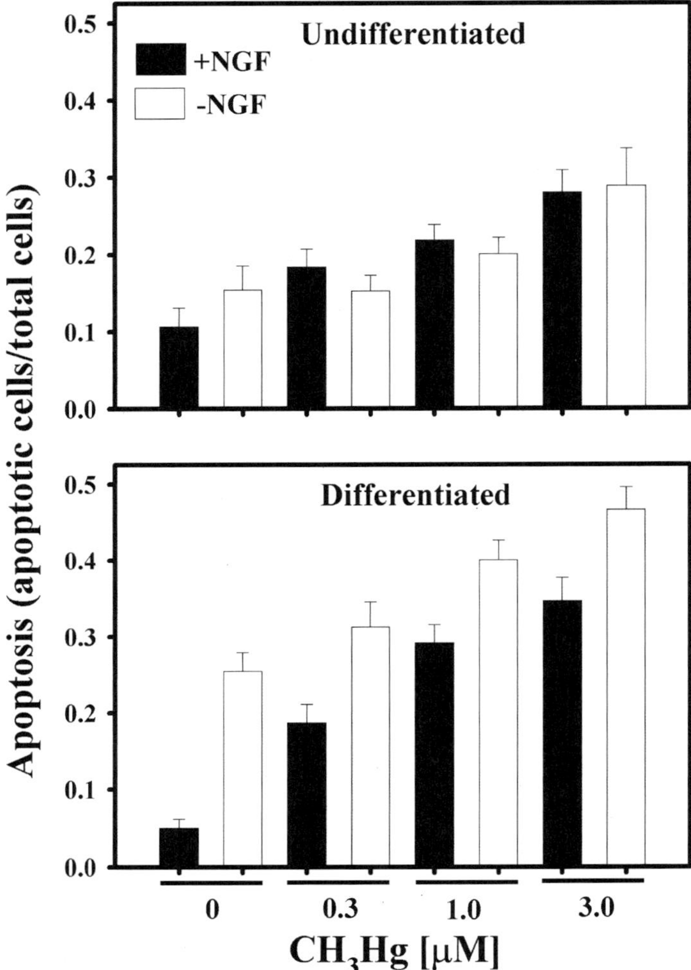

Fig. 7. Effects of methylmercury exposure in undifferentiated and differentiated PC12 cells. Undifferentiated cells have had no history of exposure to NGF. Differentiated cells have been grown in the presence of NGF for 7 d. The acute exposure to NGF under both conditions reveals short-term effects of NGF exposure on apoptosis. PC12 cells were TUNEL stained and then quantified by counting total cells and apoptotic cells. $n=6$ per dose and means are expressed with S.E. bars.

brain-derived neurotrophic factor (BDNF), and neurotrophin-3 (NT-3). Of these neurotrophins, only NGF is able to maintain the survival of the primary cortical neurons. Ethanol completely eliminated this activity; cultures treated with both NGF and ethanol have the same numbers of neurons as those treated with ethanol alone (*see* Fig. 8).

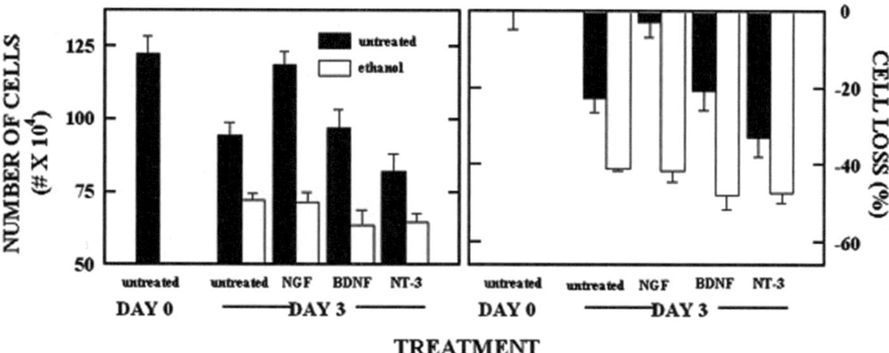

Fig. 8. Effect of neurotrophins and ethanol on the number of cortical neurons in vitro. Primary cultures of cortical neurons were exposed to one of three neurotrophins for 3 d. These neurotrophins included nerve growth factor (NGF), brain-derived neurotrophic factor (BDNF), and neurotrophin-3 (NT-3). Only NGF was able to maintain the viability of the cortical neurons. Ethanol caused cell death and it antagonized the ability of NGF to maintain neuronal survival. Bars represent the means of three pairs of independent trials and the error bars signify standard errors of the means.

The effects of ethanol on four neurotrophin receptors have been examined. These receptors include p75, the low-affinity receptor for the neurotrophins and trkA, trkB, and trkC (the high-affinity neurotrophin receptors that prefer NGF, BDNF, and NT-3/NT-4). One would predict that ethanol would have selective effects on the receptor that would be specific for NGF, which is trkA. Rather, the effects of ethanol are selective, but not for trkA. They are specific for p75. The implication is that p75 is not a promiscuous receptor that can bind any of the neurotrophins with equal affinity as some have proposed *(57)*, but, rather, p75 is selective for NGF, at least at specific developmental stages.

8.3.3. An NGF-Specific Gene

Ethanol can eliminate the expression of a gene upregulated by NGF called *neg (56)*. This gene has a 95% nucleotide identity with CC28, which is expressed by murine lymphocytes *(58)*, and a 90% nucleotide identity with KIAA0257, which is expressed by human myeloma cells *(59)*. The selective expression of *neg* has been verified by means of a ribonuclease protection assay and *in situ* hybridization. The role of the protein translated by *neg* remains unknown, however, a Prosite© analysis of KIAA0257 shows that it has transmembrane and ATP synthetase motifs. It is unclear whether the ATP synthetase segment is sufficient to imbue the protein with enzymatic activity. Nevertheless, it is appealing to speculate that *neg* codes for a mitochondrial transmembrane protein. This is intriguing in that *neg* could be an intermediary that transduces the effects of NGF to an antiapoptotic mitochondrial transmembrane protein Bcl-2.

8.3.4. In Vivo Studies of Cell Numbers

The concept that early exposure to ethanol causes neuronal death was raised well over a dozen years ago *(60,61)*. With the application of stereological methods to determine the numbers of neurons in brain regions, researchers have been able to perform longitudinal studies documenting the change in the numbers of neurons over time. Using such an approach, the occurrence of ethanol-induced neuronal death has been verified.

One structure that has been particularly instructive is the principal sensory nucleus (PSN) of the trigeminal nerve. The PSN is a small pontine nucleus in which neuronal generation occurs prenatally *(62,63)* and naturally occurring neuronal death ensues postnatally (e.g., refs. *64–66*). As with many other brain structures, the period of naturally occurring neuronal death in the PSN is simultaneous with the period of initial synaptogenesis *(65,67)*. Prenatal exposure to ethanol compromises both neuronal generation and the decline in neuronal number *(63,68)*. The negative effect of prenatal exposure on neuronal generation is twice that on neuronal loss. Furthermore, these changes in neuronal loss are mirrored by increases in the incidence of pyknotic cells.

8.3.5. ALZ-50 Immunoreactivity

A fall in neuronal number is deductive evidence for neuronal death. Ideally, these data should be matched with positive markers for neuronal death. The identification of such markers has been emerging over the last few years. One of the early identified markers was an antigen recognized by ALZ-50. ALZ-50 is a monoclonal antibody directed against an Alzheimer's-specific protein that is 68 kDa *(69)*. This ALZ-50 antigenicity is also expressed in the developing cortex *(70–72)*. In the immature cortex, an ALZ-50-positive 56-kDa protein is expressed in zones where neuronal death is particularly high, most notably the subplate. The association of ALZ-50 immunoreactivity in neuronal death is supported by a lesion study *(73)* in which transection of the infraorbital nerve, a major component of the trigeminal nerve, causes a transient and selective expression of ALZ-50 immunoreactivity in the ventral portion of the PSN. The ventral portion receives direct input from primary afferents in the infraorbital nerve. Following this transient expression of ALZ-50 immunoreactivity, there is a significant and dramatic decrease in the numbers of PSN neurons.

Prenatal exposure to ethanol affects ALZ-50 expression in the developing cerebral cortex *(74)*. In control animals, ALZ-50 immunoreactivity rises dramatically during the period from PD6 to PD15, so that in the adult, ALZ-50 immunoreactivity is virtually gone. In contrast, gestational exposure to ethanol induces increased ALZ-50 expression between PD3 and PD9 (*see* Fig. 9A). This implies that neuronal death is promoted by ethanol and that ethanol-induced neurotoxicity is, at least in part, concurrent with naturally occurring neuronal death.

Another protein that may be related to neuronal death is the oncoprotein p53 *(75–78)*, which is expressed in the cortices of control rats throughout fetal, early postnatal development, and into adulthood. Prenatal ethanol exposure affects p53 expression, particularly at times when ALZ-50 immunoreactivity is expressed in the cerebral cortex (*see* Fig. 9B). Based on an immunoprecipitation study, it appears that ALZ-50 immunologically recognizes a phosphorylated form of p53 in the developing cortex.

8.3.6. Bcl Proteins

Naturally occurring neuronal death largely exhibits the morphological features of pyknosis and apoptosis and, as mentioned earlier, there are a number of genes that are associated with this kind of death, notably the *bcl* family of genes. Prenatal exposure to ethanol affects cortical *bcl-2* expression over the fetal and early postnatal period *(79)*. In contrast, *bax* expression is not greatly affected. A key factor determining neuronal survival is the relative expression of bcl-2 and bax. The effect of ethanol on this ratio shows that the effects of ethanol are time dependent and restricted to the fetal and second postnatal weeks. Thus, these data concur with the time dependent, ethanol-induced changes in ALZ-50 and p53 immunoreactivity. An interesting counterpoint to the cortical events is the thalamus. Although both *bcl-2* and *bax* expression in the thalamus changes over time, prenatal exposure to ethanol has no effect on either protein.

8.3.7. Caspase-3

Caspase-3 is an enzyme that is activated during apoptotic death *(34,80–84)*. It is a key enzyme involved in cleaving DNA into discrete packets that are eliminated from the genome as the neuron degenerates. In the developing cortex, activated caspase-3 is transiently expressed postnataly during the period of naturally occurring neuronal death *(34)*. Prenatal ethanol exposure alters caspase-3 expression in accord with changes in the Bcl proteins *(79)*. Ethanol has no effect on caspase-3 expression in the thalamus. Thus, ethanol-induced neuronal death relies on Bcl proteins and caspase and appears to be apoptotic.

                                                                            White et al.

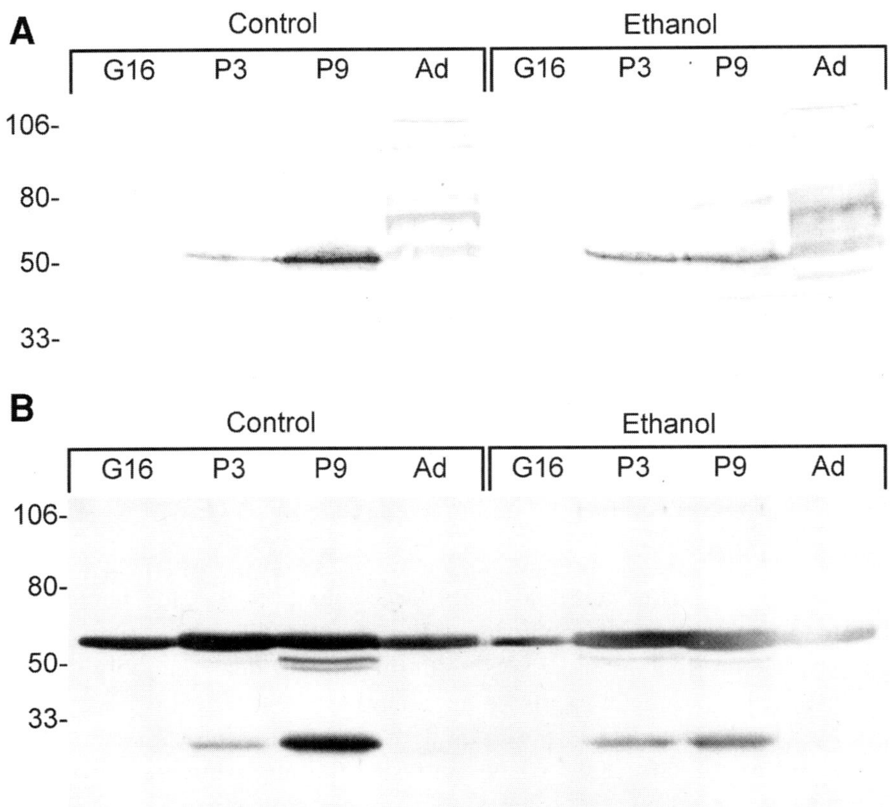

Fig. 9. Western blots of ethanol effects on protein expression in developing rat brain. (**A**) ALZ-50 expression in the developing cortex was affected by gestational exposure to ethanol. The ALZ-50-positive antigen was a 56-kDa protein that was expressed in the cortices of developing control and ethanol-treated rats. In control rats, ALZ-50 immunoreactivity was evident during the first two postnatal weeks and peaked about postnatal day 9. This pattern of expression was concurrent with the period of naturally occurring neuronal death. The timing of ALZ-50 expression was similar in ethanol-treated rats, except that peak expression occurred earlier and the amount of expression seemed to be less than that in the controls. (**B**) Prenatal exposure to ethanol affected the expression of the oncoprotein p53. These immunoblots show the expression of p53 in the cerebral cortex of control rats and rats exposed to ethanol during the latter half of gestation. p53 was evident prenatally and postnatally. Ethanol depressed the 58-kDa p53-positive peptide. A second peptide recognized by the anti-p53 antibody had a molecular weight of 56 kDa and a temporal expression profile consistent with the notion that is was the antigen recognized by ALZ-50. G, gestational day; P, postnatal day; Ad, adult. (From ref. *74*, with permission.)

8.3.8. Concordance of the Biochemical and Anatomical Data

The biochemical data support stereological anatomical studies on neuronal number in somatosensory cortex and thalamus. Following prenatal exposure to ethanol, somatosensory cortex has 33% fewer neurons *(85)*. On the other hand, the numbers of neurons in the somatosensory thalamus are unaffected by prenatal exposure to ethanol *(86)*.

Ethanol affects the survival of neurons in vivo and in vitro. The in vivo studies show that ethanol toxicity is time and place dependent. This finding is true whether the ethanol exposure occurs during the period of neuronal generation (i.e., before the period of naturally occurring neuronal death and synaptogenesis) or during the period of naturally occurring neuronal death (cf. refs. *66* and *68*). In either case, some areas of the brain are particularly affected by ethanol (e.g., somatosensory cortex), whereas others seem to be protected from ethanol-induced neuronal loss (e.g., somatosensory thalamus). The ethanol-induced effects on neuronal survival have been modeled in vitro. Using such in vitro systems has permitted us to show that ethanol-induced death is mediated by neurotrophins; specifically for cortical neurons, the critical neurotrophin is NGF. In this regard, the toxic effects of ethanol are regulated by the low-affinity neurotrophin receptor, p75, and specifically affects genes such as *neg*.

8.4. Studies of Organophosphorus Compounds

8.4.1. Effects of Chlorpyrifos and Its Metabolites on Developmental Exposure to PC12 Cells

As mentioned earlier, neural development in vitro can be examined using PC12 cells. These cells were exposed to various concentrations of chlorpyrifos [CPF: *O,O'*-diethyl *O*-(3,5,6-trichloro-2-pyridyl) phosphorothionate], two of its metabolites, chlorpyrifos-oxon and trichloropyridinol (TCP: 3,5,6-trichloro-2-pyridinol), and a fourth compound, Burroughs Wellcome (BW) 284c51, a specific acetylcholinesterase inhibitor, to determine if this developmental process could be impacted *(87)*. NGF-differentiated PC12 cells exposed to 0.1–100 nM CPF-oxon showed an increase in apoptosis in the absence of NGF, and a dose-related increase in apoptosis was observed in the presence of NGF. Differentiated PC12 cells exposed the non-cholinesterase-inhibiting metabolite, TCP, at concentrations of 0.1–100 μM showed a dose-related increase in apoptosis in the absence of NGF and at the highest dose in the presence of NGF. Similar paradigms were also used for CPF and the BW compound exposures. No effect was seen on levels of apoptosis with increasing doses of CPF. With BW compound exposure, again at 0.1–100 μM, a significant increase in apoptosis was seen in the absence of NGF. A comparison of the amount of cell death induced by these compounds in both differentiated and undifferentiated cells revealed that under all conditions, the differentiated cells had greater levels of fragmented DNA. Furthermore, the oxon induced apoptosis, with higher levels seen in differentiated cells, and NGF protected against apoptotic cell death.

Results from cell death ELISA assays were corroborated with TUNEL staining (*see* Fig. 10). Differentiated PC12 cells exposed to vehicle control, chlorpyrifos at 1 μM or 100 μM, and trichoropyridinol at 1 μM or 100 μM demonstrated increased apoptosis of primed cells with NGF withdrawal. TCP appeared to induce apoptosis at 1 μM, whereas CPF did not until concentrations of 100 μM were used.

Thus, in vitro exposure to CPF metabolites CPF-oxon or TCP in the absence of NGF resulted in a dose-dependent induction of apoptotic death with effects observed as low as 0.1 nM for CPF-oxon or I.0 μM for TCP. Exposure to NGF (10 ng/mL) protected against cell death at doses of TCP and CPF-oxon below 100 μM and 1 nM, respectively. These data suggest that differentiated PC12 cells are more vulnerable to apoptosis following NGF withdrawal than undifferentiated cells and that NGF under certain conditions can protect against this pesticide-induced apoptosis.

8.4.2. In Vivo Developmental Exposure to Chlorpyrifos Affects Apoptosis

In parallel to the above in vitro work, apoptosis in the developing brain in response to CPF exposure was determined. The exposure paradigm for this work was gavage administration of pregnant dams beginning on GD14 and continuing through GD18. Pups were then removed at various times-points following the last dose. Because earlier work from the laboratory showed that at 5 h after the last dose of CPF, cholinesterase inhibition was greatest and TCP levels were highest in fetal brain *(88)*, the 5-h time-point was used for apoptosis studies. Four doses of CPF were used: 3, 5, 7, or 10 mg/kg/d. Cell death by ELISA was used to determine that at both 7- and 10-mg/kg/d doses, levels of fragmented DNA were significantly increased in GD18 brains (*see* Fig. 11). TUNEL staining on this tissue corroborated the ELISA results, wherein control animals exposed to vehicle showed basal levels of TUNEL-stained cells at GD18. Tissue from a fetus exposed to the 7-mg/kg/d dose demonstrated apoptotic cells at levels greater than controls (*see* Fig. 12).

8.5. Contributions of Other Organophosphorus Compounds to Cell Death

Organophosphorus (OP) compounds are neurotoxic by two major pathways: inhibition of acetylcholinesterase (AChE) and induction of delayed neuropathy. AChE inhibition is the mechanism by which OP compounds exert

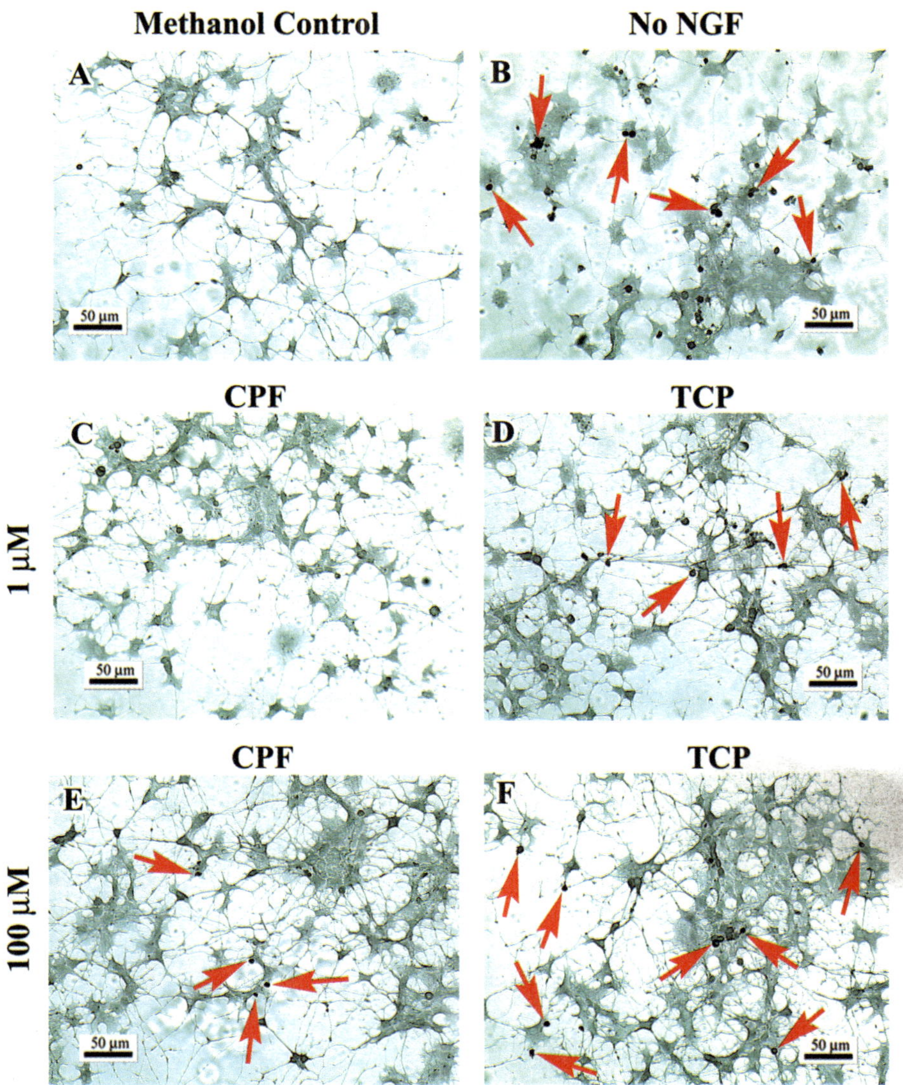

Fig. 10. Effects of chlorpyrifos or TCP exposures (1 μ*M* or 100 μ*M*) in PC12 cells in the absence and presence of NGF. Red arrows indicate apoptotic cells. Increased apoptosis is evident in TCP-exposed cells at 1 μ*M*, but is not evident in CPF-exposed cells until 100 μ*M*. Also note increased apoptosis in the absence of NGF. Scale bars = 50 μm; *n*=4 per dose.

their insecticidal effects and is far more common than OP-induced delayed neuropathy (OPIDN). OPIDN requires initial inhibition of another esterase, neuropathy target esterase (NTE, or neurotoxic esterase). NTE inhibition must

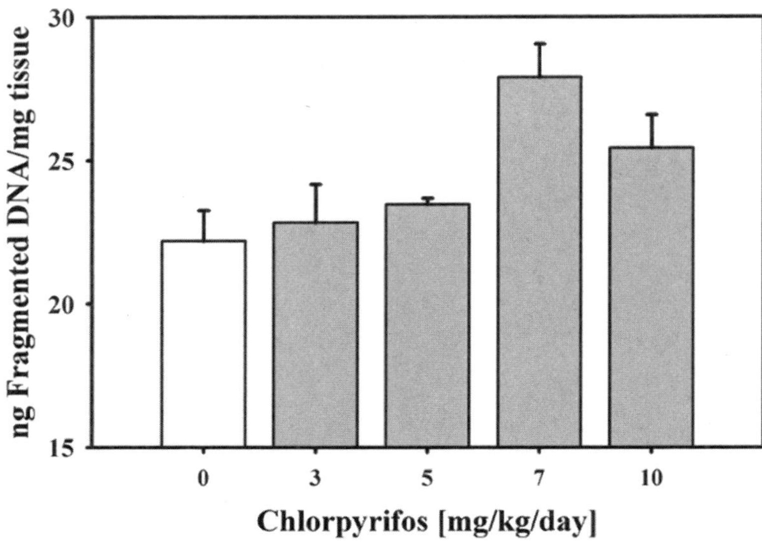

Fig. 11. Effects of gestational chlorpyrifos exposures. Cell death ELISA recognizes cytoplasmic oligonucleaosomal DNA. ELISA data from GD18 rat brains exposed to 0, 3, 5, 7, or 10 mg/kg/d CPF from GD14 until GD18. n=3 per dose.

be significant and essentially irreversible before clinical manifestations of OPIDN appear in man and susceptible animal species (e.g., chicken). OPIDN is associated with distal but not terminal degeneration of long axons in peripheral nerves and the spinal cord. OPIDN usually takes 5–21 d following a single OP exposure. There is no relationship between AChE and NTE inhibition; compounds are available that inhibit either one or both *(89)*.

Cells die if exposed to high concentrations of OP compounds. Why and how they die have been investigated but not precisely defined. Work has been initiated to investigate the contribution of apoptosis to this OP-induced cell death. This has included concentration and time–response studies with OP compounds known only to cause acute neurotoxicity via AChE inhibition (parathion and its active AChE-inhibiting metabolite paraoxon), OP compounds known for their capability to cause OPIDN because NTE inhibition is the predominant early effect (tri-*ortho*-tolyl phosphate [TOTP] and its esterase-inhibiting congener phenyl saligenin phosphate [PSP]), an OP compound that equally inhibits AChE and NTE (di-isopropyl phosphorofluoridate [DFP]), and an OP compound that causes a delayed neurotoxicity that differs clinically and morphologically from classical OPIDN (triphenyl phosphite [TPPi]) *(89)*.

Investigations on the contribution of apoptosis to OP-induced cell death were initially studied in the SH-SY5H human neuroblastoma cell line. This

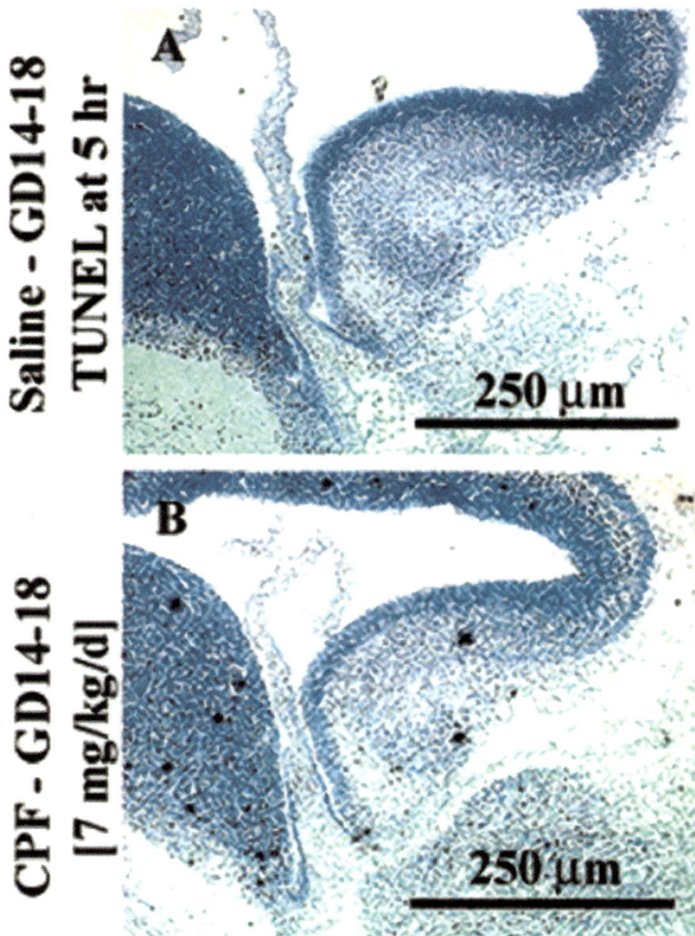

Fig. 12. Effects of gestational chlorpyrifos exposures. Apoptosis demonstrated by TUNEL staining of sagittal sections of GD18 brain exposed to either saline (**A**) or 7 mg/kg/d CPF (**B**). Brains were cut at 12 µm and stained according to kit protocols (Intergen). Tissue is counterstained with methyl green. Scale bars = 250 µm; n=4 per dose.

culture system was chosen because previous studies demonstrated its usefulness for differentiating biochemical effects of OP compounds causing acute neurotoxicity and OPIDN based on relative inhibitions of AChE and NTE, respectively, whether they were active esterase inhibitors or protoxicants *(90,91)*. Changes in nuclear morphology were used to assess the contribution of apoptosis to cell death for the six OP compounds listed.

Nuclear effects were determined by fluorescent microscopy. Results indicated that apoptotic nuclear budding occurred with parathion, paraoxon, and TPPi, but it was a relatively late event, requiring at least 16 h of exposure to 0.1 m*M* concentrations of test compounds (*see* Fig. 13). PSP and TOTP at higher concentrations (1 m*M*) induced nuclear condensation and shrinkage with little nuclear budding. Effects on the nucleus were suggestive of DNA fragmentation associated with apoptosis and were indicated by the presence of discrete bands of DNA on agarose gels of cells exposed to paraoxon, parathion, TPPi, and TOTP. Increases in subG1 DNA fragmentation detected by flow cytometry were another indication of changes in DNA integrity associated with apoptosis, with concentrations for effect similar to those needed for nuclear changes *(44)*.

The contribution of apoptosis to these alterations in nuclear morphology and DNA integrity was verified by examining OP-induced caspase activation, as this is required for apoptotic cascades. For these studies, flow cytometry was used to assess activated caspase-3 by labeling cells with antiactive caspase-3 antibodies coupled to the fluorochrome phycoerythrin. Significant caspase-3 activation was found to occur prior to DNA fragmentation and nuclear budding following exposure of neuroblastoma cells to some OP compounds (paraoxon, TOTP), but not to others (parathion, PSP, TPPi). DFP did not induce caspase-3 activation. OP-compound-induced activation of caspase-3 could be inhibited by treatment with protease inhibitors, including PMSF, a general protease inhibitor, and by more specific inhibitors of caspase-3 and caspase-8 *(44)*.

The results of the above-described in vitro studies suggest that apoptosis is the predominant form of death in neuronal cells in culture and that this occurs independent of specific esterase inhibition as protoxicants (e.g., TOTP, parathion) and both NTE and AChE inhibitors could initiate its occurrence. Additional studies suggest that dysfunctional mitochondria might be involved in determining whether cell death proceeds via apoptotic or necrotic pathways. These studies demonstrated changes in mitochondrial transmembrane potential when the neuroblastoma cell line was exposed to OP compounds *(45)*. In addition, a fluorescent dye impenetrable to undamaged mitochondria was found to enter this organelle in OP-exposed cultures of dissociated avian dorsal root ganglia neurons. In the latter, the colocalization of dyes in the mitochondria was greater in cells exposed to neuropathy-inducing OP compounds (mipafox, PSP) than it was in cells exposed to an OP only capable of inhibiting AChE (paraoxon) (*see* Fig. 14) *(46)*. Disruption of mitochondria in both culture systems was verified by electron microscopy.

Demonstration of apoptosis in OP-exposed animals has proven to be more difficult than demonstration of this mode of cell death in vitro. Attempts

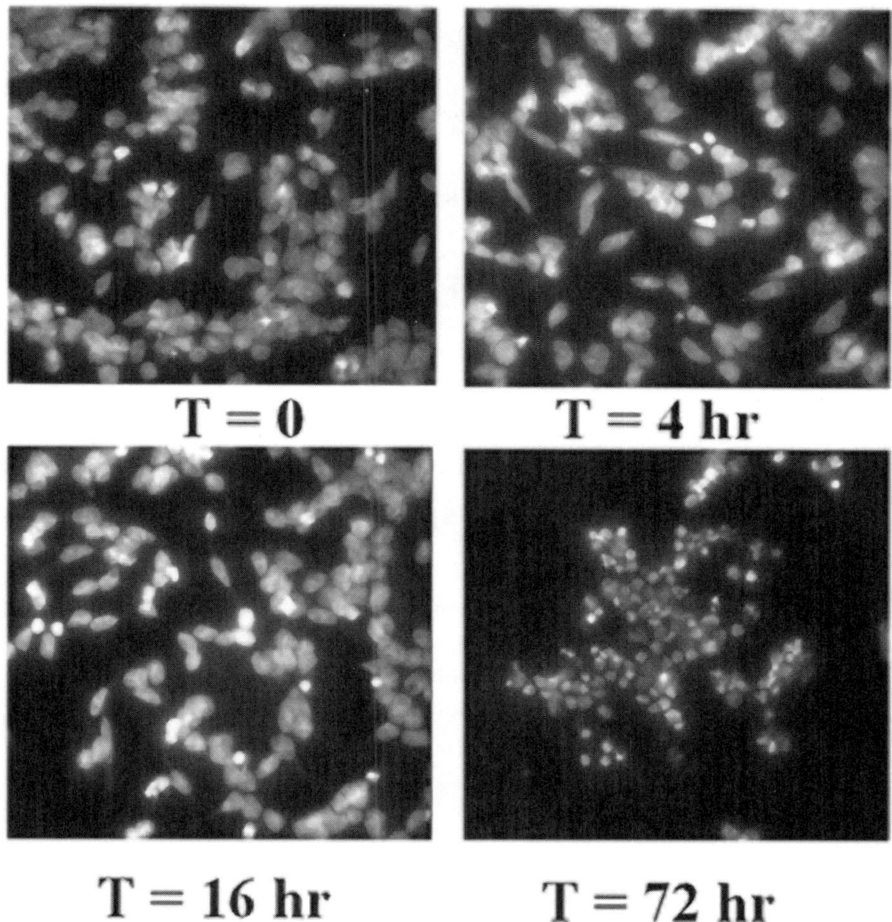

Fig. 13. Nuclear fluorescence to demonstrate apoptosis in SH-SY5Y cells. Cells were exposed to triphenyl phosphite (TPPi) for up to 72 h before acetone/ethanol fixation and staining with 10 µg/mL Hoechst 33342 solution. Increased appearance of apoptotic nuclear buds and fragments occurred as early as 4 h after exposure. Shrinkage and a loss of nuclear structure can be noted at 72 h. (Magnification = 400×.)

have been made on hens exposed to neuropathy-inducing OP compounds and rats exposed to AChE and NTE inhibitors (Carlson, Jortner, and Ehrich, unpublished). Appearance of unequivocal apoptosis has been lacking. This is to be expected, as it is not always apparent that apoptosis occurred as cells were dying if progress toward cell death is not followed over the entire time it occurs. Detection of apoptosis in vivo involves the examination of a population of cells undergoing apoptosis asynchronously. Furthermore, the body

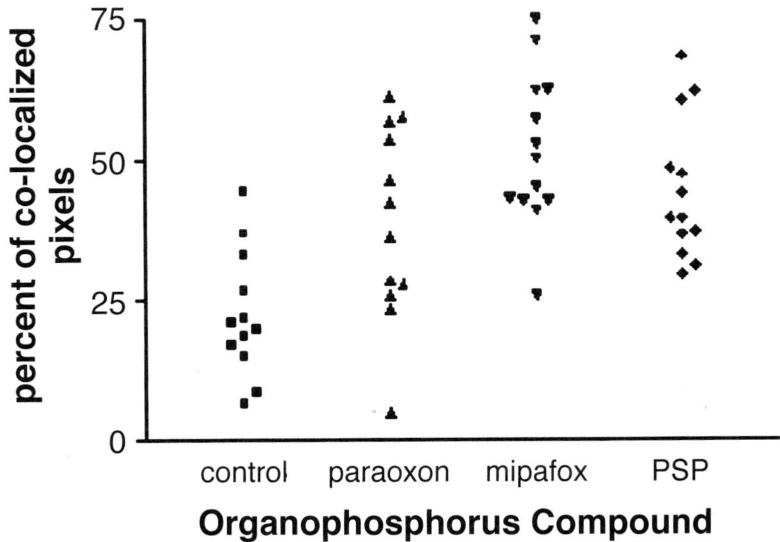

Fig. 14. Colocalization of fluorescent dyes in mitochondria of dorsal root ganglia cells isolated from 9-d-old chick embryos. The cells were exposed to 10^{-6} M concentrations of the organophosphorus compounds paraoxon, mipafox, and PSP. All are significantly different from control ($p<0.05$ for paraoxon, $p<0.001$ for mipafox, $p<0.01$ for PSP; analysis of variance followed by Tukey's multiple comparison test; $n=5$).

has mechanisms for quickly removing dying cells, making timing for detection of cells undergoing apoptosis a significant challenge. However, it is likely that the apoptosis noted in vitro is relevant to the in vivo situation. Further work is needed to improve the correlation.

9. CONCLUSIONS AND FUTURE DIRECTIONS

This review illustrates that known developmental neurotoxicants (EtOH and mercury) and compounds that are clear neurotoxicants in adults (haloacetic acids and organophosphorus agents) affect apoptosis through multiple mechanisms (*see* Fig. 15). These mechanisms include suggested alterations in neurotrophic signaling, protein phosphorylation, mitochondrial dysfunction and alterations in the balance of proapoptotic factors.

This chapter attempts to summarize the myriad methods used to detect apoptosis and describe their strengths and weaknesses with exemplar developmental neurotoxicants. It is important to note that there are methodological challenges in designing in vitro experiments that retain tissue and organismal relevance. It is not surprising that it is often difficult to detect

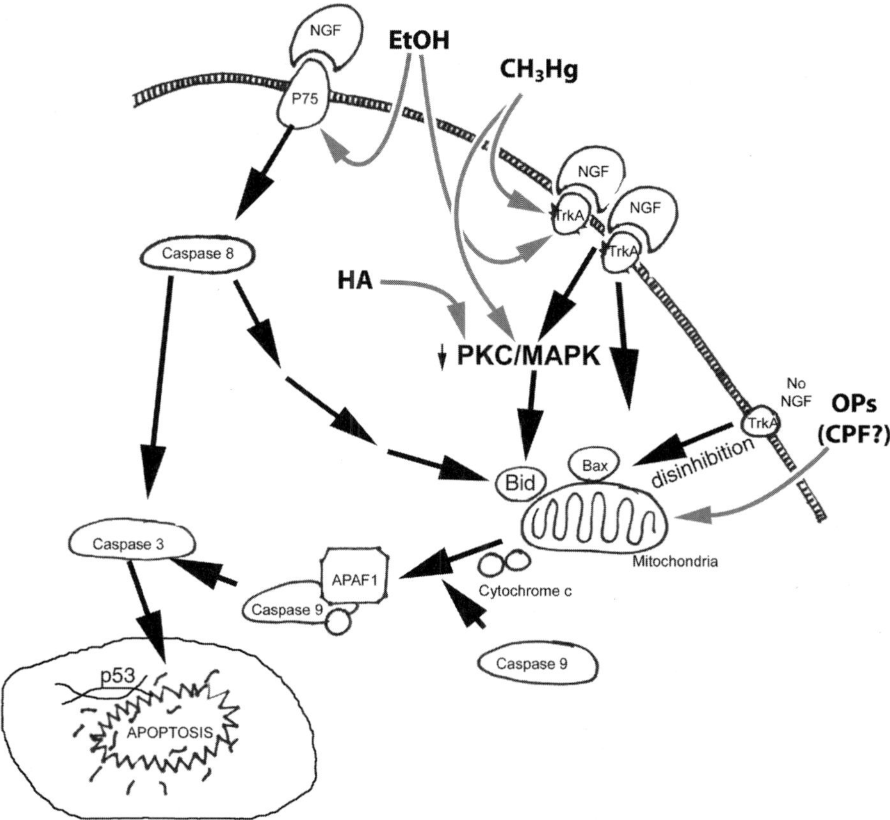

Fig. 15. Presumptive apoptotic pathways of various neurotoxicants including ethanol, organophosphates, haloacetic acids, and methylmercury. Mercury and ethanol appear to act at least partially through receptor-mediated pathways, whereas other compounds appear to act downstream, affecting cell signaling and mitochondrial function.

apoptosis in vivo in tissue, which predominantly occurs in an asynchronous fashion, versus in culture systems, in which, by design, cell death occurs in a more synchronous fashion. The methodological simplicity of in vitro systems can be a strength when dealing with issues of signal detection, but it can also be a weakness when attempting to extrapolate to a more heterogenous cell population of a specific region of the nervous system.

This review chapter illustrates both the strengths and weakness of reductionist test systems in which apoptosis can be studied. It addresses this issue from a toxicological perspective in which dose response to exogenous agents is fundamental. Regarding developmental neurotoxicology, a critical consideration that permeates the study of cell death is the time-course of effects. Whereas in vitro systems are ideal for detection of markers of apoptosis, there needs to be clear linkage of effects on apoptosis and cell number and eventual cell connectivity in the nervous system in order to more fully understand what the consequences of changes in these markers mean. It is entirely conceivable that a transient increase or decrease in apoptosis during programed cell death can lead to adverse consequences. The proof of this principle, however, remains a significant research need in order to improve extrapolation from effects observed in vitro to predicted effects in vivo in the developing nervous system. Although this task sounds gargantuan, increased evidence from in vitro systems has shed significant light on the cell biology and signaling pathways that regulate this process of cell death. Recent efforts to create mathematical models of caspase function in apoptosis could provide clues to solving some of these in vitro to in vivo extrapolation issues in a quantitative fashion *(92)*. In addition, employing such modeling efforts and validation of their predictions could help in future hypothesis testing with environmental agents that are suspected of mediating their toxicity through this process. The clinical implication of dysregulation of apoptosis in neurological, immunological diseases, and many cancers could be the study of gene and environmental interactions that are significant for not only detection but possible future treatments.

ACKNOWLEDGMENTS

For work done in the Laboratory for Neurotoxicity Studies, Virginia-Maryland Regional College of Veterinary Medicine, the contributions of Dr. Kent Carlson, Dr. Christiane Massicotte, and Dr. Bernard S. Jortner are acknowledged. Extramural support was provided by US EPA grant RA825356 and a Novartis predoctoral fellowship through the Society of Toxicology. Michael Miller thanks the many collaborators that he has had over the past dozen years, including Julie Jacobs, Jia Luo, Sandra Mooney, Gail Seabold, and the countless many in the neuroscience and alcohol research communities who continue to be his colleagues/teachers. He gratefully acknowledges the N.I.A.A.A. and the Department of Veterans Affairs for their generous support of this work. Sid Hunter acknowledges the work of Dr. Keith Ward and Ellen Rogers in the completion of his work. For work done in the Neurotoxicology Division of the US Environmental Protection Agency, the contributions of Leon Lassiter, Kaberi Das, and Damani Parran are gratefully acknowledged.

The information in this document has been funded in part by the US Environmental Protection Agency. It has been reviewed by the National Health and Environmental Effects Research Laboratory and approved for publication. Approval does not signify that the contents reflect the views of the agency nor does mention of trade names or commercial products constitute endorsement or recommendation for use.

REFERENCES

1. Kerr, J. F., Wyllie, A. H., and Currie, A. R. (1972) Apoptosis: a basic biological phenomenon with wide-ranging implications in tissue kinetics. *Br. J. Cancer* **26,** 239–257.
2. Meier, P., Finch, A., and Evan, G. (2000) Apoptosis in development. *Nature* **407,** 796–801.
3. Offen, D., Elkon, H., and Melamed, E. (2000) Apoptosis as a general cell death pathway in neurodegenerative diseases. *J. Neural Transm.* **58, Suppl.** 153–166.
4. Savill, J. and Fadok, V. (2000) Corpse clearance defines the meaning of cell death. *Nature* **407,** 784–788.
5. Bortner, C. D., Hughes, F. M., and Cidlowski, J. A. Shi (1997) Cell volume regulation, ions, and apoptosis, in *Programmed Cell Death* (Shi, Y.-B., Shi, Y., Xu, Y. and Scott, D., eds.), Plenum, New York, pp. 63–70.
6. Barrow, J. R., Stadler, H. S., and Capecchi, M. R. (2000) Roles of Hoxa1 and Hoxa2 in patterning the early hindbrain of the mouse. *Development* **127,** 933–944.
7. Oppenheim, R. W. and Cowan, W. M. (1982) Neuronal cell death and some related regressive phenomena during neurogenesis. A selective historical review and a progress report, in *Studies in Developmental Neurobiology. Essays in Honor of Victor Hamburger* (Cowan, W.M., ed.), Oxford University Press, New York, pp. 74–133.
8. Blaschke, A. J., Staley, K., and Chun, J. (1996) Widespread programmed cell death in proliferative and postmitotic regions of the fetal cerebral cortex. *Development* **122,** 1165–1174.
9. White, L. D. and Barone, S. J. (2001) Qualitatative and quantitative estimates of apoptosis from birth to senescence in the rat brain. *Cell Death Differ.* **8,** 345–356.
10. Thomaidou, D., Mione, M. C., Cavanagh, J. F., and Parnavelas, J. G. (1997) Apoptosis and its relation to the cell cycle in the developing cerebral cortex. *J. Neurosci.* **17,** 1075–1085.
11. Margolis, R. L., Chuang, D. M., and Post, R. M. (1994) Programmed cell death: implications for neuropsychiatric disorders. *Biol. Psychiatry* **35,** 946–956.
12. Busciglio, J. and Yankner, B. A. (1995) Apoptosis and increased generation of reactive oxygen species in Down's syndrome neurons in vitro. *Nature* **378,** 776–779.
13. Selemon, L. D., Rajkowska, G., and Goldman-Rakic, P. S. (1998) Elevated neuronal density in prefrontal area 46 in brains from schizophrenic patients: application of a three-dimensional, stereologic counting method. *J. Comp. Neurol.* **392,** 402–412.

14. Jarskog, L. F., Gilmore, J. H., Selinger, E. S., and Lieberman, J. A. (2000) Cortical bcl-2 protein expression and apoptotic regulation in schizophrenia. *Biol. Psychiatry* **48,** 641–650.

15. Falkai, P., Bogerts, B., and Rozumek, M. (1988) Limbic pathology in schizophrenia: the entorhinal region—a morphometric study. *Biol. Psychiatry* **24,** 515–521.

16. Beckmann, H. and Lauer, M. (1997) The human striatum in schizophrenia. II. Increased number of striatal neurons in schizophrenics. *Psychiatry Res.* **8,** 99–109.

17. Highley, J. R., Esiri, M. M., McDonald, B., Cortina-Borja, M., Herron, B. M., and Crow, T. J. (1999) The size and fibre composition of the corpus callosum with respect to gender and schizophrenia: a post-mortem study. *Brain* **122(Pt. 1),** 99–110.

18. Fidler, D. J., Bailey, J. N., and Smalley, S. L. (2000) Macrocephaly in autism and other pervasive developmental disorders. *Dev. Med. Child Neurol.* **42,** 737–740.

19. Piven, J., Arndt, S., Bailey, J., and Andreasen, N. (1996) Regional brain enlargement in autism: a magnetic resonance imaging study. *J. Am. Acad. Child Adolesc. Psychiatry* **35,** 530–536.

20. Sears, L. L., Vest, C., Mohamed, S., Bailey, J., Ranson, B. J., and Piven, J. (1999) An MRI study of the basal ganglia in autism. *Prog. Neuropsychopharmacol. Biol. Psychiatry* **23,** 613–624.

21. Hardan, A. Y., Minshew, N. J., and Keshavan, M. S. (2000) Corpus callosum size in autism. *Neurology* **55,** 1033–1036.

22. Hashimoto, T., Tayama, M., Mori, K., Fujino, K., Miyazaki, M., and Kuroda, Y. (1989) Magnetic resonance imaging in autism: preliminary report. *Neuropediatrics* **20,** 142–146.

23. Bailey, A., Luthert, P., Bolton, P., Le Couteur, A., Rutter, M., and Harding, B. (1993) Autism and megalencephaly. *Lancet* **341,** 1225–1226.

24. Hengartner, M. O. (1999) Programmed cell death in the nematode *C. elegans. Recent Prog. Horm. Res.* **54,** 213–222.

25. Lee, C. Y. and Baehrecke, E. H. (2000) Genetic regulation of programmed cell death in *Drosophila. Cell Res.* **10,** 193–204.

26. Nunez, G., Benedict, M. A., Hu, Y., and Inohara, N. (1998) Caspases: the proteases of the apoptotic pathway. *Oncogene* **17,** 3237–3245.

27. Hengartner, M. O. (2000) The biochemistry of apoptosis. *Nature* **407,** 770–776.

28. Garcia, I., Martinou, I., Tsujimoto, Y., and Martinou, J. C. (1992) Prevention of programmed cell death of sympathetic neurons by the bcl-2 proto-oncogene. *Science* **258,** 302–304.

29. Allsopp, T. E., Wyatt, S., Paterson, H. F., and Davies, A. M. (1993) The proto-oncogene bcl-2 can selectively rescue neurotrophic factor-dependent neurons from apoptosis. *Cell* **73,** 295–307.

30. Chao, D. T. and Korsmeyer, S. J. (1998) BCL-2 family: regulators of cell death. *Annu. Rev. Immunol.* **16,** 395–419.

31. Vekrellis, K., McCarthy, M. J., Watson, A., Whitfield, J., Rubin, L. L., and Ham, J. (1997) Bax promotes neuronal cell death and is downregulated during the development of the nervous system. *Development* **124,** 1239–1249.

32. van Lookeren, C. M. and Gill, R. (1998) Tumor-suppressor p53 is expressed in proliferating and newly formed neurons of the embryonic and postnatal rat brain: comparison with expression of the cell cycle regulators p21Waf1/Cip1, p27Kip1, p57Kip2, p16Ink4a, cyclin G1, and the proto-oncogene Bax. *J. Comp. Neurol.* **397,** 181–198.

33. Shimohama, S., Fujimoto, S., Sumida, Y., and Tanino, H. (1998) Differential expression of rat brain bcl-2 family proteins in development and aging. *Biochem. Biophys. Res. Commun.* **252,** 92–96.

34. Mooney, S. M. and Miller, M. W. (2000) Expression of bcl-2, bax, and caspase-3 in the brain of the developing rat. *Dev. Brain Res.* **123,** 103–117.

35. Krammer, P. H. (2000) CD95's deadly mission in the immune system. *Nature* **407,** 789–795.

36. Rabizadeh, S., Oh, J., Zhong, L. T., et al. (1993) Induction of apoptosis by the low-affinity NGF receptor. *Science* **261,** 345–348.

37. Casaccia-Bonnefil, P., Kong, H., and Chao, M. V. (1998) Neurotrophins: the biological paradox of survival factors eliciting apoptosis. *Cell Death Differ.* **5,** 357–364.

38. Li, H., Zhu, H., Xu, C. J., and Yuan, J. (1998) Cleavage of BID by caspase 8 mediates the mitochondrial damage in the Fas pathway of apoptosis. *Cell* **94,** 491–501.

39. Luo, X., Budihardjo, I., Zou, H., Slaughter, C., and Wang, X. (1998) Bid, a Bcl2 interacting protein, mediates cytochrome c release from mitochondria in response to activation of cell surface death receptors. *Cell* **94,** 481–490.

40. Yin, X. M. (2000) Signal transduction mediated by Bid, a pro-death Bcl-2 family proteins, connects the death receptor and mitochondria apoptosis pathways. *Cell Res.* **10,** 161–167.

41. Rich, T., Allen, R. L., and Wyllie, A. H. (2000) Defying death after DNA damage. *Nature* **407,** 777–783.

42. Zucker, R. M., Hunter, S., and Rogers, J. M. (1998) Confocal laser scanning microscopy of apoptosis in organogenesis-stage mouse embryos. *Cytometry* **33,** 348–354.

43. Charriaut-Marlangue, C. and Ben-Ari, Y. (1995) A cautionary note on the use of the TUNEL stain to determine apoptosis. *NeuroReport* **7,** 61–64.

44. Carlson, K., Jortner, B. S., and Ehrich, M. (2000) Organophosphorus compound-induced apoptosis in SH-SY5Y human neuroblastoma cells. *Toxicol. Appl. Pharmacol.* **168,** 102–113.

45. Carlson, K. and Ehrich, M. (1999) Organophosphorus compound-induced modification of SH-SY5Y human neuroblastoma mitochondrial transmembrane potential. *Toxicol. Appl. Pharmacol.* **160,** 33–42.

46. Massicotte, C. (2001) The effects of neuropathy-inducing organophosphate esters on energy metabolism: a biochemical and morphological assessment, Ph.D. dissertation, Virginia Tech, Blacksburg, VA.

47. van Engeland, M., Nieland, L. J., Ramaekers, F. C., Schutte, B., and Reutelingsperger, C. P. (1998) Annexin V-affinity assay: a review on an

apoptosis detection system based on phosphatidylserine exposure. *Cytometry* **31,** 1–9.

48. Hunter, E. S., III, Rogers, E. H., Schmid, J. E., and Richard, A. (1996) Comparative effects of haloacetic acids in whole embryo culture. *Teratology* **54,** 57–64.

49. Ward, K. W., Rogers, E. H., and Hunter, E. S., III (1998) Dysmorphogenic effects of a specific protein kinase C inhibitor during neurulation. *Reprod. Toxicol.* **12,** 525–534.

50. Ward, K. W., Rogers, E. H., and Hunter, E. S., III (2000) Comparative pathogenesis of haloacetic acid and protein kinase inhibitor embryotoxicity in mouse whole embryo culture. *Toxicol. Sci.* **53,** 118–126.

51. Levi, A., Biocca, S., Cattaneo, A., and Calissano, P. (1988) The mode of action of nerve growth factor in PC12 cells. *Mol. Neurobiol.* **2,** 201–226.

52. Parran, D. K., White, L. D., and Barone, S., Jr. (2000) Methylmercury and mercuric chloride affect neuronal apoptosis in PC12 cell in a dose- and NGF-dependent fashion. *Toxicol. Soc.* **545,** 115.

53. Nagashima, K. (1997) A review of experimental methylmercury toxicity in rats: neuropathology and evidence for apoptosis. *Toxicol Pathol.* **25,** 624–631.

54. Seabold, G. K., Luo, J., and Miller, M. W. (1998) Effect of ethanol on neurotrophin-mediated cell survival and receptor expression in cultures of cortical neurons. *Dev. Brain Res.* **108,** 139–145.

55. Miller, M. W. (2003) Describing the balance of cell proliferation and death: a mathematical model. *J. Neurobiol.*, in press.

56. Jacobs, J. S. and Miller, M. W. (2001) Neg, a nerve growth factor-promoted gene expressed by fetal neorcortical neurons that is down-regulated by ethanol. *J. Comp. Neurol.* **460,** 212–222.

57. Chao, M. V. (1994) The p75 neurotrophin receptor. *J. Neurobiol.* **25,** 1373–1385.

58. Tscharke, D. C., Wilkinson, R., and Simmons, A. (2000) Use of mRNA differential display to study the action of lymphocyte subsets in vivo and application to a murine model of herpes simplex virus infection. *Immunol. Lett.* **74,** 127–132.

59. Nagase, T., Seki, N., Ishikawa, K., Ohira, M., et al. (1996) Prediction of the coding sequences of unidentified human genes. VI. The coding sequences of 80 new genes (KIAA0201–KIAA0280) deduced by analysis of cDNA clones from cell line KG-1 and brain. *DNA Res.* **3,** 321–354.

60. West, J. R. (1987) Fetal alcohol-induced brain damage and the problem of determining temporal vulnerability: a review. *Alcohol Drug Res.* **7,** 423–441.

61. Ward, G. R. and West, J. R. (1992) Effects of ethanol during development on neuronal survival and plasticity, in *Development of the Central Nervous System: Effects of Alcohol and Opiates* (Miller, M.W., ed.), Wiley–Liss, New York, pp. 109–138.

62. Nornes, H. O. and Morita, M. (1979) Time of origin of the neurons in the caudal brain stem of rat. An autoradiographic study. *Dev. Neurosci.* **2,** 101–114.

63. Miller, M. W. and Muller, S. J. (1989) Structure and histogenesis of the principal sensory nucleus of the trigeminal nerve: effects of prenatal exposure to ethanol. *J. Comp. Neurol.* **282,** 570–580.

64. Ashwell, K. W. and Waite, P. M. (1991) Cell death in the developing trigeminal nuclear complex of the rat. *Dev. Brain Res.* **63,** 291–295.

65. Miller, M. W. and Al-Ghoul, W. M. (1993) Numbers of neurons in the developing principal sensory nucleus of the trigeminal nerve: enhanced survival of early-generated neurons over late-generated neurons. *J. Comp. Neurol.* **330,** 491–501.

66. Miller, M. W. (1995) Effect of pre- or postnatal exposure to ethanol on the total number of neurons in the principal sensory nucleus of the trigeminal nerve: cell proliferation and neuronal death. *Alcohol Clin. Exp. Res.* **19,** 1359–1363.

67. Al-Ghoul, W. M. and Miller, M. W. (1993) Development of the principal sensory nucleus of the trigeminal nerve of the rat and evidence for a transient synaptic field in the trigeminal sensory tract. *J. Comp. Neurol.* **330,** 476–490.

68. Miller, M. W. (1999) A longitudinal study of the effects of prenatal ethanol exposure on neuronal acquisition and death in the principal sensory nucleus of the trigeminal nerve: interaction with changes induced by transection of the infraorbital nerve. *J. Neurocytol.* **28,** 999–1015.

69. Wolozin, B. L., Pruchnicki, A., Dickson, D. W., and Davies, P. (1986) A neuronal antigen in the brains of Alzheimer patients. *Science* **232,** 648–650.

70. Wolozin, B., Scicutella, A., and Davies, P. (1988) Reexpression of a developmentally regulated antigen in Down syndrome and Alzheimer disease. *Proc. Natl. Acad. Sci. USA* **85,** 6202–6206.

71. Al-Ghoul, W. M. and Miller, M. W. (1989) Transient expression of Alz-50 immunoreactivity in developing rat neocortex: a marker for naturally occurring neuronal death? *Brain Res.* **481,** 361–367.

72. Valverde, F., Lopez-Mascaraque, L., and de Carlos, J. A. (1990) Distribution and morphology of Alz-50-immunoreactive cells in the developing visual cortex of kittens. *J. Neurocytol.* **19,** 662–671.

73. Miller, M. W., Al-Ghoul, W. M., and Murtaugh, M. (1991) Expression of ALZ-50 immunoreactivity in the developing principal sensory nucleus of the trigeminal nerve: effect of transecting the infraorbital nerve. *Brain Res.* **560,** 132–138.

74. Kuhn, P. E. and Miller, M. W. (1998) Expression of p53 and ALZ-50 immunoreactivity in rat cortex: effect of prenatal exposure to ethanol. *Exp. Neurol.* **154,** 418–429.

75. Zhan, Q., Carrier, F., and Fornace, A. J., Jr. (1993) Induction of cellular p53 activity by DNA-damaging agents and growth arrest. *Mol. Cell Biol.* **13,** 4242–4250.

76. Mosner, J., Mummenbrauer, T., Bauer, C., Sczakiel, G., Grosse, F., and Deppert, W. (1995) Negative feedback regulation of wild-type p53 biosynthesis. *EMBO J.* **14,** 4442–4449.

77. Morrison, R. S., Wenzel, H. J., Kinoshita, Y., Robbins, C. A., Donehower, L. A., and Schwartzkroin, P. A. (1996) Loss of the p53 tumor suppressor gene protects neurons from kainate-induced cell death. *J. Neurosci.* **16,** 1337–1345.

78. Miller, M. W. and Kuhn, P. E. (1997) Neonatal transection of the infraorbital nerve increases the expression of proteins related to neuronal death in the principal sensory nucleus of the trigeminal nerve. *Brain Res.* **769,** 233–244.

79. Mooney, S. M. and Miller, M. W. (2001) Effects of prenatal exposure on the expression of bcl-2, bax, and caspase-3 in the developing rat trigeminal/somatosensory system. *Brain Res.* **911,** 71–81.

80. Keane, R. W., Srinivasan, A., Foster, L. M., et al. (1997) Activation of CPP32 during apoptosis of neurons and astrocytes. *J. Neurosci. Res.* **48,** 168–180.

81. Armstrong, R. C., Aja, T. J., Hoang, K. D., et al. (1997) Activation of the CED3/ICE-related protease CPP32 in cerebellar granule neurons undergoing apoptosis but not necrosis. *J. Neurosci.* **17,** 553–562.

82. Harada, J. and Sugimoto, M. (1999) Activation of caspase-3 in beta-amyloid-induced apoptosis of cultured rat cortical neurons. *Brain Res.* **842,** 311–323.

83. Kirsch, D. G., Doseff, A., Chau, B. N., et al. (1999) Caspase-3-dependent cleavage of Bcl-2 promotes release of cytochrome c. *J. Biol. Chem.* **274,** 21,155–21,161.

84. Liu, X. and Zhu, X. Z. (1999) Roles of p53, c-Myc, Bcl-2, Bax and caspases in serum deprivation-induced neuronal apoptosis: a possible neuroprotective mechanism of basic fibroblast growth factor. *NeuroReport* **10,** 3087–3091.

85. Miller, M. W. and Potempa, G. (1990) Numbers of neurons and glia in mature rat somatosensory cortex: effects of prenatal exposure to ethanol. *J. Comp. Neurol.* **293,** 92–102.

86. Mooney, S. M. and Miller, M. W. (1999) Effects of prenatal exposure to ethanol on systems matching: the number of neurons in the ventrobasal thalamic nucleus of the mature rat. *Dev. Brain Res.* **117,** 121–125.

87. Das, K. P., Barone, S., Jr., and White, L. D. (2000) Metabolites of chlorpyrifos induce apoptosis in PC12 cells. *Toxicol. Soc.* **545,** 117.

88. Hunter, D. L., Lassiter, T. L., and Padilla, S. (1999) Gestational exposure to chlorpyrifos: comparative distribution of trichloropyridinol in the fetus and dam. *Toxicol. Appl. Pharmacol.* **158,** 16–23.

89. Ehrich, M. and Jortner, B. S. (2001) Organophosphorus-induced delayed neuropathy, in *Handbook of Pesticide Toxicology* (Krieger, R., ed.), Academic, San Diego, CA, pp. 987–1012.

90. Ehrich, M., Correll, L., and Veronesi, B. (1997) Acetylcholinesterase and neuropathy target esterase inhibitions in neuroblastoma cells to distinguish organophosphorus compounds causing acute and delayed neurotoxicity. *Fundam. Appl. Toxicol.* **38,** 55–63.

91. Barber, D., Correll, L., and Ehrich, M. (1999) Comparative effectiveness of organophosphorus protoxicant activating systems in neuroblastoma cells and brain homogenates. *J. Toxicol. Environ. Health A* **57,** 63–74.

92. Fussenegger, M., Bailey, J. E., and Varner, J. (2000) A mathematical model of caspase function in apoptosis. *Nature Biotechnol.* **18,** 768–774.

6

Impairment of Neurotransmitter Metabolism and Function by Neurotoxicants

Enzyme Pathways in Neurons and Astroglia

Michael Aschner and Ursula Sonnewald

1. INTRODUCTION

In order to perform neurotoxicological studies, model systems have to be established and techniques developed to analyze relevant parameters. The present chapter describes the in vitro effects of the neurotoxicants aminooxyacetic acid (AOAA), 3-nitropropionic acid (3-NPA), and methylmercury (MeHg) on glial cell neurotransmitters, and for 3-NPA, we also describe the effects on cultured neurons. Major emphasis is directed at the effects of these compounds on glutamate metabolism.

2. CELL CULTURES

Cells taken directly from the organism and subsequently grown for at least 24 h in vitro are considered to be primary cultures. Different procedures have been used, often in combination, to enable the establishment of monotypic cultures from mixed-cell suspensions. They are obtained after an initial mechanical and/or enzymatic dissociation of the nervous tissue of neonatal or newborn rat, mouse, or chick. Because of the relative abundance of cells, magnetic resonance spectroscopy (MRS) studies are often performed on cultures consisting of excitatory cerebellar granule cells or inhibitory γ-aminobutyric-acid-(GABA)ergic cerebral cortex neurons prepared as described by Schousboe et al. *(1)* and Hertz et al. *(2)*. The choice of these particular preparations of cultured neurons should be viewed in light of the fact that 90% of the synapses in the brain utilize either glutamate or

From: *Methods in Pharmacology and Toxicology: In Vitro Neurotoxicology: Principles and Challenges*
Edited by: E. Tiffany-Castiglioni © Humana Press Inc., Totowa, NJ

GABA as the neurotransmitter. As counterparts for the neurons, typically astrocytes from the same brain region can be maintained in culture as detailed by Hertz et al. *(3)*.

Appreciation of the essential role of astrocytes in aiding neuronal metabolism and maintaining and modifying the biochemical milieu of the central nervous system (CNS) has grown greatly in the last decades *(4–6)*. Included among these interdependent processes between astrocytes and neurons are guidance of neuronal migration *(7)*, the release of neurotrophic factors *(8)*, as well as glutamate uptake and its metabolism to glutamine *(6,9–11)*. Because neurons are not capable of anaplerosis, it is essential that they obtain precursors from astrocytes for transmitter synthesis *(6)*. Observations of additional astrocyte and neuron interactions include the description of an obligatory role for astrocytes in providing precursor molecules for neuronal glutathione (GSH) synthesis *(12–15)*. More recent studies demonstrate that few synapses form in the absence of glial cells and that the few synapses that do form are functionally immature *(16)*. As suggested by Ullian et al. *(16)*, astrocytes increase the number of mature functional synapses on the CNS neurons by sevenfold and are required for synaptic maintenance in vitro. Thus, astrocytes are invoked to induce and stabilize synapses, raising the possibility that glia could actively participate in synaptic plasticity. Astrocytes also actively participate in synaptic integration by releasing glutamate via a calcium-regulated, exocytosis like process *(17)*. This process follows activation of the receptor CXCR4 by the chemokine stromal cell-derived factor 1 (SDF-1). An extraordinary feature of the ensuing signaling cascade is the rapid extracellular release of tumor necrosis factor (TNF). Bezzi et al. *(17)* also demonstrated that altered glial communication has direct neuropathological consequences, identifying a new pathway for glia–glia and glia–neuron communication that is relevant to both normal brain function and neurodegenerative diseases.

3. MAGNETIC RESONANCE SPECTROSCOPY (MRS)

^{13}C-MRS is a powerful tool for the analysis of brain metabolism and metabolic trafficking between different brain compartments *(18–20)* and it is also useful in studying the effects of neurotoxicants on metabolism in vivo *(21,22)* and in vitro *(23–26)*. The nuclei that are most commonly used in MRS for metabolic studies are ^{1}H, ^{31}P, and ^{13}C. ^{1}H and ^{31}P are naturally abundant isotopes and, therefore, the most common methods of study involves examining differences in the natural abundance spectra under various metabolic states. In contrast, ^{13}C has a natural abundance of 1.1%. This disadvantage normally makes detection difficult and ^{13}C-MRS is thus of limited use for studies on endogenous metabolites, unless they occur in large amounts. However, the low natural abundance can be an advantage in that ^{13}C-enriched precursors can be used for metabolic pathway mapping with little or no background interference from endogenous metabolites.

^{13}C-MRS and [U-^{13}C]glutamate have been used extensively for metabolic studies in astrocytes *(11,24,27–29)* and cerebellar granule neurons *(30)*. It could be shown that exogenous glutamate was metabolized in cultured astrocytes to a great extent. Labeled glutamine, aspartate, and glutathione synthesized from [U-^{13}C]glutamate were detected in cell extracts, whereas in medium, in addition to the added [U-^{13}C]glutamate, labeled glutamine, aspartate, and lactate were also observed. In cerebellar granule neurons (glutamatergic) [U-^{13}C]glutamate is metabolized to aspartate, glutathione, and, to a small extent, lactate *(30)*. In both cell types, glutamate is also synthesized via the tricarboxylic acid (TCA) cycle from labeled glutamate. The schematic presentation of the distribution of label in different metabolites derived from TCA cycle intermediates is shown in Fig. 1. After uptake by astrocytes, [U-^{13}C]glutamate can be either converted to [U-^{13}C]glutamine directly by glutamine synthetase or enter the TCA cycle after conversion to 2-oxoglutarate for energy production and/or the synthesis of other metabolites. [U-^{13}C]oxaloactate is formed after several steps, and [U-^{13}C]aspartate can be synthesized thereafter. [U-^{13}C]lactate can be derived after several steps of gluconeogenesis from [U-^{13}C]oxaloacetate or directly via malic enzyme from [U-^{13}C]malate. In the presence of unlabeled glucose, unlabeled pyruvate can be converted to acetyl-coenzyme A. The condensation of labeled oxaloacetate and unlabeled acetyl-coenzyme A will lead to the synthesis of [1,2-^{13}C]/ [3,4-^{13}C]aspartate, [1,2,3-^{13}C]glutamate, and [1,2,3-^{13}C]glutamine via TCA cycle intermediates (*see* Fig. 1).

4. IMPAIRMENT OF NEUROTRANSMITTER METABOLISM AND FUNCTION BY NEUROTOXICANTS

4.1. Aminooxyacetic

An increasing number of observations suggest that neurodegenerative diseases might be associated with aberrations in energy metabolism and the handling of glutamate *(31)*. Glutamate metabolism is thus a central issue in several of the major brain pathologies. In order to obtain animal models of neurodegenerative diseases, inhibitors of mitochondrial energy metabolism have been used. The transaminase inhibitor aminooxyacetic acid (AOAA)

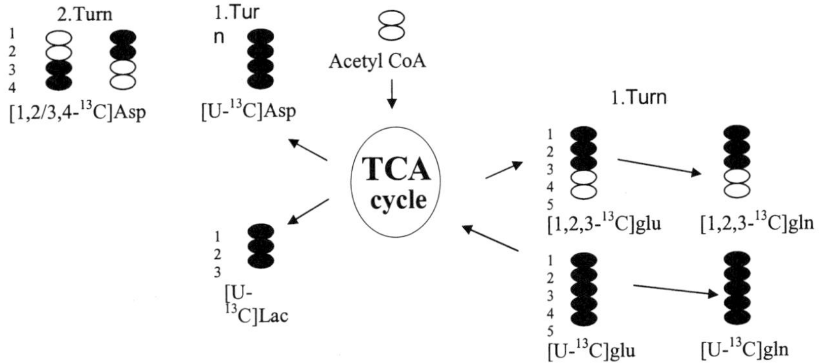

Fig. 1. The distribution of label in different metabolites derived form tricarboxylic acid cycle intermediates.

induces striatal lesions characteristic of neurodegenerative diseases *(32)*. AOAA inhibits the major transaminases, aspartate aminotransferase (AAT) and alanine aminotransferase (ALAAT), both in cytosol and in mitochondria. AAT is an essential component of the malate–aspartate shuttle, which is important also in brain. This shuttle transports reduction equivalents of NADH from the cytosol into mitochondria. The lesions produced by AOAA are attenuated by NMDA antagonists or prior decortication. This and other observations have led to the formulation of an excitotoxic hypothesis for neurodegenerative disorders *(33)*.

4.1.1. Effect of AOAA on [U-^{13}C]Glutamate Metabolism in Astrocytes

Extracellular glutamate is very efficiently taken up into astrocytes *(34)*. In keeping with this, a fourfold increase in the intracellular glutamate content was observed when the cells were incubated in a glutamate-containing medium *(29)*. Conversion of extracellular glutamate to glutamine is a part of the so-called "glutamate–glutamine cycle" *(35,36)*. Previous studies of glutamate metabolism in astrocytes have clearly shown that oxidative metabolism in the TCA cycle takes place in astrocytes *(37–39)*. However, different conclusions with regard to the significance and mechanism of oxidation through the TCA cycle have been reached. In one study, it was demonstrated that the extent of oxidation is coupled to the glutamate concentration *(28)*. A prerequisite for entry of exogenous glutamate into the TCA cycle is the conversion of glutamate to 2-oxoglutarate (2-OG), which can take place via a transamination or a deamination. In order to probe the significance of transamination for the oxidative metabolism of glutamate, the transaminase inhibitor AOAA has been used *(37–39)*. It has been shown that transamination played a minor role for formation of 2-OG from glutamate *(29)*. It appears, however, to be the major pathway for the opposite reaction (i.e., formation of glutamate from 2-OG). Formation of [1,2,3-^{13}C]glutamate and glutamine (a sign of TCA cycle activity) was strongly reduced in the presence of AOAA. An explanation for the great decrease of these isotopomers is that transamination is the major pathway for glutamate formation from 2-OG, which is in accordance with the low affinity of glutamate dehydrogenase (GDH) for ammonia *(40)*. However, the importance of GDH for normal brain function is underlined by the demonstration that the neurodegenerative disorder olivopontocerebellar atrophy is linked to impairment of GDH activity *(41)*.

4.2. 3-Nitropropionic Acid

3-Nitropropionic acid (3-NPA) is an irreversible inhibitor of succinate dehydrogenase, which is part of both the TCA cycle and complex II of the mitochondrial electron transport chain. Accidental ingestion of 3-NPA in humans or systemic administration to experimental animals results in selective striatal lesions *(42,43)*. 3-NPA showed an age-dependent neurotoxicity in young adult rodents, which is similar to the late age of onset for Huntington's disease and other neurodegenerative diseases *(42,43)*. It has been shown that 3-NPA inhibited synaptosomal respiration in a dose-dependent manner *(44)*. In the absence of glutamine, 3-NPA caused a decrease in internal concentrations of aspartate and glutamate, whereas GABA increased. No increase was found in the external levels of these amino acids. With glutamine and 3-NPA in the medium, both glutamate and GABA increased inside the synaptosomes while the external concentration of glutamate rose also *(44)*, lending further evidence for an excitotoxic mechanism in neurodegeneration. In mice injected subcutaneously with 3-NPA, an increased GABA concentration was observed, whereas glutamate was slightly decreased *(21)*. Furthermore, using [1-^{13}C]glucose or [2-^{13}C]acetate in combination with MRS, it could be shown that 3-NPA inhibited neurons more than glial cells *(21)*.

4.2.1. Effect of 3-NPA on [U-^{13}C]Glutamate Metabolism in Neurons

In cerebellar granule neurons, TCA cycle activity was efficiently blocked by 3 m*M* of 3-NPA *(27)*; the metabolism of [U-^{13}C]glutamate was restricted to the formation of succinate. Only the uniformly labeled isotopomer of glutamate could be detected by MRS and the amount of labeled glutamate within the cells was decreased compared to the control *(29)*, which agrees well with observations in synaptosomes *(44)*. Lactate labeling through the TCA cycle has been observed previously in cell culture *(27)* and mouse *(21)*. This formation of labeled lactate in cerebellar granule neurons was abolished by 3 m*M* of 3-NPA *(30)*.

4.2.2. Effect of 3-NPA on [U-¹³C]Glutamate Metabolism in Astrocytes

3-Nitropropionic acid intoxication has also been studied in murine astrocytes receiving 0.5 mM of [U-¹³C]glutamate in all cases and two different concentrations of 3-NPA (3 and 10 mM) *(25)*. 3-NPA intoxication clearly affected glutamate metabolism in astrocytes. Succinate accumulated intracellularly and extracellularly, and intracellular glutamate and glutamine concentrations were reduced. In the control group, the succinate concentration was too small to be detected by ¹³C-MRS or, alternatively, succinate was not labeled from glutamate. After 3-NPA treatment, no label was detected in aspartate. However, label appeared in lactate in astrocytes receiving 3 mM of 3-NPA, and intracellular [1,2,3-¹³C]glutamate and extracellular [1,2,3-¹³C]glutamine were also still present in cells receiving 3 mM of 3-NPA, although both were significantly reduced. Such labeling from [U-¹³C] glutamate is only possible using precursors from the TCA cycle, indicating that 3 mM of 3-NPA was not sufficient to achieve a complete TCA cycle inhibition. With 10 mM of 3-NPA, the TCA cycle conversion of [U-¹³C]glutamate to metabolites was restricted to the formation of succinate *(25)*.

4.2.3. Effect of 3-NPA on Uptake and Degradation of Glutamate

Uptake and degradation of glutamate was not impaired, because no accumulation of extracellular or intracellular glutamate was observed with 3-NPA *(25)*. To the contrary, intracellular glutamate was significantly reduced, consistent with previous findings both in cerebellar granule cells *(30)* and synaptosomes *(44)*. In synaptosomes incubated in medium without glutamine, 3-NPA caused a small drop in internal concentrations of glutamate and an overall decline in the sum of aspartate, glutamate, and GABA concentrations, suggesting that the glutamate dehydrogenase reaction was stimulated. There is evidence for stimulation of GDH activity also in astrocytes *(25)* because intracellular glutamate concentrations decreased in the presence of 3-NPA, a reduction not related to inhibition of the uptake of glutamate, as there was no accumulation of extracellular glutamate *(27)*. In the same study, it was shown that intracellular glutamine also decreased after 3-NPA treatment. Thus, the decrease in glutamate was not related to an increase in glutamine synthetase activity. Stimulation of glutamine synthetase is also unlikely because proportionally less glutamate was metabolized directly to glutamine in the presence of 3-NPA, whereas there was massive accumulation of succinate. Together, these data suggest that GDH activity was stimulated by 3-NPA both in astrocytes and neurons.

4.2.4. Energy Metabolism in the Presence of 3-NPA

A significant fall in ATP has been observed, both in synaptosomes [1–2 mM of 3-NPA for 5–30 min, *(44)*] and in neuronal cultures of murine frontal cortex [0.25–1 mM of 3-NPA for 2–4 h *(30)*]. Intrastriatal injection of 3-NPA has also been reported to result in a reduced ATP content within 3 h in the area close to the injection site *(45)*. In cortical astrocytes, only a small, statistically not significant decrease in ATP was observed after administration of 3-NPA *(25)*. These results suggested that astrocytic ATP stores were less vulnerable to 3-NPA intoxication than neuronal ATP stores. A possible explanation is the glial localization of pyruvate carboxylase, which is essential for *de novo* synthesis of glutamine in astrocytes and subsequently glutamate and GABA in neurons *(46)*. Thus, astrocytes have the ability to fuel the TCA cycle with intermediates from glucose via pyruvate and oxaloacetate, a pathway not present in neurons *(46)*. Indeed, there are indications of an increased pyruvate carboxylase activity in 3-NPA-treated astrocytes because glucose consumption was increased although lactate production was decreased in media from cells that had received a high glutamate concentration *(25)*. In synaptosomes, where pyruvate carboxylase is not present, lactate concentration increased after 3-NPA treatment *(44)*.

4.2.5. Conclusions

In conclusion, astrocyte metabolism is clearly modified by 3-NPA. However, higher concentrations are necessary in order to elicit a complete inhibition of the astrocytic TCA cycle when compared to the TCA cycle of cerebellar granule cells. Astrocytes managed remarkably well in the presence of high concentrations of 3-NPA, because ATP levels and energy-demanding processes such as glutamate uptake and glutamine synthesis were largely maintained. This was probably the result of the fact that astrocytes have the ability to produce oxaloacetate from glucose via pyruvate. The results support the hypothesis that 3-NPA can be used in animal models for Huntington's disease, as neurons appear to be more sensitive to this compound than astrocytes.

4.3. Methylmercury

Methylmercury (MeHg) is a highly neurotoxic compound producing neuronal death that can be at least in part attributable to glutamate *(47,48)* and overproduction of reactive oxygen species (ROS) *(49–51)*. Although MeHg produces neuronal death and alters neuronal function *(4,52)*, mercurials localize predominantly within astrocytes *(53,54)*. Earlier studies by us and others have shown that MeHg produces astrocytic swelling both in cultured primary astrocytes *(55)* and in vivo *(53,54)*, stimulates astrocytic efflux of excitatory amino acids (EAA) and inhibits the uptake of EAA *(55,56)*. Combined, these data suggest that MeHg-induced neuronal toxicity is, at least in part, mediated by astrocytes.

4.3.1. Effects of MeHg on Glumatergic Systems

As alluded to earlier, a common finding upon exposure to MeHg is the overproduction of ROS and alterations in glutamatergic function *(49–51)*. Excess extracellular glutamate, such as that seen during inhibition of astrocytic uptake, might generate excess ROS *(57)*, and it is well established that overproduction of ROS inhibits glutamate uptake *(58–60)*. In addition, excess extracellular glutamate concentrations lead to inhibition of the uptake of cystine, a GSH precursor *(61)*, and decreased intracellular GSH content, thus rendering cells more susceptible to both the toxic sequelae of MeHg and ROS. The effect of MeHg on cystine uptake were addressed because cystine uptake might involve the same family of transporters, X_{AG-}, which are inhibited by MeHg. Studies were designed to distinguish whether the primary toxic mechanism of MeHg-induced neurodegeneration is the result of the effects on the glutamatergic system or direct production of ROS. The interactions among glutamate, ROS, GSH, and MeHg are shown in Fig. 2.

Overproduction of ROS is a common feature of MeHg toxicity, especially in neuronal cultures *(62)*. Neurons contain approx 10-fold lower GSH levels compared with astrocytes *(63)* and, therefore, are likely more susceptible to MeHg toxicity that coincides with decreased intracellular GSH concentrations. Previous studies have suggested that neurons rely exclusively on astrocytes for providing GSH precursors *(12,13,15)*. Thus, it was reasoned that if MeHg inhibited cystine transport in astrocytes, neurons would be disadvantaged as well, given the deprivation of astrocyte-derived GSH precursors.

Evaluation of ^{35}S-cystine accumulation revealed that astrocytes as well as neurons readily transported ^{35}S-cystine *(64)*. These data corroborate work by others who have demonstrated high-affinity ^{35}S-cystine transport in cultured neurons *(14,61)*, yet are inconsistent with reports in which cultured neurons displayed no ^{35}S-cystine transport *(12,13)*. The factors associated with the apparent differences between these findings are unclear, but they may relate to culture conditions, such as the choice of medium supplements or source of serum. In addition, the cell types in the various experiments were obtained by different isolation methods, which might have influenced their physiological properties. Hippocampal neurons, such as those used in the present study, have relatively high levels of GSH compared to those

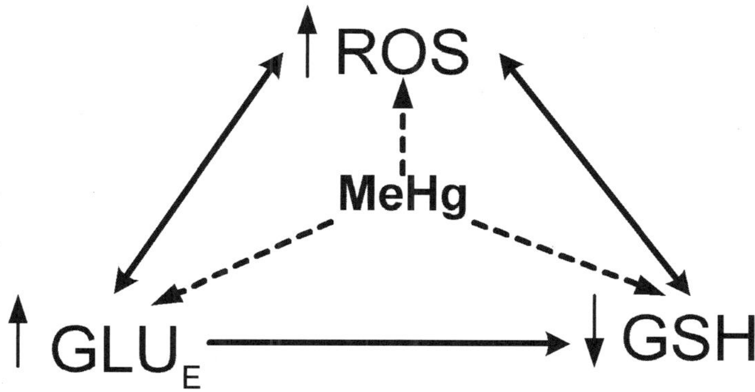

Fig. 2. Interactions among increased extracellular glutamate (GLU$_E$), GSH, ROS, and MeHg. Increased GLU$_E$ increases ROS production leading to decreased GSH levels. Increased GLU$_E$ also inhibits uptake of the GSH precursor cystine, leading to decreased GSH levels. Decreased GSH levels lowers intracellular antioxidant levels, thus decreasing the ability to detoxify ROS. Increased ROS (H$_2$O$_2$) inhibit glutamate uptake, producing increased GLU$_E$. MeHg interacts with each of these systems, magnifying the detrimental effects and resulting in increased toxicity.

found in other brain regions *(63)* and, therefore, might posses a more efficient transport mechanism for GSH precursor uptake.

Recent studies *(64)* established that ^{35}S-cystine uptake was temperature dependent, demonstrating an active transport process in both astrocytes and neurons. Pretreatment with MeHg produced a concentrate-dependent decrease in ^{35}S-cystine uptake in astrocytes, but had no effect on ^{35}S-cystine uptake in neurons. These data suggest that cortical astrocyte and hippocampal neuron cultures utilize differential cystine transport mechanisms *(64)*. Allen et al. *(64)* concluded that in astrocytes, uptake of ^{35}S-cystine was approx 30% Na$^+$ dependent. Interestingly, omission of Na$^+$ from the assay buffer had no effect on ^{35}S-cystine transport in neurons *(64)*.

A well-characterized cystine transporter is the Na$^+$-independent System X$_{C-}$ *(65)*. The system is driven by the intracellular to extracellular glutamate gradient to transport cystine into the cell. It is inhibited by high levels of extracellular glutamate *(65)*. Treatment of astrocytes with glutamate produced a decrease in ^{35}S-cystine uptake, suggesting a role for System X$_{C-}$ *(64)*. However, it has also been suggested that the Na$^+$-dependent excitatory amino acid transporter (EAAT) family (System X$_{AG-}$) is also capable of transporting cystine *(61,66)* and that the transport of ^{35}S-cystine by the same system may be competitively inhibited by elevated concentrations of glutamate. As a first step in determining the contribution of the two transporters to the overall uptake of cystine, cells were treated with quisqualate, a specific inhibitor of

System X_{C-}, or threo-β-hydroxyaspartate (THA), a specific inhibitor of System X_{AG-}. These studies revealed that in both neurons and astrocytes, System X_{C-} transports cystine and that astrocytes also transport cystine by System X_{AG-}. No change in neuronal cystine uptake was apparent following removal of Na^+. Accordingly, the Na^+-dependent System X_{AG-} was ruled out as a contributor to cystine uptake in neurons.

MeHg potently inhibits the uptake of ^3H-D-aspartate via System X_{AG-} (EAAT1) in cultured astrocytes *(47,55)*. Because System X_{AG-} is also capable of transporting cystine, it is likely that the inhibitory effects of MeHg are the result of the inhibition of System X_{AG-} function. To test this hypothesis, astrocytes were incubated with a System X_{AG-} blocker THA, MeHg, or THA plus MeHg. The addition of MeHg to the uptake buffer produced no further inhibition of THA-mediated decrease in cystine uptake, suggesting that THA and MeHg are acting upon the same target. Thus, MeHg's inhibition of cystine transport was the result of actions on System X_{AG-} *(64)*.

Intracellular glutathione (GSH) levels *(67,68)* are known to modulate MeHg toxicity. MeHg decreases intracellular GSH levels because of increased efflux and oxidation, and thus increases in the synthesis of GSH are required to maintain adequate reducing power within astrocytes. Allen et al. *(64)* report that buthionine sulfoximine (BSO), a GSH-depleting agent, induced increases in cystine transport, and this effect was abolished by the addition of MeHg in a dose-dependent manner. Given that MeHg appears to selectively blocks cystine transport via system X_{AG-}, these data suggest that the increased transport of cystine was largely the result of the increased function of System X_{AG-}. The consequences of these effects are that MeHg not only decreases cystine uptake in astrocytes with normal GSH levels but also prevents a compensatory increase in cystine transport induced by decreased GSH levels. MeHg decreases intracellular astrocyte GSH levels both as a result of increased GSH efflux and ROS production. Lowered intracellular GSH levels further increase the toxic effects of MeHg by decreasing intracellular antioxidant levels, propagating a feedforward system that likely continues unabated, producing ROS and, ultimately, cell death.

Decreases in cystine transport, and thus GSH levels, are also seen with high levels of extracellular glutamate, because of the inhibition of the cystine : glutamate heteroexchange System X_{C-} *(69)*. Thus, decreased function of the EAA System X_{AG-} transporter by MeHg will not only induce a direct decrease in cystine transport but also an indirect inhibition of its transport because of disruption of the intracellular/extracellular glutamate gradient.

A recent study published by Bender et al. *(66)* corroborates the above findings, namely that cystine is transported via System X_{AG-} in cultured astrocytes. System X_{AG-} accounted for nearly 95% of cystine uptake in cultured astrocytes *(66)*, whereas in our hands, System X_{AG-} represented approx 25% of astrocytic cystine uptake. However, they treated cells with a cell-permeable cyclic AMP analog prior to studies of cystine uptake *(66)*. The cyclic AMP analog is known to dramatically increase levels of both EAAT1 and EAAT2 *(70)*, thus increasing the System X_{AG-} to System X_{C-} ratio, resulting in decreased contribution of System X_{C-} to cystine transport.

The mechanisms of MeHg-mediated inhibition of System X_{AG-} remain unknown. Acute (5-min) coincubation with MeHg and cystine produced no inhibitory effects on cystine uptake, suggesting a lack of direct interaction between MeHg and the EAA transporter *(64)*. Studies examining the effects of mercurials on D-aspartate transport suggest that intracellular GSH levels are important mediators of MeHg toxicity *(68)*. However, it is unclear whether these effects are the result of antioxidant actions of GSH or to GSH acting as an intracellular buffer of MeHg that would have the effect of lowering "free" MeHg concentrations within the cells.

To examine possible mechanisms of MeHg-mediated inhibition of glutamate transport, an additional series of studies were conducted *(71)*. As alluded to earlier, two leading hypotheses for mechanisms of MeHg toxicity invoke overproduction of ROS *(50,51)* and direct interactions of MeHg with protein thiol. Electrophysiological studies suggest that both the thiol redox state and ROS might mediate glutamate-induced glutamate transporter current *(60)*.

To investigate the role of the thiol redox state on glutamate transporter function in cultured primary astrocytes, cells were incubated with a thiol-reducing agent, dithiothreitol (DTT), or a thiol-oxidizing agent, 5,5'-dithio-bis(2-nitrobenzoic) acid (DTNB) *(71)*. In contrast to the effects seen on glutamate-induced EAA transporter current *(60)*, no changes in the actual transport of the glutamate analog, ^{3}H-D-aspartate, were noted. MeHg-mediated inhibition of ^{3}H-D-aspartate uptake was found to be time dependent. No changes in ^{3}H-D-aspartate uptake were noted after acute 5-min cotreatment with MeHg and ^{3}H-D-aspartate. However, ^{3}H-D-aspartate uptake was inhibited following 60-min MeHg pretreatment. This lack of an acute effect argues against an inhibitory action of MeHg on ^{3}H-D-aspartate that is directly mediated by the transport protein.

Although not specifically determined, the mechanism of MeHg-induced ROS-mediated inhibition of EAA transport is hypothesized to be the result of the inhibition of Na^+/K^+-ATPase and the activation of a Na^+/H^+ exchanger *(72)*. The net effect of these actions is to increase intracellular Na^+ levels *(72)*. Because glutamate transport relies on the extracellular/intracellular Na^+

gradient to provide the driving force for a transport of glutamate against a 10,000 : 1 intracellular to extracellular glutamate gradient, changes in intracellular Na^+ levels might dramatically inhibit EAA function.

Taken together, these studies suggest a major role for inhibition of the EAA transporter (System X_{AG-}; EAAT1) in mediating MeHg toxicity in cultured astrocytes (*see* Fig. 2). Inhibition of this transporter results in diminished uptake of the GSH precursor cystine *(73)*. This, in turn, will diminish astrocytic GSH levels and increase MeHg toxicity, either as a result of diminished release of MeHg that is complexed with GSH or the result of reduced antioxidant capacity, enabling MeHg to target sensitive cellular sites. Given that GSH of astrocytic origin is degraded extracellularly and is vital in providing precursors for GSH synthesis in at least some neuronal types *(12,15)*, the effect of MeHg on astrocytes will also indirectly lead to reduced neuronal GSH levels. The resultant decreased GSH levels increase neuronal vulnerability to ROS that are generated either as the result of excess NMDA receptor activation or by MeHg. It is noteworthy that a good correlation exists between areas of MeHg toxicity, such as cerebellar granule cells and visual association cortex, and high levels of glutamatergic innervation and NMDA receptors *(74,75)*.

4.3.2. Metabolic Effects of MeHg

The effect of methylmercury on glutamate metabolism has been studied by ^{13}C-MRS *(76)*. Cerebral cortical astrocytes were pretreated with MeHg, 1 μM for 24 h or 10 μM for 30 min, and subsequently with 0.5 mM of [U-^{13}C]glutamate for 2 h. High-performance liquid chromatography (HPLC) analysis of amino acids showed no changes in concentrations between groups. Furthermore, the amounts of most metabolites synthesized from [U-^{13}C]glutamate were also unchanged in the presence of MeHg. However, the formation of [U-^{13}C]lactate was decreased in the 10-μM group. This was not observed for labeled aspartate. It should be noted that both [U-^{13}C]lactate and [U-^{13}C]aspartate can only be derived from [U-^{13}C]glutamate via mitochondrial metabolism. [U-^{13}C]glutamate enters the tricarboxylic acid cycle after conversion to 2-[U-^{13}C]oxoglutarate, and [U-^{13}C]aspartate is formed from [U-^{13}C]oxaloacetate, as is [U-^{13}C]lactate. [U-^{13}C]lactate can also be formed from [U-^{13}C]malate. This differential effect on labeled aspartate and lactate indicated cellular compartmentation, as also shown in other studies *(77)*, and thus selective vulnerability of mitochondria within the astrocytes to the effects of MeHg. The decreased lactate production from glutamate might be detrimental for the surrounding cells because lactate has been shown to be an important substrate for neurons.

4.3.3. Conclusions

The above-detailed studies suggest multiple directions for future studies. Consequences of decreased cystine uptake in vivo as a result of MeHg are unknown. Given the ability of neurons to readily transport cystine and the specific effects of MeHg on astrocytic cystine transport, the cumulative effects on neuronal GSH levels present an unanswered question. The ability of catalase to reverse the inhibitory effects of MeHg on cystine transport, such as that seen with aspartate transport, is hypothesized but untested in the present set of experiments. The studies described herein only examined acute effects of MeHg on cystine and aspartate transport. Longer exposure times with lower concentrations of MeHg might provide mechanisms of toxicity that are different from those induced by acute MeHg treatment. Another unanswered question pertains to the selective inhibition of EAAT1 by MeHg or H_2O_2. To date, all studies have only examined astrocytic EAA transporters. MeHg may differentially affect neuronal EAA transporters, and their ability to transport cystine has not been studied. Although MeHg and H_2O_2 inhibit EAA transport in astrocytes, the molecular mechanisms underlying these inhibitory actions remain elusive.

REFERENCES

1. Schousboe, A., Meier, E., Drejer, J., and Hertz, L. (1989) Preparation of primary cultures of mouse (rat) cerebellar granule cells, in *A Dissection and Tissue Culture Manual of the Nervous System* (Shahar, A., De Vellis, J., Vernadakis, A., and Haber B., eds.), Alan R. Liss, New York, pp. 183–186.
2. Hertz, E., Yu, A. C. H., Hertz, L., Juurlink, B. H. J., and Schousboe, A. (1989) Preparation of primary cultures of mouse (rat) neurons, in *A Dissection and Tissue Culture Manual of the Nervous System* (Shahar, A., De Vellis, J., Vernadakis, A., and Haber, B, eds.), Alan R Liss, New York, pp. 183–186.
3. Hertz, L., Juurlink, B. H. J., Hertz, E., Fosmark, H., and Schousboe, A. (1989) Preparation of primary cultures of mouse (rat) astrocytes, in *A Dissection and Tissue Culture Manual of the Nervous System* (Shahar, A., De Vellis, J., Vernadakis, A., and Haber, B., eds.), Alan R. Liss, New York, pp. 105–108.
4. Aschner, M. and Kimelberg, H. K. (eds.) (1996) *The Role of Glia in Neurotoxicology*, CRC, Boca Raton, FL.
5. Kettenmann, H. and Ransom, B. R. (eds.) (1995) *Neuroglia*, Oxford University Press, New York.
6. Schousboe, A., Westergaard, N., Sonnewald, U., Peterson, S. B., Yu, A. C. H., and Hertz, L. (1992) Regulatory role of astrocytes for neuronal biosynthesis and homeostasis of glutamate and GABA. *Prog. Brain Res.* **94,** 199–211.
7. Rakic, R. (1971) Neuron–glia relationship during granule cell migration in developing cerebellar cortex. A Golgi and electronmicroscopic study in Macacus Rhesus. *J. Comp. Neurol.* **141,** 283–312.

8. Rudge, J. S. (1993) Astrocyte-derived neurotrophic factors, in *Astrocytes: Pharmacology and Function* (Murphy, S., ed.), Academic, San Diego, CA, pp. 267–308.

9. Martinez-Hernandez, A., Bell, K. P., and Norenberg, M. D. (1977) Glutamine synthetase: glial localization in brain. *Science* **195,** 1356–1358.

10. Schousboe, A., Westergaard, N., Sonnewald, U., Peterson, S. B., Huang, R., and Peng, L. (1993) Glutamate and glutamine metabolism and compartmentation in astrocytes. *Dev. Neurosci.* **15,** 359–366.

11. Sonnewald, U., Westergaard, N., and Schousboe, A. (1997) Glutamate transport and metabolism in astrocytes. *Glia* **21,** 56–63.

12. Dringen, R., Pfeiffer, B., and Hamprecht, B. (1999) Synthesis of the antioxidant glutathione in neurons: supply by astrocytes of CysGly as precursor for neuronal glutathione. *J. Neurosci.* **19,** 562–569.

13. Sagara, J., Miura, K., and Bannai, S. (1993) Maintenance of neuronal glutathione by glial cells. *J. Neurochem.* **61,** 1672–1676.

14. Sagara, Y. and Schubert, D. (1998) The activation of metabotropic glutamate receptors protects nerve cells from oxidative stress. *J. Neurosci.* **18,** 6662–6671.

15. Wang, X. F. and Cynader, M. S. (2000) Astrocytes provide cysteine to neurons by releasing glutathione. *J. Neurochem.* **74,** 1434–1442.

16. Ullian, E. M., Sapperstein, S. K., Christopherson, K. S., and Barres, B. A. (2001) Control of synapse number by glia. *Science* **291,** 657–661.

17. Bezzi, P., Domercq, M., Brambilla, L., et al. (2001) CXCR4-activated astrocyte glutamate release via TNFalpha: amplification by microglia triggers neurotoxicity. *Nature Neurosci.* **4,** 702–710.

18. Hassel, B. and Sonnewald, U. (1995) Glial formation of pyruvate and lactate from TCA cycle intermediates: implications for the inactivation of transmitter amino acids. *J. Neurochem.* **65,** 2227–2234.

19. Hassel, B., Sonnewald, U., and Fonnum F (1995) Glial–neuronal interactions as studied by cerebral metabolism of [2-^{13}C]acetate and [1-^{13}C]glucose: an ex vivo ^{13}C NMR spectroscopy study. *J. Neurochem.* **64,** 2773–2782.

20. Håberg, A., Qu, H., Haraldseth, O., Unsgård, G., and Sonnewald, U. (1998) *In vivo* injection of [1-^{13}C]glucose and [1,2-^{13}C]acetate combined with ex vivo ^{13}C nuclear magnetic resonance spectroscopy: a novel approach to the study of middle cerebral artery occlusion in the rat. *J. Cereb. Blood Flow Metab.* **18,** 1223–1232.

21. Hassel, B. and Sonnewald, U. (1995) Selective inhibition of the TCA cycle of GABAergic neurons with 3-nitropropionic acid in vivo. *J. Neurochem.* **65,** 1184–1191.

22. Hassel, B., Bachelard, H., Fonnum, F., and Sonnewald, U. (1997) Trafficking of amino acids between neurons and glia *in vivo*. Effects of inhibition of glial metabolism by fluoroacetate. *J. Cereb. Blood Flow Metab.* **17,** 1230–1238.

23. Hassel, B., Sonnewald, U., Unsgård, G., and Fonnum, F. (1994) NMR spectroscopy of cultured astrocytes; synthesis of citrate and glutamine by different

TCA cycles. Effects of glutamine and the gliotoxin fluorocitrate. *J. Neurochem.* **62,** 2187–2194.

24. Bakken, I. J., White, L. R., Unsgård, G., Aasly, J., and Sonnewald, U. (1998) [U-^{13}C]glutamate metabolism in astrocytes during hypoglycemia and hypoxia. *J. Neurosci. Res.* **51,** 636–645.

25. Bakken, I. J., Johnsen, S. F., White, L. R., Unsgård, G., Åsly, J., and Sonnewald, U. (1997) NMR spectroscopy study of the effect of 3-nitropropionic acid on glutamate metabolism in cultured astrocytes. *J. Neurosci. Res.* **47,** 642–649.

26. Westergaard, W., Drejer, J., Schousboe, A., and Sonnewald, U. (1996) Evaluation of the importance of transamination versus deamination in astrocytic metabolism of (U-^{13}C(glutamate. *Glia* **17,** 160–168.

27. Sonnewald, U., Westergaard, N., Petersen, S. B., Unsgård, G., and Schousboe, A. (1993) Metabolism of [U-^{13}C]glutamate in astrocytes studied by ^{13}C NMR spectroscopy: incorporation of more label into lactate than into glutamine demonstrates the importance of the TCA cycle. *J. Neurochem.* **61,** 1179–1182.

28. McKenna, M. C., Sonnewald, U., Huang, X., Stevenson, J., and Zielke, R. H. (1996) Exogenous glutamate concentration regulates the metabolic fate of glutamate in astrocytes. *J. Neurochem.* **66,** 386–393.

29. Sonnewald, U., Westergaard, N., Drejer, J., and Schousboe, A. (1996) Evaluation of the importance of transamination versus deamination in astrocytic metabolism of [U-^{13}C]glutamate: implications for neurodegenerative diseases. *Glia* **17,** 160–168.

30. Sonnewald, U., White, L., Ødegård, E., et al. (1996) MRS study of glutamate metabolism in cultured neurons/glia. *Neurochem. Res.* **21,** 987–993.

31. Beal, M. F., Hyman, B. T., and Koroshetz, W. (1993) Do defects in mitochondrial energy metabolism underlie the pathology of neurodegenerative diseases? *Trends Neurosci.* **16,** 125–131.

32. Urbanska, E., Ikonomidou, C., Sieklucka, M., and Turski, W. A. (1991) Aminooxyacetic acid produces excitotoxic lesions in rat striatum. *Synapse* **9,** 129–135.

33. Beal, M. F., Swartz, K. J., Hyman, B. T., Storey, E., Finn, S. F., and Koroshetz, W. (1991) Aminooxyacetic acid results in excitotoxin lesions by a novel indirect mechanism. *J. Neurochem.* **57,** 1068–1073.

34. Gegelashvili, G. and Schousboe, A. (1998) Cellular distribution and kinetic properties of high-affinity glutamate transporters. *Brain Res. Bull.* **45,** 233–238.

35. Hertz, L., Dringen, R., Schousboe, A., and Robinson, S. R. (1999) Astrocytes: glutamate producers for neurons. *J. Neurosci. Res.* **57,** 417–428.

36. Shank, R. P. and Aprison, M. H. (1977) Glutamine uptake and metabolism by the isolated toad brain: evidence pertaining to its proposed role as a transmitter precursor. *J. Neurochem.* **28,** 1189–1196.

37. Farinelli, S.E. and Nicklas, W. J. (1992) Glutamate metabolism in rat cortical astrocyte cultures. *J. Neurochem.* **58,** 1905–1915.

38. Yu, A. C., Fisher, T. E., Hertz, E., Tildon, J. T., Schousboe, A., and Hertz, L. (1984) Metabolic fate of [^{14}C]-glutamine in mouse cerebral neurons in primary cultures. *J. Neurosci. Res.* **11,** 351–357.
39. Yudkoff, M., Nissim, I., Hummeler, K., Medow, M., and Pleasure, D. (1986) Utilization of [^{15}N]glutamate by cultured astrocytes. *Biochem. J.* **234,** 185–192.
40. Cooper, A. J. and Plum, F. (1987) Biochemistry and physiology of brain ammonia. *Physiol. Rev.* **67,** 440–519.
41. Plaitakis, A. and Berl, S. (1988) Pathology of glutamate dehydrogenase, in *Glutamine and glutamate in mammals* (Kvamme, E., ed.), CRC, Boca Raton, FL, pp. 128–140.
42. Wullner, U., Young, A. B., Penney, J. B., and Beal, M. F. (1994) 3-Nitropropionic acid toxicity in the striatum. *J. Neurochem.* **63,** 1772–1781.
43. Brouillet, E., Jenkins, B. G., Hyman, B. T., et al. (1993) Age-dependent vulnerability of the striatum to the mitochondrial toxin 3-nitropropionic acid. *J. Neurochem.* **60,** 356–359.
44. Erecinska, M. and Nelson, D. (1994) Effects of 3-nitropropionic acid on synaptosomal energy and transmitter metabolism: relevance to neurodegenerative brain diseases. *J. Neurochem.* **63,** 1033–1041.
45. Beal, M. F, Brouillet, E., Jenkins, B., Henshaw, R., and Hyman B. T. (1993) Age-dependent striatal excitotoxic lesions produced by the endogenous mitochondrial inhibitor malonate. *J. Neurochem.* **61,** 1147–1150.
46. Yu, A. C. H, Drejer, J., Hertz, L., and Schousboe, A. (1983) Pyruvate carboxylase activity in primary cultures of astrocytes and neurons. *J. Neurochem.* **41,** 1484–1487.
47. Brookes, N. and Kristt, D. A. (1989) Inhibition of amino acid transport and protein synthesis by HgCl$_2$ and methylmercury in astrocytes: selectivity and reversibility. *J. Neurochem.* **53,** 1228–1237.
48. Kim, S. U., Park, S. T., Lim, K. T., and Chung, Y. T. (1996) Methylmercury-induced neurotoxicity in cerebral neuron culture is blocked by antioxidants and NMDA receptor antagonists. *Neurotoxicology* **17,** 37–45.
49. Ali, S. F., LeBel, C. P., and Bondy, S.C. (1992). Reactive oxygen species formation as a biomarker of methylmercury and trimethyltin neurotoxicity, *Neurotoxicology* **13,** 637–648.
50. Ganther, H. E., Goudie, C., Sunde, M. L., et al. (1972) Selenium: relation to decreased toxicity of methyl mercury added to diet containing tuna. *Science* **75,** 1122–1124.
51. Yee, S. and Choi, B. H. (1996) Oxidative stress in neurotoxic effects of methylmercury poisoning. *Neurotoxicology* **17,** 17–26.
52. Atchison, W. D. and Hare, M. F. (1994) Mechanisms of methylmercury-induced neurotoxicity, *FASEB J.* **8,** 622–629.
53. Charleston, J. S., Body, R. L., Mottet, N. K., Vahter, M. E., and Burbacher, T. M. (1995) Autometallographic determination of inorganic mercury distribution in the cortex of the carlacrine sulcus of the monkey *Macaca fascicularis* following long-term subclinical exposure to methylmercury and mercuric chloride. *Toxicol. Appl. Pharmacol.* **132,** 325–333.

54. Garman, R. H., Weiss, B., and Evans, H. L. (1975) Alkylmercurial encephalopathy in the monkey (*Saimiri sciureus* and *Macaca arctoides*): a histopathologic and autoradiographic study. *Acta Neuropathol.* **32,** 61–74.

55. Aschner, M., Eberle, N. B., Miller, K., and Kimelberg, H. K. (1990) Interactions of methylmercury with rat primary astrocyte cultures: inhibition of rubidium and glutamate uptake and induction of swelling. *Brain Res.* **530,** 245–250.

56. Aschner, M., Yao, C. P., Allen J. W., and Tan, K. H. (2000) Methylmercury alters glutamate transport in astrocytes. *Neurochem. Int.* **37,** 199–206.

57. Coyle, J. T. and Puttfarken, P. (1993) Oxidative stress, glutamate, and neurodegenerative disorders. *Science* **262,** 689–695.

58. Volterra, A., Trotti, D., Tromba, C., Floridi, S., and Racagni, G. (1994) Glutamate uptake inhibition by oxygen free radicals in rat cortical astrocytes. *J. Neurosci.* **14,** 2924–2932.

59. Volterra, A., Trotti, D., and Racagni, G. (1994) Glutamate uptake is inhibited by arachidonic acid and oxygen radicals via two distinct and additive mechanisms. *Mol. Pharm.* **46,** 986–992.

60. Trotti, D., Nussberger, S., Volterra, A., and Hediger, M. A. (1997) Differential modulation of the uptake currents by redox interconversion of cysteine residues in the human neuronal glutamate transporter EAAC1. *Eur. J. Neurosci.* **9,** 236–124.

61. Murphy, T. H., Schnaar, R. L., and Coyle, J. T. (1990) Immature cortical neurons are uniquely sensitive to glutamate toxicity by inhibition of cystine uptake. *FASEB J.* **4,** 1624–1633.

62. Sarafian, T. A., Vartavarian, L., Kane, D. J., Bredesen, D. E., and Verity, M. A. (1994) Bcl-2 expression decreases methyl mercury-induced free-radical generation and cell killing in a neural cell line. *Toxicol. Lett.* **74,** 149–155.

63. Philbert, M. A., Beiswanger, C. M., Waters, D. K., Reuhl, K. R., and Lowndes, H. E. (1991) Cellular and regional distribution of reduced glutathione in the nervous system of the rat: histochemical localization by mercury orange and *o*-phthaldialdehyde-induced histofluorescence. *Toxicol. Appl. Pharmacol.* **107,** 215–227.

64. Allen, J. W., Shanker, G., and Aschner, M. (2001) Methylmercury inhibits the in vitro uptake of the glutathione precursor, cystine, in astrocytes but not in neurons. *Brain Res.* **891,** 148–157.

65. Bannai, S. (1984) Transport of cystine and cysteine in mammalian cells. *Biochim. Biophys. Acta* **779,** 289–306.

66. Bender, A. S., Reichelt., W., and Norenberg, M. D. (2000) Characterization of cystine uptake in cultured astrocytes. *Neurochem. Int.* **37,** 269–276.

67. Miura, K. and Clarkson, T. W. (1993) Reduced methylmercury accumulation in a methylmercury-resistant rat pheochromocytoma PC12 cell line. *Toxicol. Appl. Pharmacol.* **118,** 39–45.

68. Aschner, M., Mullaney, K. J., Wagoner, D, Lash, L. H., and Kimelberg, H. K. (1994) Intracellular glutathione (GSH) levels modulate mercuric chloride

(MC)- and methylmercuric chloride (MeHgCl)-induced amino acid release from neonatal rat primary astrocytes cultures. *Brain Res.* **664,** 133–140.

69. Bannai, S. and Kitamura, E. (1980) Transport interaction of L-cystine and L-glutamate in human diploid fibroblasts in culture. *J. Biol. Chem.* **255,** 2372–2376.

70. Schlag, B. D., Vondrasek, J. R., Munir, M., et al. (1998) Regulation of the glial Na$^+$-dependent glutamate transporters by cyclic AMP analogs and neurons. *J. Neurosci.* **53,** 355–369.

71. Allen, J. W., Mutkus, L. A., and Aschner, M. (2001) Methylmercury-mediated inhibition of ^{3}H-D-aspartate transport in cultured astrocytes is reversed by the antioxidant catalase. *Brain Res.* **902,** 97–100.

72. Vitarella, D., Kimelberg, H. K., and Aschner, M. (1996) Inhibition of regulatory volume decrease in swollen rat primary astrocyte cultures by methylmercury is due to increased amiloride-sensitive Na$^+$ uptake. *Brain Res.* **732,** 169–178.

73. Kranich, O., Dringen, R., Sandberg, M., and Hamprecht, B. (1998) Utilization of cysteine and cysteine precursors for the synthesis of glutathione in astroglial cultures: preference for cystine. *Glia* **22,** 11–18.

74. Monaghan, D. T., Holets, V. R., Toy, V. W., and Cotman, C. W. (1983) Anatomical distributions of four pharmacologically distinct ^{3}H-L-glutamate binding sites. *Nature* **306,** 176–179.

75. Monaghan, D. T. and Cotman, C. W. (1985) Distribution of NMDA-sensitive ^{3}H-L-glutamate binding sites in rat brain as determined by quantative autoradiography. *J. Neurosci.* **5,** 2909–2919.

76. Sonnewald, U., Hertz, L., and Schousboe, A. (1998) Mitochondrial heterogeneity in the brain at the cellular level. *J. Cereb. Blood Flow Metab.* **18,** 231–237.

77. Allen, J. W., El-Oqayli, H., Aschner, M., Syversen, T., and Sonnewald, U. Methylmercury has a selective effect on mitochondria in cultured astrocytes in the presence of [U-^{13}C]glutamate. *Brain Res.* **908,** 149–154.

7

Cell-Type Specific Responses of the Nervous System to Lead

Evelyn Tiffany-Castiglioni and Yongchang Qian

1. CELLULAR BASIS FOR THE NEUROTOXICITY OF LEAD

Cells that make up the nervous system interact in complex, dynamic structural and biochemical contexts to generate organ function. A neurotoxicant that alters the activities of a particular cell type also induces secondary changes in the interactions between this cell and other cells. All types of cell in the nervous system are potential primary or secondary targets for damage by neurotoxic substances. The purpose of this chapter is to examine the reported cell-specific effects of an archetypal environmental neurotoxicant, inorganic lead (Pb), on neurons and neuroglia. Pb is an archetype in the broad sense that, like several environmental neurotoxicants, it affects multiple cell types, employs multiple mechanisms of toxic action, produces sublethal functional impairment to cells at low doses, is widespread in the environment, and is metabolically nonessential. Pb was perhaps the earliest environmental contaminant to be recognized as a neurotoxicant and is the most thoroughly studied to date in vitro. Pb neurotoxicologists have charted their own courses, often guided by progress in neuroscience and cell biology and sometimes pointing out new directions for neurobiology. The approaches that Pb neurotoxicologists have taken or not taken, the roads, paths, and blind alleys, will be discussed in this chapter, in the hope that telling the story will facilitate in vitro studies with other neurotoxicants. This work will be limited to effects of Pb on neurons, astroglia, and myelinating glia (oligodendroglia and Schwann cells), as the effects of Pb on microglia are virtually unstudied.

From: *Methods in Pharmacology and Toxicology: In Vitro Neurotoxicology: Principles and Challenges*
Edited by: E. Tiffany-Castiglioni © Humana Press Inc., Totowa, NJ

Lead ranks second of 275 on the ATSDR/EPA Priority List of Hazardous Substances for 2001 *(1)*. The severity of its detrimental effects on the human nervous system is associated with the degree by which blood Pb concentrations are elevated. Thus, Pb encephalopathy occurs at blood Pb levels in excess of 80 µg/dL and peripheral neuropathies at greater than 50 µg/dL. Slowed nerve conduction velocity occurs at levels of 30 µg/dL or higher *(2,3)*. Because of the reduction of Pb content in gasoline and paint and stricter regulation of occupational exposures, both the number and severity of these types of Pb-induced effects have declined over the past 20 yr. Nevertheless, Pb continues to be a pervasive contaminant in the environment, with significant health risks. Extensive epidemiologic evidence shows that low-level Pb exposure causes developmental neurotoxicity in children *(3,4)*, characterized in part by reduced attention span, deficits in school performance *(5)*, reduced IQ scores (0.25–0.5 units per 1 µg/dL in blood above 10 µg/dL) *(6,7)*, and increased aggression *(8)*. The Centers for Disease Control have defined 10 µg/dL as a screening blood Pb level of pediatric health concern *(9)*, yet, in the United States from 1992 to 1994, approx 4% of children aged 1–5 yr had blood Pb levels greater than 10 µg/dL *(10)*. In addition, long-term occupational exposure (> 20 yr) to Pb has been suggested as a risk factor in the development of Parkinson's disease *(11–14)*.

1.1. Relative Sensitivities of Cell Types

The cellular bases for toxic effects of Pb on the central nervous system (CNS) are likely to be complex and involve several cell types, as well as multiple toxicologic mechanisms. Both neurons and neuroglia show morphologic and functional abnormalities after Pb exposure. Neuronal effects include alterations in morphology, neurite growth, ion channels, and both presynaptic and postsynaptic neuronal function *(15–28)*. Many of these effects are discussed in other chapters of this volume. Effects on Schwann cells include partial inhibition of myelination *(29)* and ultrastructural abnormalities *(30)*. Oligodendrocyte progenitor cells show delayed differentiation as a result of exposure to Pb *(31)*. Pb-induced effects on cultured astroglia or glial cell line models include intracellular accumulation of Pb *(32)*, altered glutamate metabolism *(33,34)*, altered homeostasis of calcium and copper ions *(32,35–40)*, oxidative or mitochondrial stress *(41–44)*, and a reduced basal respiratory rate *(45,46)*. The breadth of cellular effects indicates that Pb interacts with diverse proteins to impair cell function.

Figure 1 depicts the relative sensitivities of various cell types to morphological changes and cell death induced by Pb and lists characteristic responses of each cell type. The idea that myelinating cells and neurons are more sensitive than astroglia to Pb-induced morphological alterations or cell

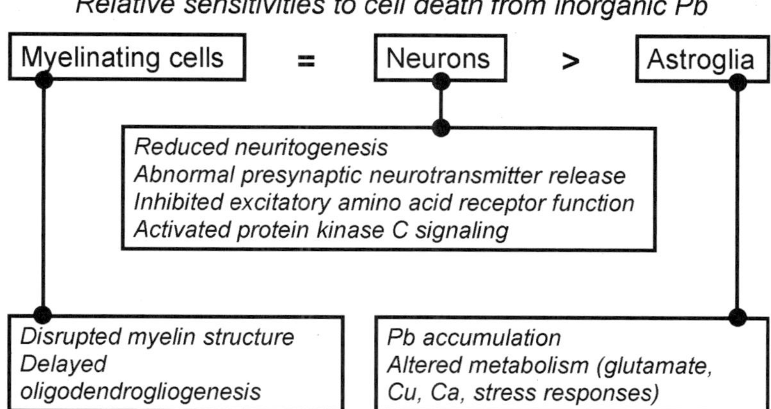

Fig. 1. Relative sensitivities of neural cells to damage by inorganic Pb. Collective in vivo and in vitro data suggest that myelinating cells (oligodendroglia and Schwann cells) and neurons are more sensitive to lead-induced morphological changes or cell death than are astroglia. The major reported effects of subcytotoxic lead exposure on the various cell types are shown in this figure.

death was first proposed in 1993 *(47)* based on a comparison of all available in vitro findings at that time. No single study had compared all three cell types under identical conditions; therefore, relative sensitivities were deduced from several studies in which two cell types were compared. This ranking continues to be supported by newer data, for example, the finding by Tang et al. *(30)* that Schwann cells are 10-fold more sensitive than astroglia to Pb-induced ultrastructural alterations. However, sensitivity based on morphologic changes or cell death does not predict relative sensitivities of critical unique cell functions to damage by Pb, and such comparisons cannot be extracted readily from existing studies. The difficulty in comparing different in vitro studies is that they are usually carried out under nonequivalent conditions that have been optimized in individual laboratories for the cell type and/or end points to be measured. As useful as these conditions are for the examination of circumscribed questions about the cell type, they obstruct rigorous comparisons between cell types.

Many of the above-listed cellular effects have been observed both in vivo and in vitro. These parallel observations help establish the relevancy of the in vitro results obtained and validate the utility of the in vitro system for further mechanistic explorations of the phenomenon. The caveat is that parallel observations in vivo/in vitro are obtained under different exposure conditions and regimens, and although the end point affected might be the same, the mechanisms may be different. In vitro neurotoxicology is practiced under this weight of uncertainty, which only the counterweight of sufficient data will offset.

1.2. Lead Exposure Regimens In Vitro

One of the most difficult validation problems facing in vitro neurotoxicology is the replication of toxicologically relevant exposure regimens to the toxicant. This subject has been reviewed previously with regard to Pb *(47,48)* and is further considered in Chapter 9. Ideally, basal conditions such as the developmental stage at time of exposure, duration and intensity of exposure, and biological availability of the toxicant should be reproduced in the in vitro system. Some approaches with which in vitro neurotoxicologists have attempted to replicate these conditions are presented in this chapter. Early developmental stages can be modeled, as will be described for effects of Pb on oligodendroglial and astroglial development, but effects of Pb on the aging nervous system in culture remain to be explored. One-time or repeated exposure can also be carried out in cell culture, as will be illustrated for several cell types; however, the incremental or sporadic nature of childhood exposure to Pb is typically ignored in vitro.

Biological availability is the most complex problem in vitro of the three conditions outlined, as the availability of Pb to target cells is dependent on many factors. Pb availability in vivo is dependent on diet, nutritional status, and age *(49–51)*, which are just beginning to be explored in vitro. Biological availability of Pb is also dependent on the poorly understood dynamics of Pb transport across the blood–brain barrier, its levels in interstitial fluid in the brain, and its potential for uptake by brain cells. These facets have been roughly approximated in vitro in the absence of sufficient information, but they are confounded by in vitro artifacts. Even when known total amounts of Pb are added to cultures, the biological availability of Pb is decreased by such factors as precipitation in culture medium *(38)* and the presence of serum in the medium *(37,52,53)*, which detract from the achievement of precise, relevant exposure conditions in vitro. The species of Pb that is biologically relevant could hold the key to this dilemma, but it is a matter of continued debate. Several investigators view the free-Pb cation (Pb^{2+}) as the principal species of interest *(21,54–57)*, although it has not been ruled out that Pb bound to other molecules is also biologically active. Free-Pb ion concentrations can be closely regulated in short-term experiments by the use of appropriate buffers or chlelating agents *(56,58)*, but these methods are not suitable for long-term exposures in vitro because of the toxicity of the chelators and the lack of nutrients in the buffers.

2. EFFECTS OF LEAD ON NEURONS

Neuronal activities and properties that are vulnerable to disruption by Pb in the developing brain include morphological differentiation of neurites, synaptogenesis, presynaptic neurotransmitter release, postsynaptic receptor function, intracellular signaling, and gene expression. This section will address neuritogenesis (morphology) and molecular mechanisms of differentiation. A detailed discussion of the effects of Pb on synaptic function can be found in Chapter 9. Audesirk and Tjalkens consider intracellular signaling in detail in Chapter 4 and Barone et al. offer an additional perspective on the effects of Pb on neurite extension in Chapter 8.

2.1. Neuronal Morphology

Several studies in vivo have shown that low to moderate levels of Pb exposure alter the morphology of neurons in experimental animals. Earlier work on neuronal morphology in lead encephalopathy is omitted from this discussion. Whereas other cells in the body lack polarity or have simple cytoarchitecture characterized by apical, basal, and lateral surfaces, neurons have an extremely complex morphology. The dendritic tree of a multipolar neuron receives both excitatory and inhibitory inputs from the efferent processes of as many as 150 other neurons, entailing the maintenance of postsynaptic membrane domains, each responsive to a specific neurotransmitter. The neuron's axon can be millimeters or centimeters in length, depending on its function, and can be specifically targeted during development to form part of a fiber tract or nerve. The establishment of neuronal connectivity adds another dimension to development that includes four events: neurite extension, synapse formation, the pruning of overproduced synapses, and the development of synaptic strength through activity. The neuron thus presents numerous sites of vulnerability through which toxicants might alter its morphology and, hence, its function.

The earliest studies reporting effects of moderate Pb levels on neuronal morphology were those of Crofton, McCauley, and colleagues *(15,17)*. These investigators showed that prenatal exposure (69.2 µg/dL blood Pb at birth) in rats results in perturbation of normal cortical synaptic overproduction and pruning. They found a depressed rate of synaptic density accumulation from postnatal days 11–15 but normal synaptic density on d 21. However, behavioral deficits were evident on d 15–21, suggesting that neuronal circuitry could have been improperly established as a result of the loss of synapses that should have been available for pruning. Several subsequent in vivo studies reported abnormal dendritic morphology in a variety of species exposed to Pb. Alfano and Petit *(16)* reported increased dendritic branching close to the cell body and decreased total number of branches in hippocampal dentate granule cells of rats exposed postnatally to moderately high Pb levels. Reuhl et al. *(19)* found that arborization and volume density of dendrites are decreased in pyramidal neurons in monkey visual cortex after moderate Pb exposure from birth to 6 yr. Legare et al. *(59)* found increased dendritic branching in cortical pyramidal neurons of guinea pigs prenatally exposed to low Pb levels (10–30 µg/dL in blood). In addition, Patrick and Anderson *(20)* found hyperspinous distal apical dendrites in the cortical pyramidal neurons of kittens postnatally exposed to low Pb levels.

In most of the above studies, the search for statistically significant morphological alterations was laborious and painstaking, as many parameters measured appeared unaffected. Comparisons of dendritic morphology are subject to technical limitations, rather like comparing the branching patterns of trees on the horizon in winter. Some types of analysis, such as Scholl analysis, are so labor intensive that sufficient sample size and statistical power are difficult to acquire *(59)*. A major obstacle is that differences might be masked by the large variation in neuronal morphology that occurs in the normal brain. However, taken together, these studies show morphological alterations in dendrites from several brain regions and species, supporting the idea that Pb is a developmental teratogen, as originally proposed by Regan and colleagues *(18,60–62)*.

Two elegant in vivo studies further support the teratogenic hypothesis, although in reference to axons rather than dendrites. In the first study, Cline et al. *(23)* used a technically sophisticated approach to measure the effects of Pb on the developing retinotectal system of *Rana pipiens* tadpoles. A matrix material (Elvax40P) was prepared in Pb acetate and surgically implanted over the dorsal surface of each tectal lobe to expose the developing optic tecta. Topographic measurements of arbor morphology showed no effect on the organization of the retinotectal projection but a 25–90% stunting of axonal arbor area and branch tip number after exposure to 0.1 nM to 1 µM Pb for 6 wk. The data suggest that Pb does not interfere with branch tip additions or arbor migration, but increases branch retractions. In a second study, Wilson et al. *(28)* examined a discreet anatomical unit, the rat barrel field cortex, for Pb-induced effects. Cortical barrels in the rat somatosensory cortex are functional units comprised of neuronal aggregates that receive their input from the vibrissae of a rodent's whisker pad. These large whiskers are arranged in five rows that map topographically through the thalamus to the cortical barrels. The authors compared areas of the barrel field and individual barrels between controls and rat pups exposed to Pb from postnatal days 0 through 10, a time period during which target neurons cluster into barrels. The organization of the topographic map was not altered by Pb treatment. However, the authors found a 10–12% reduction in cortical barrel field area in neonatal rats with low Pb exposure (20–30 μg/dL in blood). These results suggest stunting of the arborization of thalamocortical axons in columnar processing units of the immature neocortex. The two studies are in good agreement that low-level Pb exposure during development alters axonal morphology in a manner that could impair connectivity and behavior.

In vitro models theoretically offer opportunities for examining the specific targets and mechanisms by which Pb alters neuronal morphology. Several such studies have been carried out that demonstrate a variety of effects on neurite development. As these models are refined, they should offer valuable insight into the chronology and mechanisms of Pb-induced alterations. Audesirk and colleagues *(63,64)* demonstrated a significant decrease in neurite initiation by cultured rat hippocampal neurons exposed to 25–100 n*M* Pb chloride. Axonal elongation and branching were not affected at these concentrations. The latter finding is at variance with the above-described in vivo effects and might reflect the lack of three-dimensional tissue interactions that exist in vivo. However, Kern and Audesirk *(21)* replicated their findings by showing a 25% reduction of neurite initiation, but not "axon" or "dendrite" length or branching by cultured rat hippocampal neurons exposed to 100 n*M* Pb for 2 d. An axon was descriptively identified as the process twofold longer than any other process on the cell. These authors provided evidence by the use of specific inhibitors that Pb might act by stimulating protein phosphorylation by Ca^{2+}/calmodulin-dependent protein kinase or protein kinase A. In contrast to these studies with cultured rat hippocampal neurons, studies with the PC12 rat pheochromocytoma cell line show that comparable Pb levels stimulate neurite outgrowth in cells treated with nerve growth factor (NGF) *(65,66)*. These differences might reflect differential responses of various types of neuron to Pb exposure, an area that merits further investigation. The differences also reflect a molecular effect, specifically a role for NGF and its receptor in responses of PC12 cells to Pb. NGF was not added to the primary cultures used by Audesirk and colleagues. Studies of molecular mechanisms by which Pb induces alterations in neuronal morphology and function are described in the next subsection.

2.2. Molecular Mechanisms in Neurons

The mechanisms by which Pb affects neuritogenesis have been examined both in vivo and in vitro. As diagrammed in Figure 2, neurite extension, the establishment of connectivity, and synaptosomal structuring are complex

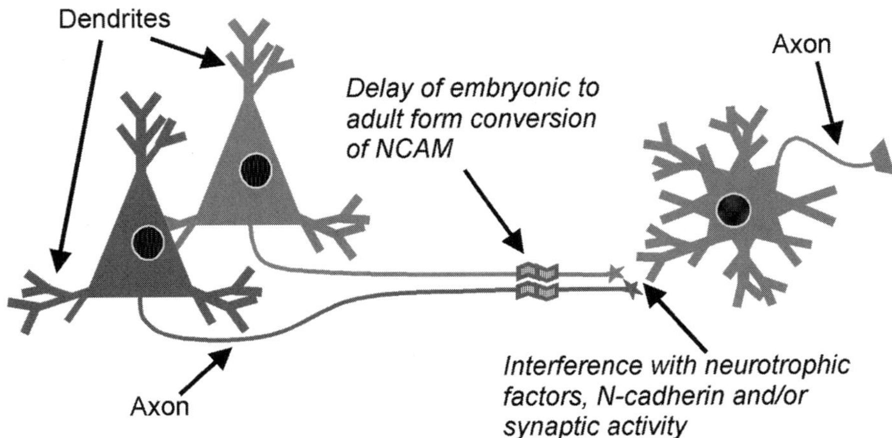

Fig. 2. Possible mechanisms of impairment of neurite growth and differentiation by lead. Shown are two pyramidal cells extending axons toward an interneuron. Growth cones at the tips of extending axons are guided along substrates to target cells by cell–substrate adhesion molecules, such as *N*-cadherin. Neurites form bundles by homophilic binding between neuronal cell adhesion molecules (NCAMs) on the plasma membranes of adjacent parallel axons. Neurotrophic factors and/or neurotransmitters attract growth cones of the developing axons to targets for synapse formation. Homophilic binding between synaptic *N*-cadherin molecules on presynaptic and postsynaptic membranes structurally stabilizes the synapse. Lead interferes with most or all of these molecular signaling mechanisms in neuritogenesis.

processes that require the coordinate function of appropriate adhesion and signaling molecules. Cell adhesion molecules are cell surface proteins that serve as mechanical links for cell–cell or cell–substrate attachment *(67)*. Pb is known to interfere with the expression of two of these molecules: the neuronal cell adhesion molecule (NCAM) and *N*-cadherin *(18,68)*. Both NCAM and *N*-cadherin are integral plasma membrane proteins of neurons that interact through homophilic binding to regulate cell–cell adhesion during development. NCAM and cadherins are viewed as potential targets for several neurotoxic metals, including Pb, Cd, and Hg *(69)*. Other possible targets are developmental proteins, including growth-associated protein 43 (GAP-43) and ornithine decarboxylase (ODC) *(70–72)*.

The neuronal cell adhesion molecule has been studied as a reporter molecule of synaptic elaboration in rats and birds exposed postnatally to Pb *(18,68)*. NCAM consists of several isoforms derived from alternative splicing of one gene *(73)*. Three major forms have been identified: NCAM-180, -140, and -120 *(74)*. NCAM-120 is the predominant isoform in glial cells *(75)*.

NCAM-180 and -140 are associated with neurite outgrowth. The embryonic form of NCAM is heavily sialylated with polysialic acid (PSA) residues connected by an α2,8 linkage, which are added to the protein core by sialyltransferase (ST) enzymes in the Golgi apparatus. The large negatively charged volume formed by the PSAs prevents premature homophilic interaction with other NCAMs and subsequent contact-mediated events in neuritogenesis. Conversion of the embryonic to adult form occurs via desialylation to coincide with synaptogenesis *(76–78)*. The conversion of the embryonic to the adult form of NCAM is delayed in the cerebellum of rats exposed postnatally to low levels of Pb through the dams' drinking water *(18,60,61)*. Similarly, the expression of synaptosomal PSA–NCAM (i.e., the embryonic form) is slightly increased on posthatching day 34 in herring gulls exposed to a single high dose of Pb acetate (100 mg/kg body weight) on posthatching day 2, but returns to the control level by d 44 *(68)*. Both Pb treatment regimens are associated with behavioral deficits without weight loss in their respective animal models. These findings suggest that the conversion of the embryonic to the adult form of NCAM is delayed by Pb, reflecting either direct stimulation of the enzyme that sialylates NCAM, inhibition of desialylation, or some other primary effect of Pb. In both the rat and herring gull studies, ST activity was stimulated in the Pb-treated animals to coincide with the prolonged appearance of PSA–NCAM expression.

Davey and Breen *(79)* examined the stimulation of ST activity by Pb in two neuronal cell lines that model different developmental stages, designated HN9 and HN25. HN9 and HN25 cells were generated respectively by the fusion of mouse N18TG2 neuroblastoma cells with hippocampal cells from an embryonic day 9 or a postnatal day 25 mouse. Both cell lines showed a twofold or greater stimulation of ST activity from continuous exposure to Pb acetate, although at different concentrations. In HN9 cells, stimulation occurred at 10^{-14} and 10^{-12} M Pb, but not at 10^{-10}, 10^{-8}, or 10^{-6} M. In contrast, ST activity was stimulated in HN25 cells to similar degrees by 10^{-10}, 10^{-8}, and 10^{-6} M Pb, but not by lower concentrations. Zinc had no effect on ST activity. The authors showed that in HN9 cells, the increase in ST activity was primarily from an increase in the protein level of α2,3(N) ST and not α2,6(N) ST, that an exponential increase in enzyme activity occurred between 48 and 96 h of Pb exposure, and that *de novo* protein synthesis was required for stimulation of enzyme activity. The lag time for enzyme induction was attributed to the gradual intracellular accumulation of Pb, although these levels were too low to be detectable. The cell lines used do not express PSA–NCAM, but rather the desialylated forms. Therefore, Pb effects on the expression of embryonic and adult forms of NCAM could not be measured. Nevertheless, this cell culture study is in agreement with the conclusion of in vivo studies that ST activity is stimulated by Pb in neural cells. The cell lines provide models for further study of detailed cellular mechanisms by which Pb can impair the development of neuronal connectivity.

In the herring gull study discussed earlier, synaptosomal *N*-cadherin levels were significantly decreased on posthatching days 34 and 44, recovering to control levels on d 55 *(68)*. *N*-Cadherin has two roles in the establishment of neuronal connectivity. First, during the outgrowth of neurites, *N*-cadherin mediates the movement of growth cones along extracellular substrates (e.g., the surfaces of axon bundles) *(80,81)*. *N*-Cadherin is expressed at high levels on neurites during axonal elongation and diminishes after the axon has synapsed with its target *(82)*. Second, *N*-cadherin is localized within synapses, forming adherens junctions that frame the neurotransmitter release zone *(67,83,84)*. The finding that Pb treatment decreases *N*-cadherin levels highlights an additional target for the disruption of neuronal development. This target has not yet been examined in a cell culture model.

A number of other mechanisms by which Pb might disrupt normal neuritogenesis or synaptogenesis have been identified, including processes involving neurotrophic factors. These mechanisms might be important not only in development but throughout life, because neurites are constantly remodeled in adulthood. Two studies provide evidence for an interaction between Pb and NGF on neurons. Zhou et al. *(85)* found that nerve growth factor (NGF) protects rats pups exposed to Pb (0.2% in dams' drinking water) from the Pb-induced loss of cholinergic neurons in the septum. NGF conferred complete protection only if administered on postnatal day 2, but not on d 4, 11, or 18. This finding implies a critical period of vulnerability of the developing rat septum that is amenable to rescue by NGF. The mechanism of rescue is unknown. In an in vitro study, Crumpton et al. *(66)* have shown that Pb acetate (0.025–1.0 μM) or recombinant human NGF (0.3–50 ng/mL) each stimulates similar increases in binding of the transcription factor Sp1 to DNA in PC12 nuclear extracts, and their effects are not additive when administered concurrently. The authors report temporal evidence that Sp1 DNA binding is mechanistically linked to the stimulation of neurite outgrowth by NGF or Pb and speculate that Pb may possess neurotrophic activity.

Additional studies indicate that Pb can interfere with other growth-associated proteins, including GAP-43 and ODC. GAP-43 is a major component of neuronal growth cones that is expressed by neurons during neurite elongation *(86)*. GAP-43 expression is repressed when neuronal process extension is completed. Zawia and Harry *(70)* found that mRNA expression for GAP-43 is significantly stimulated in the cerebellum of rat pups postnatally exposed to Pb via the dam's drinking water (0.2% Pb acetate) on postnatal day 9. This finding suggests a disruption of the normal pattern of neuronal elongation. ODC is a critical growth-specific enzyme associated with brain damage and disease. ODC carries out the decarboxylation of L-ornithine to form putrescine, which is the precursor to the natural polyamines spermidine and spermine. These polyamines are critical for numerous metabolic processes in the developing and mature nervous systems. ODC is localized to neurons in the nervous system, although astroglial expression occurs in reactive astrocytes *(87)*. In rats exposed to Pb via the dams' drinking water (0.2% Pb acetate), prenatal exposure (gestational day 13 to birth) to Pb alters the specific activity of ODC in the hippocampus, neocortex and cerebellum, whereas postnatal exposure (1–15 d after birth) stimulates ODC activity in the cerebellum *(71,72)*. The observation that ODC activity is stimulated in the hippocampus following prenatal exposure is of interest because an increase in ODC gene expression has been suggested as a prognostic factor for predicting recurrence in meningiomas *(88)*. The mechanism of Pb-induced ODC activity remains to be explored, although it has been observed that 0.01 and 0.1 μM Pb stimulate but 1 μM inhibits ODC activity in vitro *(72)*. Studies with PC12 cells suggest that ODC activity can be regulated by protein kinase C *(89)*, which is activated by Pb, as reviewed in Chapter 4.

3. EFFECTS OF LEAD ON MYELINATING CELLS

Lead has been known for decades to induce morphological changes in the myelin sheath of axons in both the central and peripheral nervous systems. Hypomyelination or demyelination occurs in rats exposed to high lead levels during neonatal or early postnatal development *(90–93)*, and peripheral neuropathies in occupationally exposed adults *(94)*. In addition, both humans and animal models show reduced nerve conduction velocity with Pb exposure, suggesting damage to the myelin sheath *(95)*. As described in the next sections, cell-specific responses of Schwann cells have been studied very little in vitro, although oligodendroglia have been the focus of a number of recent studies from one team of investigators.

3.1. Schwann Cell Myelination and Morphology

The direct effects of Pb on Schwann cells have received little study in cell culture models, probably because of the lack of good models for myelination in vitro *(96)*. However, two studies indicate that Schwann cells are sensitive primary targets for Pb-induced damage. In the first study, it was shown that partial inhibition of myelination in embryonic rat dorsal root ganglion explants occurs in cultures exposed to 0.1 μM Pb for 28 d *(29)*. Evidence from a second study shows ultrastructural abnormalities in rat Schwann cells exposed in culture to 1 μM Pb acetate for 24–96 h. Alterations include an increase of cell surface blebs, mitochondrial swelling, enlargement of rough endoplasmic reticulum cisternae, cytoplasmic vacuolization, and formation of myelinoid bodies. In contrast, cultured rat astroglia do not show comparable changes below 10 μM Pb *(30)*. The latter study supports the idea that myelinating cells are more sensitive than astrocytes to Pb- induced damage.

3.2. Oligodendroglial Development

Structural alterations of myelin in the CNS are associated with moderate and high lead exposure. For example, ultrastructural abnormalities occur in 90% of the myelin in juvenile rats chronically exposed to low lead levels that produce an average blood lead level of 38.2 µg/dL *(97)*. In vitro models offer a means for testing the possibility that these alterations represent a direct, rather than a secondary, effect of Pb on oligodendroglia. An early study showed the reduction of glycerol phosphate dehydrogenase (GPDH) activity in cultured oligodendroglia from a single exposure to a high concentration (100 μM) of Pb acetate *(98)*. This finding is paralleled by the reduction of GPDH activity in fetal guinea pigs and their dams exposed to low lead levels that produced blood lead levels of 11–39 µg/dL in blood *(99)*. Whereas GPDH is a developmental enzyme of oligodendroglia *(100)*, these findings suggest delayed development.

More recent work by Poretz and co-workers *(31)* clearly shows that Pb delays the progression of oligodendrocyte precursor cells through differentiation. The results of their work are summarized in Fig. 3. These investigators used well-characterized oligodendroglial cell cultures in which differentiation was experimentally controlled and various stages of differentiation were distinguished by immunofluorescence labeling for the stage-specific markers A2B5, O4, galactocerebroside (GC), 2', 3'-cyclic nucleotide 3'-phosphohydrolase (CNP), and myelin basic protein (MBP), listed in order of developmental appearance. Pb concentrations over a range comparable to low and moderate exposure in rats were tested. Oligodendrocyte progenitor (OP) cells were prepared from neonatal rat mixed glial cultures and maintained in the presence of basic fibroblast growth factor (bFGF) and platelet derived growth factor (PDGF) to prevent their differentiation. When bFGF and PDGF were no longer added to the medium, the OPs differentiated into oligodendrocytes (OLs). The investigators found that a single treatment with 1 μM Pb acetate 24 h before removal of the growth factors delays progression of OP cells from A2B5+ progenitor cells to O4+ late progenitor cells. However, by d 4 after withdrawal of growth factors, control and Pb-treated cells achieve the same stage of differentiation. Furthermore, this level

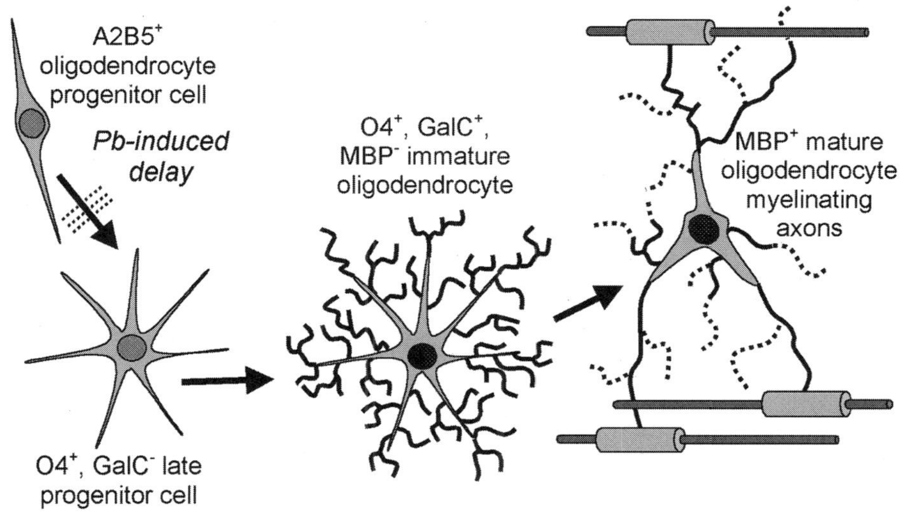

Fig. 3. Effects of lead on the developmental potential of oligodendrocyte lineage cells. Shown are four morphologically distinct stages of oligodendrocyte differentiation. A2B5+ is a surface ganglioside expressed by oligodendrocyte progenitor cells. The O4 antigen is a marker for late oligodendrocyte progenitors, galactocerebrocide (GalC) is expressed by postmitotic differentiated oligodendrocytes at both immature (premyelinating) and mature stages, and myelin basic protein (MPB) is a structural myelin protein of mature oligodendrocytes. Low-level Pb exposure has been shown in vitro to delay the differentiation of oligodendrocyte progenitor cells, as evidenced by the delayed appearance of both a multibranched morphology and O4. However, the cells eventually differentiate, even in the continued presence of Pb. Postmitotic immature oligodendrocytes progress at the normal rate through differentiation in the presence of Pb.

of Pb has no effect on subsequent maturation of postmitotic young oligodendrocytes, indicating that differentiated oligodendrocytes are resistant to the effects of Pb.

Poretz' group also showed that Pb-exposed oligodendroglia in culture have reduced cell numbers, an effect that is dependent on degree of differentiation *(31)*. OP cells continue to divide in culture, whereas OLs cease dividing. Total cell numbers in OP cultures are reduced by exposure to 1 μM Pb acetate for 3–7 d, suggesting a decrease of proliferation or survival. Total cell numbers are also reduced in nonproliferating OL cultures, although higher Pb concentrations and longer exposures are needed, supporting the idea that mature oligodendrocytes become resistant to some of the deleterious effects of Pb. Protein kinase C activation appears to be required for both the inhibition of differentiation and proliferative capacity in OP cells by Pb *(101)*.

The same investigators examined the developmental levels of myelin-specific galactolipids and their metabolic enzymes in several experiments. In a cell culture experiment, galactolipids in cultured cells were metabolically radiolabeled with ^{3}H-D-galactose and ratios between pairs of galactolipids were determined. The cell type examined was a central glia-4-like (CG-4-like) cell line, which is a propagating cell line established from primary OP cultures by repeated passage in medium containing a high percentage of neuroblastoma B104-conditioned medium. The ratio of nonhydroxy fatty acid galactocerebroside to glucocerebroside normally increases during differentiation in untreated cells *(102)*, but this increase was significantly less in cultures treated with 5 μ*M* Pb for 6 d *(31)*. The ratio of hydroxy fatty acid to nonhydroxy fatty acid galactocerebroside and the ratio of galactocerebrosides to sulfatides were also depressed. These findings suggest that Pb interferes with developmentally regulated galactolipid expression in oligodendroglia. Similar reductions occur in brain tissue of rats developmentally exposed to Pb, which substantiates the cell culture finding. However, the animals in the in vivo study were exposed to Pb levels so high as to cause significant weight loss, an important confounding factor (500 or 2000 ppm Pb in the dams' drinking water during gestation and lactation, as well as pups' drinking water after weaning). The blood lead levels in the pups were 62 and 63 μg/dL on d 7 in the two groups, respectively, rising to 58 and 152 μg/dL on d 14 *(103)*. This study has not been repeated with lower Pb doses in vivo.

Changes in specific activities of galactolipid metabolic enzymes in brain tissue of rats exposed to Pb during development *(103)* and in Pb-treated OL cells *(104)* confirm that Pb perturbs the galactolipid pathway. Rat pups exposed to Pb as described in the preceding paragraph show dose-dependent decreases in CNP specific activity on postnatal days 14–56. This finding suggests a reduced number of mature oligodendrocytes. Biosynthetic and catabolic enzymes in the galactolipid pathway likewise show reduced activities. As mentioned earlier, weight loss in the pups is a confounding factor. However, an in vitro study by the same investigators shows similar reductions in galactolipid metabolic enzymes and CNP in OP cultures treated with 1 μ*M* Pb acetate 24 h before removal of the growth factors. After 6 d of differentiation in the presence of Pb, enzyme levels recover to those of Na-treated controls, with the exception of arylsulfatase A (ARSA), which remains depressed *(104)*. This finding is of interest, as Poretz and colleagues *(105,106)* reported that Pb causes a missorting of ARSA in human fibroblasts and speculate that humans with an inherited deficiency in ARSA could have enhanced susceptibility to Pb-induced neurotoxicity.

The significance of delays in the progression of oligodendrocyte progenitor cells through differentiation may extend beyond probable delays in the onset or extent of myelination. Evidence has recently been presented from in vitro studies that oligodendrocytes enhance axonal growth *(107)* and neuronal survival *(108)*, and stimulate Na^+ channel clustering in neurons *(109)*. There is also evidence in the demyelinating "twitcher" mutant mouse that perineuronal oligodendroglia protect against neuronal apoptosis by upregulation of lipocalcin-type prostaglandin D synthase, an enzyme expressed in mature oligodendrocytes *(110)*. These intercellular dependencies emphasize the importance of understanding the effects of Pb on specific cell types in order to understand the mechanisms of Pb-induced developmental neurotoxicity.

3.3. Oligodendroglial Gene Expression

The delay in oligodendrocyte progenitor differentiation found by Poretz and colleagues *(31)* would not have been predicted from the early onset of myelin gene expression found by Zawia and Harry *(70,111)* and, indeed, the opposite was predicted (i.e., accelerated oligodendroglial development). Zawia and Harry used an in vivo rat pup model that differed in some respects from that of Deng and Poretz *(103)*, the most important being the developmental stage of exposure. In the Zawia and Harry model, rats were exposed to 0.2% Pb acetate in the dams' drinking water from birth to postnatal day 20, and therefore were not exposed during gestation. In the first of two studies with rats *(111)*, a developmental pattern for gene expression in the brain frontal lobes of control pups was established for MPB, CNP, and proteolipid protein (PLP), a structural myelin protein. In controls, all three mRNA levels peaked on postnatal day 20, followed by a sharp decline. However, the mRNA level for PLP significantly increased on d 20 in Pb-treated rats, but not at other time-points (postnatal days 6, 9, 12, 15, and 25). Pb treatment did not significantly alter expression of the other two myelin mRNAs at any time-point.

In a second study, Zawia and Harry performed a similar study of MPB mRNA expression in rat cerebellum, again finding a peak of mRNA levels on postnatal day 20, followed by a reduction on d 25 that remained level through day 50 *(70)*. Pb-treated animals differed in two respects from controls: the level of MBP mRNA expression was much lower than controls from d 20 to d 50, and an early onset of gene expression was noted, beginning on postnatal day 9. These findings again suggest transiently accelerated oligodendroglial development, rather than delayed development. On the other hand, the finding that cerebellar mRNA levels for MBP were depressed after weaning and into adulthood by Pb treatment is consistent with the loss of myelin markers observed in the study by Deng and Poretz *(103)*. The developmental period of Pb exposure probably is a key factor in responses of oligodendroglial linage cells to Pb exposure, and further investigation will be required to clearly identify the targets that are affected by Pb during each developmental event. Aside from its potential developmental implications, the finding that postnatal Pb exposure induces MBP and PLP gene expression offers intriguing evidence to support the proposal that Pb is a carcinogen. MBP and PLP have been suggested as molecular markers to identify human astrocytomas or oligodendrogliomas *(112)*. Pb is classified as a possible carcinogen *(113–115)*.

Zawia and colleagues have continued their investigation of mechanisms by which Pb may alter the gene expression of MPB and PLP in oligodendroglia through studies of the zinc-finger protein Sp1. Sp1 is a component of a transcriptional complex that participates in the regulation of genes rich in GC elements. Some genes under Sp1 control are MBP *(116)*, PLP *(117)*, ODC *(118)*, and NMDA receptor 1 *(119)*. Sp1 levels are 100-fold higher in differentiating cells than mature cells *(120)*, supporting the idea that this protein has an important role in cell differentiation. MBP and PLP genes contain multiple Sp1 promoter regions, and Sp1 plays a critical role during oligodendrocyte development in the human brain *(117)*. In cerebellar tissue from rats exposed to 0.2% Pb acetate in the dams' water from birth to weaning, the peak developmental period of increased binding of the Sp1 consensus sequence to nuclear extracts is shifted from postnatal days 20–30 to d 5–10. This shift corresponds temporally with the premature expression of mRNAs for MBP and PLP *(70,121)*. Neither DNA binding of the transcription factor necrosis factor (NF)-κB nor expression of the tubulin gene is affected in Pb-treated animals, suggesting specificity of Pb for Sp1 and genes it regulates. In PC12 cell cultures, 0.1 μM Pb acetate added to the medium shifts maximal NGF-stimulated Sp1–DNA binding from about 48 h to 0.5 h *(66,121)*, which is congruent with in vivo results. The effect of Pb on Sp1 binding has not been studied as yet in oligodendroglial cultures. Studies with a recombinant peptide of the human Sp1 active domain containing a Zn-finger motif show that Pb, Hg, and Cd, but not Ca, can modulate Sp1 function through selective binding to the Zn-finger motif *(122,123)*. A diagram of a possible interaction of Pb with Sp1 leading to upregulation of MPB and PLP expression is given in Fig. 4. An additional consideration is that the transcription factor activating protein-1 (AP-1) is probably involved in the modulation of Sp1- regulated

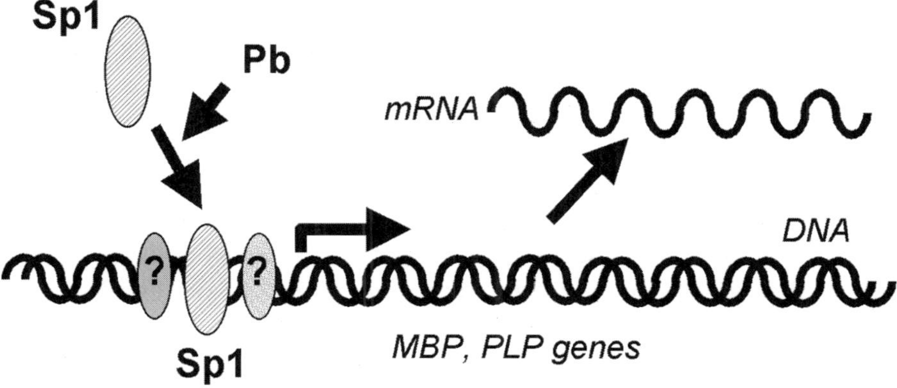

Fig. 4. Modulation of gene expression by lead in oligodendroglia. Pb may alter brain development through modulation of the zinc-finger protein Sp1. Sp1 is a component of a transcriptional complex for gene regulation. It targets *MBP*, *PLP*, and other genes. Sp1 levels are 100-fold higher in differentiating cells than mature cells. Premature Sp1–DNA binding and MBP and PLP mRNA expression occur in cerebella of rat pups exposed postnatally to Pb.

MBP gene expression, because an AP-1-like binding site has been identified in the promoter of the MBP gene *(124)*.

4. LEAD STORAGE AND NEUROTOXICITY IN ASTROGLIA

Astroglia are generally considered the most resistant cell type in the nervous system to morphological and cytocidal effects of Pb and are the presumed repositories for Pb deposition in the brain. Toxic effects of Pb to astroglia have been reviewed regularly over the past 20 yr, and the reader is referred to these reviews for work prior to 1998. Among the effects reported are minimal pathology or cell death at low and moderate exposure levels, minimal or slight elevations in glial fibrillary acidic protein, alterations in glutamine synthetase activity, alterations in calcium ion homeostasis, and Cu accumulation *(45,47,48,125–128)*. More recently, the view has been taken that some responses of astroglia of Pb are stress responses, including induction of heat shock proteins (HSPs) *(129–132)* and the 78-kDa glucose regulated protein (GRP78) *(42–44)*. The upregulation of glial fibrillary acidic protein (GFAP), which is the major intermediate filament cytoskeletal protein of mature astrocytes, can also be viewed as a response to stress, as it is a hallmark of reactive gliosis. The subjects will be considered in the remainder of the chapter.

4.1. Lead Deposition in Astroglia

The brain accumulates Pb when the blood Pb level is elevated *(133)*, but has no known mechanisms for its removal. Astroglia are a key cell type in understanding Pb deposition and neurotoxicity in the brain because they are the major site for Pb accumulation *(45,134)*. Three seminal in vivo studies support the concept that Pb is selectively deposited in astroglia after it crosses the blood–brain barrier. First, Thomas et al. *(135)* observed that 72 h after 1-d-old rat pups are injected with ^{210}Pb, Pb is localized autoradiographically to capillary endothelium and astroglial footplates in the cerebellum. Second, Shirabe and Hirano *(136)* demonstrated the presence of cytoplasmic and intranuclear inclusions in macrophages and astroglia by energy-dispersive X-ray (EDX) microanalysis with transmission electron microscopy in adult rats 6 mo after implantation of Pb acetate pellets into their forebrains. Third, Holtzman et al. *(45)* showed that in weanling rats dosed daily with high amounts of Pb, a Pb-sequestering property is exhibited by astroglia in more differentiated brain tissue, but not in less mature brain tissue. The subcellular distribution of Pb in cerebral tissue was found by EDX microanalysis to be in astroglial cytoplasm, lysosomes, and nuclei, but not in neurons. In contrast, Pb was distributed throughout the organelles of both astroglia and neurons in the cerebellum. From these observations arose the hypothesis *(45)*, subsequently dubbed the "lead sink hypothesis" *(125)*, that astroglia *in situ*, when they are sufficiently mature, have the capacity to take up Pb into nontoxic subcellular sites, potentially protecting neurons. The study by Holtzman et al. *(45)* did not address long-term distribution (and possible redistribution) of Pb in brain nor did it address distribution of Pb in low-level exposure conditions.

Cell culture studies have been carried out to test the Pb sink hypothesis, with conflicting results. Early cell culture work from our laboratory with atomic absorption spectroscopy (AAS) showed that rat astroglia in culture take up Pb from the surrounding medium and concentrate it up to 10,000-fold the extracellular level *(32,38,125)*. This finding tended to support the Pb sink hypothesis, although Pb accumulation was not examined in neurons. On the other hand, Zurich et al. *(137)* found that neuron-enriched aggregating cell cultures from fetal rat brain accumulated twice as much Pb as glial-enriched cultures when both were treated with low Pb levels. A confounding factor in the latter study was that only the neuron-enriched cultures were exposed to depolarizing levels of K$^+$ during Pb treatment. The depolarization of the cultures by the high K^+ concentration was considered by the authors to be a possible influence on Pb accumulation, and indeed depolarization has been shown to greatly enhance Pb uptake by a voltage-regulated Ca^{2+} channel *(59)*.

In another study, we addressed the question of whether the apparent ability of astroglia to serve as a Pb sink in the mature brain tissue might result either from the strategic location of astroglia between the blood–brain barrier and neurons or from intrinsic differences between the ability of astroglia and neurons to take up this metal *(134)*. We compared Pb accumulation, as measured by AAS, in the SY5Y human neuroblastoma cell line with that of primary cultures of astroglia established from neonatal rats. After treatment with 1 μM Pb daily for up to 1 wk, astroglia accumulated up to 14-fold more intracellular Pb than did neuroblastoma cells. Furthermore, astroglial cells were stimulated to accumulate more Pb by treatment with conditioned medium from SY5Y cultures. In contrast, SY5Y cells differentiated by human recombinant β-NGF took up significantly less Pb than did undifferentiated SY5Y cells, suggesting that differentiated neurons either lose the ability the take up Pb or develop the capacity to exclude most of it. These findings were further explored in a bicameral coculture (Millipore® filter) system in which astroglia were cocultured with SY5Y cells and both were exposed to Pb in shared medium. In coculture, astroglia accumulated at least 14-fold more Pb than did SY5Y cells. It appears that astroglia have an intrinsic ability to take up substantially more Pb than do neuronal cells, an ability that is enhanced by interactions with neuronal cells. The idea that the Pb-sequestering property of astroglia is specifically inducible in neuronal cells strongly supports and further refines the original Pb sink hypothesis.

4.2. Interactions of Lead with Other Metals

Several characteristics of astroglia suggest that they have the capacity to serve as depots or distribution sites for metals in the brain. First, astroglia are histoarchitecturally positioned on the abluminal side of blood vessels to be the first cells of the brain parenchyma that encounter metals crossing the blood–brain barrier *(138)*. Second, astroglia have high cytosolic levels of metallothioneins I and II, in contrast to low levels in neurons *(139,140)*. Metallothionein III has been localized to hippocampal neurons *(141,142)* and astrocytes *(143)*. Through their high binding affinities for metals, metallothioneins could allow astroglia to chelate certain free metals in the brain as a neuroprotective action *(144)*. Metallothionein mRNA and protein are inducible in cultured astrocytes by Cd^{2+}, Hg^{2+}, and Zn^+, although not by Pb^{2+} *(145)*. Third, astroglia have higher cytosolic levels of the redox buffering molecule glutathione (GSH) than do neurons *(146–148)*. Fourth, astroglia have metal transport proteins, including ceruloplasmin *(149,150)*, ATP7a (Cu-ATPase or Menkes protein) *(151,152)*, and divalent cation transporter-1 (DCT-1) *(44)*. Potential interactions between Pb and the mechanisms by which cells handle essential metals emphasize the importance of examining metal interactions when studying the mechanisms of action of neurotoxic metals. This topic has recently been reviewed *(127)*.

The metal-handling machinery of astroglia presents numerous possible sites for interactions with Pb, some of which may be mechanisms for metabolic damage. Among them is interference with metal transport proteins. The idea that Pb might disrupt the normal physiological balance of trace metals in brain tissue is supported by animal studies showing an elevation of Cu in brain tissue of Pb-exposed animals *(99,153,154)*. An effect of Pb accumulation in astroglia that has been observed in cell cultures is the transient accumulation of Cu *(38)*. We have further examined this phenomenon in the C6 rat glioma cell line, which expresses the astroglial property of Pb accumulation *(155)*, and found that Pb blocks Cu efflux, apparently by inhibiting the Cu efflux pump ATP7a, also known as Menkes protein *(39,40)*.

These observations regarding Cu have led our laboratory to a more general consideration of astroglia as key cells that accumulate several metals, including Cu and Mn, a property that gives these cells roles as either metal depots, relay stations for metals, or sites for toxic damage. A predominant astroglial localization of Mn in the brain has been inferred from observations that 80% of the Mn in brain is associated with glutamine synthetase *(156)*, which is localized primarily to astroglia *(157)*. However, Mn localization has not been confirmed by comparisons of age-matched neurons and astrocytes, either in vivo or in vitro. Astroglia have an emerging role in the maintenance of brain Cu homeostasis, based on observations with brindled and macular mouse models for Menkes disease. Astroglia are hypothesized to transport Cu from the endothelial cells forming the blood–brain barrier to neurons. Neurons in patients with Menkes disease are deficient in Cu, leading to neuronal death *(158,159)*. Figure 5 depicts a hypothetical model in which Pb accumulation by astroglia could result in Cu accumulation and impaired astroglial function. Whereas a role of astroglia might be to supply neurons with Cu, their reduced ability to do so would compromise neuronal function *(160)*. Also shown in the figure is signaling activity whereby neurons stimulate the capacity for astrocytes to accumulate Pb *(134)*.

4.3. Stress Responses in Astroglia

Since recognition in the 1980s that astroglia apparently function as a depot for Pb and possibly other metals, studies have focused on the role of stress

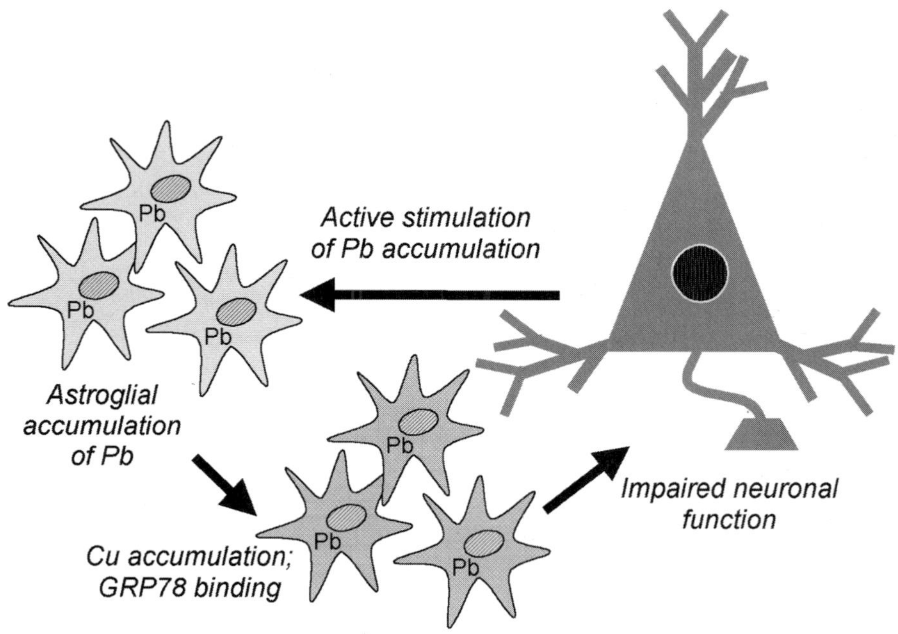

Fig. 5. Functional effects of lead accumulation by astroglia. Mature astrocytes accumulate Pb intracellularly to a much higher concentration than do mature neurons. Pb accumulation in glia is associated with the inhibition of Cu efflux via the ATP7a (Menkes) protein and transient intracellular accumulation of Cu. Cu transport from astrocytes to neurons during development might, therefore, be impaired. Neurons provide a soluble signal to developing astrocytes that stimulates their ability to accumulate Pb.

proteins in Pb tolerance in these cells. Cultured astroglia exposed to low levels of Pb in culture show multiple indications of oxidative stress or endoplasmic reticulum (ER) stress, including transient depletion and subsequent elevation of intracellular GSH levels *(41)*, loss of mitochondrial membrane potential *(41)*, increased binding of the ROS-activated transcription factors AP-1 *(161)* and NF-κB to DNA *(43)*, and induction of stress proteins. Opanashuk and Finkelstein *(129,130)* found that Pb concentrations of 5 and 50 μ*M* induce *de novo* biosynthesis of a set of stress proteins, including HSP70, in cultured rat astroglia. The transient induction of HSP70 protein was subsequently observed in brain tissue of 21- to 45-d-old rats exposed to a moderately high Pb dose (1% in dams' drinking water, as well as pups' drinking water after weaning) during gestation and up to postnatal day 160 *(131)*.

Li and Rossman *(132)* showed that gene expression of HSP90 is increased after treatment of wild-type C6 rat glioma cells with very high concentrations of Pb nitrate (100–600 µ*M*) for 24 h. As previously mentioned, the C6 cell line is an astroglialike cell line that takes up and stores large quantities of Pb *(155)*. They also noted that HSP90 was one of seven genes upregulated or overexpressed in a Pb-resistant variant of C6 cells, PbR11, which is about sixfold more resistant to Pb-induced cytotoxity than wild-type C6 cells. However, other genes that are upregulated in PbR11 cells compared to wild-type cells, which include thrombospondin-1, heparin sulfate 6-sulfotransferase, neuropilin-1, ubiqitinlike activating enzyme E1C, and rat endogenous retrovirus, were not induced by Pb in wild-type C6 cells. The selective sensitivity of HSP90 suggests that HSP90 may be particularly responsive to Pb, even in Pb-tolerant cells. HSP90 is a molecular chaperone that is required for the proper folding of certain proteins *(162,163)*. The Pb-resistant clone may be a useful model in which to study induction of HSP90 by Pb.

Like HSP90, GRP78 is a molecular chaperone required for protein folding and is induced by stress. We have reported the induction of gene expression of GRP78 at both the mRNA and protein levels in C6 cells exposed to 1 µ*M* Pb acetate for 1 wk *(42,43)*. Induction also occurs in rat primary astroglia *(44)*. GRP78 is one of several ER-resident proteins, others being a 94-kDa glucose-regulated protein (GRP94), protein disulfide isomerase (PDI), and calreticulin, that have been identified as ER stress markers *(164–167)*. Under conditions of oxidative or chemical stress, the ER undergoes a stress response termed the unfolded (or misfolded) protein response (UPR) *(168,169)*. GRP78 gene expression is highly inducible in a delayed fashion (e.g., 12 h) at the transcriptional level by chemicals that disrupt redox potential *(170)*, organelle Ca^{2+} homeostasis *(169)*, and protein phosphorylation *(171)*. Our finding that Pb exposure upregulates gene and protein expression of GRP78 in C6 cells *(42,43)* is in agreement with upregulation of gene expression seen in Pb-exposed HepG2 hepatoma cells *(172)*. The mechanism for GRP78 induction is unknown. However, Pb can specifically bind to GRP78 in vitro *(42)*. It remains to be clarified whether the induction of GRP78 by Pb exposure provides tolerance to Pb or is a pathological response, as GRP78 is overexpressed in malignant human breast lesions *(173)*. We also note that C6 cells have much higher GRP78 mRNA and protein levels than rat primary astroglia in culture (Qian et al., unpublished data). Furthermore, an increase of tumor necrosis factor-α (TNF-α) gene expression by Pb has been reported in a human U-373MG glioma cell line *(174)*. These observations suggest mechanisms for the potential carcinogenicity of Pb.

The mechanisms by which Pb induces oxidative and ER stress in astroglia are open to speculation, as Pb has no redox potential, but exists in biological tissues at a single +2 valence state. The cellular homeostatic mechanisms perturbed by Pb that result in oxidative stress to the cell are probably multiple. As yet, studies have not provided direct evidence to link a primary effect of Pb exposure with secondary alterations in the cellular redox state. Whereas Cu is highly redox reactive because of its shifts between the cuprous and cupric ionic forms, Cu accumulation might be the primary effect of Pb exposure that leads to oxidative stress. Alternatively, the binding of Pb to GRP78 might be sufficient to produce ER stress and subsequent oxidative stress.

As a result of stress conditions such as trauma, infection, some diseases, and some types of toxic exposure, astrocytes could exhibit a unique morphological stress response known as gliosis *(175)*. Gliosis is characterized by several features: astroglial proliferation, astroglial hypertrophy, scar formation involving astrocytes and meningeal fibroblasts, and an increase in cytoskeletal intermediate filaments, specifically GFAP. In vivo and in vitro studies tend to show little correlation with regard to gliotic responses of astrocytes to Pb exposure. Gliosis does not occur in vitro in purified astroglial cultures treated with either low or high concentrations of Pb *(46,125)*. In vivo, responses are more varied and appear to depend on duration and developmental window of exposure, as well as brain region. For example, gene expression for GFAP is decreased from d 30 to d 50 in the cerebellum of rats exposed from birth to postnatal day 20 via 0.2% Pb acetate in the dams' drinking water *(70)*. A similar finding has been reported in hippocampus *(176)*. GFAP protein expression is elevated in young rats chronically exposed to moderately high Pb levels *(177,178)*. Acute exposure of adult rats to Pb acetate (25 mg/kg body weight intraperitoneally for 3 d) results in enhanced GFAP protein expression in the hippocampus and cerebral cortex but not in cerebellum *(179)*. One explanation for these results is that mature astrocytes become gliotic in response to primary damage to neurons *(126,179)*. It should be possible to clarify the signals required for Pb-induced astrogliosis in cell culture models through the use of cocultures with other cell types, including neurons, cerebrovascular endothelial cells, and microglia.

5. SUMMARY AND RESEARCH NEEDS

Information generated from in vitro studies is beginning to yield an improved understanding of the effects of Pb on neuronal and glial cells, if not of complete mechanisms, then at least of their complexity. Among the general conclusions from these studies and parallel in vivo studies are the following:

- Lead affects neurons, oligodendroglia, Schwann cells, and astroglia at toxicologically relevant concentrations in vivo and in vitro.
- Myelinating cells and neurons are more sensitive to Pb-induced structural damage or cytotoxicity than are astroglia, but functional sensitivities might be similar among cell types.
- Developmental windows of cellular vulnerability to Pb are highly relevant but poorly understood.
- Accumulation of Pb by astroglia is associated with sublethal alterations in metabolism and gene expression. However, the mechanistic significance of astroglial Pb accumulation with respect to Pb neurotoxicity is poorly understood.
- Deleterious effects of Pb on neuronal development and function involve numerous mechanisms, including some mediated by direct effects upon glia.

These conclusions suggest an abundance of fruitful areas for further investigation that should bring about a better understanding not only of cellular mechanisms of neurotoxicity but also of intercellular interactions in the nervous system. Pb may be considered a tool for probing some of these interactions. Some suggested areas for further research are the following: a mechanistic integration of the effects of lead on behavior with molecular effects of Pb on neurons and glia; the morphologic, physiologic, and molecular effects of Pb on synaptogenesis; the complete chronological fate of Pb distribution in brain (early vs late distribution in cell types); the mechanisms of Pb uptake, storage and release by astroglia; the basis for differences in Pb handling between immature and mature astroglia; linkage of neurobehavioral deficits Pb-delayed development of oligodendroglia; and metabolic interactions of Pb with essential metals.

ACKNOWLEDGMENTS

The authors' work is supported by National Institutes of Health grants P42 ES04917, P30 ES09106 and T32 ES07273 and by ATSDR grant U61/ATU684505. We thank Dr. Ronald Poretz for his helpful comments on the section on oligodendroglia.

REFERENCES

1. ATSDR (2001) *CERCLA List of Priority Hazardous Substances*, ATSDR Information Center, Division of Toxicology, Agency for Toxic Substances and Disease Registry, US Department of Health and Human Services, Atlanta, GA.
2. Banks, E. C., Ferretti, L. E., and Shucard, D. W. (1997) Effects of low level lead exposure on cognitive function in children: a review of behavioral, neuropsychological and biological evidence. *Neurotoxicology* **18,** 237–282.
3. Markowitz, M. (2000) Lead poisoning: a disease for the new millennium. *Curr. Probl. Pediatr.* **30,** 62–70.

4. Tong, S., von Schirnding, Y. E., and Prapamontol, T. (2000) Environmental lead exposure: a public health problem of global dimensions. *Bull. World Health Organ.* **78,** 1068–1077.

5. Needleman, H. L., Gunnoe, C., Leviton, A., et al. (1979) Deficits in psychologic and classroom performance of children with elevated dentine lead levels. *N. Engl. J. Med.* **300,** 689–695.

6. Stiles, K. M. and Bellinger, D. C. (1993) Neuropsychological correlates of low-level lead exposure in school-age children: a prospective study. *Neurotoxicol. Teratol.* **15,** 27–35.

7. Schwartz, J. (1994) Low-level lead exposure and children's IQ: a meta-analysis and search for threshold. *Environ. Res.* **65,** 42–6555.

8. Needleman, H. L., Riess, J. A., Tobin, M. J., Biesecker, G. E., and Greenhouse, J.B. (1996) Bone lead levels and delinquent behavior. *J. Am. Med. Assoc.* **275,** 363–369.

9. Centers for Disease Control and Prevention (1991) Preventing lead poisoning in young children: a statement by the Centers for Disease Control. US Department of Health and Human Services, Atlanta, GA.

10. United States Environmental Protection Agency (2000) *America's Children and the Environment: A First View of Available Measures*, US EPA, Research Triangle Park, NC.

11. Duckett, S., Galle., P., and Kradin, R. (1977) The relationship between Parkinson syndrome and vascular siderosis: an electron microprobe study. *Ann. Neurol.* **2,** 225–229.

12. Gorell, J. M., Johnson, C. C., Rybicki, B. A., et al. (1999) Occupational exposure to manganese, copper, lead, iron, mercury and zinc and the risk of Parkinson's disease. *Neurotoxicology* **20,** 239–248.

13. Gorell, J. M., Rybicki, B. A., Johnson, C. C., and Peterson, E. L. (1999) Occupational metal exposures and the risk of Parkinson's disease. *Neuroepidemiology* **18,** 303–308.

14. Kuhn, W., Winkel, R., Woitalla, D., Meves, S., Przuntek, H., and Müller T. (1998) High prevalence of parkinsonism after occupational exposure to lead-sulfate batteries. *Neurology* **50,** 885–1886.

15. Crofton, K. M., Taylor, D. H., Bull, R. J., Sivulka, D. J., and Lutkenhoff, S. D. (1980) Developmental delays in exploration and locomotor activity in male rats exposed to low level lead. *Life Sci.* **26,** 823–831.

16. Alfano, D. P. and Petit, T. L. (1982) Neonatal lead exposure alters the dendritic development of hippocampal dentate granule cells. *Exp. Neurol.* **75,** 275–288.

17. McCauley, P. T., Bull, R. J., Tonti, A. P., et al. (1982) The effect of prenatal and postnatal lead exposure on neonatal synaptogenesis in rat cerebral cortex. *Toxicol. Environ. Health* **10,** 639–651.

18. Cookman, G. R., King, W., and Regan, C. M. (1987) Chronic low-level lead exposure impairs embryonic to adult conversion of the neural cell adhesion molecule. *J. Neurochem.* **49,** 399–403.

19. Reuhl, K. R., Rice, D. C, Gilbert, S. G., and Mallett, J. (1991) Effects of chronic developmental lead exposure on monkey neuroanatomy: visual system. *Toxicol. Appl. Pharmacol.* **99,** 501–509.

20. Patrick, G. W. and Anderson, W. J. (1995) Dendritic alterations of cortical pyramidal neurons in postnatally lead-exposed kittens: a Golgi–Cox study. *Dev. Neurosci.* **17,** 219–229.

21. Kern, M. and Audesirk, G. (1995) Inorganic lead may inhibit neurite development in cultured rat hippocampal neurons through hyperphosphorylation. *Toxicol. Appl. Pharmacol.* **134,** 111–123.

22. Ishihara, K., Alkondon, M., Montes, J. G., and Albuquerque, E. X. (1995) Ontogenically related properties of NMDA receptors in rat hippocampal neurons and the age-specific sensitivity of developing neurons to lead. *J. Pharm. Exp. Ther.* **273,** 1459–1470.

23. Cline, H. T., Witte, S., and Jones, K. W. (1996) Low lead levels stunt neuronal growth in a reversible manner. *Proc. Natl. Acad. Sci. USA* **93,** 9915–9920.

24. Gilbert, M. E., Mack, C. M., and Lasley, S. M. (1996) Chronic developmental lead exposure increases threshold for long-term potentiation in the rat dentate gyrus in vivo. *Brain Res.* **736,** 118–124.

25. Gilbert, M. E. and Mack, C. M. (1998) Chronic developmental lead exposure accelerates decay of long-term potentiation in rat dentate gyrus in vivo. *Brain Res.* **789,** 139–149.

26. Omelchenko, I. A., Nelson, C. S., Marino, J. L., and Allen, C. N. (1996) The sensitivity of NMDA receptors to lead inhibition is dependent on the receptor subunit composition. *J. PET* **278,** 15–20.

27. Omelchenko, I. A., Nelson, C. S., and Allen, C. N. (1997) Lead inhibition of NMDA receptors containing NR2A, NR2C and NR2D subunits. *J. PET* **282,** 1458–1464.

28. Wilson, M. A., Johnston, M. V., Goldstein, G. W., and Blue, M. E. (2000) Neonatal lead exposure impairs development of rodent barrel field cortex. *Proc. Natl. Acad. Sci. USA* **97,** 5540–5545.

29. Windebank, A. J. (1986) Specific inhibition of myelination by lead in vitro; comparison with arsenic, thallium, and mercury. *Exp. Neurol.* **94,** 203–212.

30. Tang, H.-W., Yan, H.-L., Hu, X.-H., Liang, Y.-X., and Shen, X.-Y. (1996) Lead cytotoxicity in primary cultured rat astrocytes and Schwann cells. *J. Appl. Toxicol.* **16,** 187–196.

31. Deng, W., McKinnon, R. D., and Poretz, R. D. (2001) Lead exposure delays the differentiation of oligodendroglial progenitors in vitro. *Toxicol. Appl. Pharmacol.* **174,** 235–244.

32. Tiffany-Castiglioni, E., Zmudzki, J., Wu, J.-N., and Bratton, G. R. (1987) Effects of lead treatment on intracellular Cu and Fe in cultured astroglia. *Metab. Brain Dis.* **2,** 61–79.

33. Engle, M. J. and Volpe, J. J. (1990) Glutamine synthetase activity of developing astrocytes is inhibited in vitro by very low concentrations of lead. *Dev. Brain Res.* **55,** 283–287.

34. Sierra, E. M. and Tiffany-Castiglioni, E. (1991) Reduction of glutamine synthetase activity in astroglia exposed in culture to low levels of inorganic lead. *Toxicology* **65,** 295–304.
35. Dave, V., Vitarella, D., Aschner, J. L., Fletcher, P., Kimelberg, H. K., and Aschner, M. (1993) Lead increases inositol 1,4,5-trisphosphate levels but does not interfere with calcium transients in primary rat astrocytes. *Brain Res.* **618,** 9–18.
36. Kerper, L. E. and Hinkle, P. M. (1997) Cellular uptake of lead is activated by depletion of intracellular calcium stores. *J. Biol. Chem.* **272,** 8346–8352.
37. Legare, M. E., Barhoumi, R., Hebert, E., Bratton, G. R., Burghardt, R. C., and Tiffany-Castiglioni, E. (1998) Analysis of Pb^{2+} entry into cultured astroglia. *Toxicol. Sci.* **46,** 90–100.
38. Rowles, T. K., Womac, C., Bratton, G. R., and Tiffany-Castiglioni, E. (1989) Interaction of lead and zinc in cultured astroglia. *Metab. Brain Dis.* **4,** 187–201.
39. Qian, Y., Tiffany-Castiglioni, E., and Harris, E. D. (1995) Copper transport and kinetics in cultured C6 rat glioma cells. *Am. J. Physiol.* **269,** C892–C898.
40. Qian, Y., Mikeska, G., Harris, E. D., Bratton, G. R., and Tiffany-Castiglioni, E. (1999) Effect of lead exposure and accumulation on copper homeostasis in cultured C6 rat glioma cells. *Toxicol. Appl. Pharmacol.* **158,** 41–49.
41. Legare, M. E., Barhoumi, R., Burghardt, R. C., and Tiffany-Castiglioni, E. (1993) Low-level lead exposure in cultured astroglia: identification of cellular targets with vital fluorescent probes. *Neurotoxicology* **14,** 267–272.
42. Qian, Y., Harris, E. D., Zheng, Y., and Tiffany-Castiglioni, E. (2000) Lead targets GRP78, a molecular chaperone, in C6 rat glioma cells. *Toxicol. Appl. Pharmacol.* **163,** 260–266.
43. Qian, Y., Falahatpsheh, M. H., Zheng, Y., Ramos, K. S., and Tiffany-Castiglioni, E. (2001) Induction of 78 kD glucose-regulated protein (GRP 78) expression and redox-regulated transcription factor activity by lead and mercury in C6 rat glioma cells. *Neurotox. Res.* **3,** 581– 589.
44. Qian, Y. and Tiffany-Castiglioni, E. (2003) Lead-induced endoplasmic reticulum (ER) stress responses in the nervous system. *Neurochem. Res.* **28,** 153–162.
45. Holtzman, D., de Vries, C., Nguyen, H., Olson, J., and Bensch, K. (1984) Maturation of resistance to lead encephalopathy: cellular and subcellular mechanisms. *Neurotoxicology* **5,** 97–124.
46. Holtzman, D., Olson, J., de Vries, C., and Bensch, K. (1987) Lead toxicity in primary cultured cerebral astrocytes and cerebellar granule neurons. *Toxicol. Appl. Pharmacol.* **89,** 211–235.
47. Tiffany-Castiglioni, E. (1993) Cell culture models for lead toxicity in neuronal and glial. *Neurotoxicology* **4,** 513–536.
48. Tiffany-Castiglioni, E., Legare, M.E., Schneider, L. A., Hanneman, W. H., Zenger, E., and Hong, S. J. (1996) Astroglia and neurotoxicity, in *The Role of*

Glia in Neurotoxicity (Aschner, M. and Kimelberg, H. K., eds.) CRC, Boca Raton, FL, pp. 175–200.

49. Yip, R. and Dallman, P. R. (1984) Developmental changes in erythrocyte protoporphyrin: the roles of iron deficiency and lead toxicity. *J. Pediatr.* **104,** 710–730.

50. Yip, R. (1990) Multiple interactions between childhood iron deficiency and lead poisoning: evidence that childhood lead poisoning is an adverse consequence of iron deficiency, in *Recent Knowledge on Iron and Folate Deficiencies in the World* (Hercberg, S., Galan, P., and Dupin, H., eds.), Colloque INSERM, Paris, pp. 523–532.

51. O'Flaherty, E. J. (1995) Physiologically based models for bone-seeking elements. V. Lead absorption and disposition in childhood. *Toxicol. Appl. Pharmacol.* **131,** 297–308.

52. Scortegagna, M., Chikhale, E., and Hanbauer, I. (1998) Lead exposure increases oxidative stress in serum deprived E14 mesencephalic cultures. Role of metallothionein and glutathione. *Restor. Neurol. Neurosci.* **12,** 95–101.

53. Liu, M. Y., Hsieh, W. C., and Yang, B. C. (2000) In vitro aberrant gene expression as the indicator of lead-induced neurotoxicity in U-373MG cells. *Toxicology* **147,** 59–64.

54. Long, G. J., Rosen, J. F., and Schanne, F. A. X. (1994) Lead activation of protein kinase C from rat brain. *J. Biol. Chem.* **269,** 834–837.

55. Srivastava, D., Hurwitz, R. L., and Fox, D. A. (1995) Lead- and calcium-mediated inhibition of bovine rod cGMP phosphodiesterase: interactions with magnesium. *Toxicol. Appl. Pharmacol.* **134,** 43–52.

56. Tomsig, J. L. and Suszkiw, J. B. (1995) Multisite interactions between Pb^{+2} and protein kinase C and its role in norepinephrine release from bovine adrenal chromaffin cells. *J. Neurochem.* **64,** 2667–2773.

57. Westerink, R. H. S. and Vijverberg, H. P. M. (2002) Ca^{+2}-independent vesicular catecholamine release in PC12 cells by nanomolar concentrations of Pb^{+2}. *J. Neurochem.* **80,** 861–873.

58. Tomsig, J. L. and Suszkiw, J. B. (1990) Pb-induced secretion from bovine chromaffin cells: fura-2 as a probe for Pb^{2+}. *Am. J. Physiol.* **259,** C762–C768.

59. Legare, M. E., Castiglioni, A. J., Jr., Rowles, T. K., Calvin, J. A., Snyder-Armstead, C., and Tiffany-Castiglioni, E. (1993) Morphological alterations of neurons and astrocytes in guinea pigs exposed to low levels of inorganic lead. *NeuroToxicology* **14(1),** 77–80.

60. Breen, K. and Regan, C. M. (1988) Developmental control of N-CAM sialylation state by Golgi sialyltransferase isoforms. *Development* **104,** 147–154.

61. Breen, K. and Regan, C. M. (1988) Lead stimulates Golgi sialyltransferase at times coincident with the embryonic to adult conversion of the neural cell adhesion molecule. *Toxicology* **49,** 71–76.

62. Regan, C. M. (1993) Neural cell adhesion molecules, neuronal development, and lead toxicity. *Neurotoxicology* **14,** 69–74.

63. Audesirk, T., Audesirk, G., Ferguson, C., and Shugarts, D. (1991) Effects of inorganic lead on the differentiation and growth of cultured hippocampal and neuroblastoma ce.. *Neurotoxicology* **12,** 529–538.

64. Kern, M., Audesirk, T., and Audesirk, G. (1993) Effects of inorganic lead on the differentiation and growth of cortical neurons in culture. *Neurotoxicology* **14,** 319–328.

65. Williams, T. M., Ndifor, A. M., Neary, J. T., and Reams-Brown, R. R. (2000) Lead enhances NGF-induced neurite outgrowth in PC12 cells by potentiating ERK/MAPK activation. *Neurotoxicology* **21,** 1081–1090.

66. Crumpton, T., Atkins, D., Zawia, N., and Barone, S. (2001) Lead exposure in pheochromocytoma (PC12) cells alters neural differentiation and Sp1 DNA-binding. *Neurotoxicology* **22,** 49–62.

67. Tepass, U., Truong, K., Godt, D., Ikura, M., and Peifer, M. (2000) Cadherins in embryonic and neural morphogenesis. *Nature Rev.* **1,** 91–100.

68. Dey, P. M., Burger, J., Gochfeld, M., and Reuhl, K. R. (2000) Developmental lead exposure disturbs expression of synaptic neural cell adhesion molecules in herring gull brains. *Toxicology* **146,** 137–147.

69. Prozialeck, W. C., Grunwald G. B., Dey, P. M., Reuhl, K. R., and Parrish, A. R. (2002) Cadherins and NCAM as potential targets in metal toxicity. *Toxicol. Appl. Pharmacol.* **182,** 255–265.

70. Zawia, N. H. and Harry, G. J. (1996) Developmental exposure to lead interferes with glial and neuronal differential gene expression in the rat cerebellum. *Toxicol. Appl. Pharmacol.* **138,** 43–47.

71. Zawia, N. H., Evers, L. B., and Harry, G. J. (1994) Developmental profiles of ornithine decarboxylase activity in the hippocampus, neocortex and cerebellum: modulation following lead exposure. *Int. J. Dev. Neurosci.* **12,** 25–30.

72. Zawia, N. H., Evers, L. B., Kodavanti, P. R., and Harry, G. J. (1994) Modulation of developmental cerebellar ornithine decarboxylase activity by lead-acetate. *Neurotoxicology* **15,** 903–911.

73. Murray, B. A., Hemperly, J. J., Prediger, E. A., Edelman, G. M., and Cunningham, B. A. (1986) Alternatively spliced mRNAs code for different polypeptide chains of the chicken neural cell adhesion molecule (N-CAM). *J. Cell Biol.* **102,** 189–193.

74. Jorgensen, O. S. (1995) Neural cell adhesion molecule (NCAM) as a quantitative marker in synaptic remodeling. *Neurochem. Res.* **20,** 533–547.

75. Noble, M., Albrechtsen, M., Moller, C., et al. (1985) Glial cells express N-CAM/D2-CAM-like polypeptides *in vitro. Nature* **316,** 725–748.

76. Moran, N. M. and Bock, E. (1988) Characterization of the kinetics of neural cell adhesion molecule homophilic binding. *FEBS Lett.* **242,** 121–124.

77. Edelman, G. M. and Chuong, C.-M. (1982) Embryonic to adult conversion of neural cell adhesion molecules in normal and staggerer mice. *Proc. Natl. Acad. Sci. USA* **79,** 7036–7040.

78. Ronn, L. C. B., Hartz, B. P., and Bock, E. (1998) The neural cell adhesion molecule (NCAM) in development and plasticity of the nervous system. *Exp. Gerontol.* **33,** 853–864.

79. Davey, F. D. and Breen, K. C. (1998) Stimulation of sialyltransferase by subchronic low-level lead exposure in the developing nervous system. A potential mechanism of teratogen action. *Toxicol. Appl. Pharmacol.* **151,** 16–21.

80. Riehl, R., Johnson, K., Bradley, R., et al. (1996) Cadherin function is required for axon outgrowth in retinal ganglion cells in vivo. *Neuron* **17,** 837–848.

81. Inoue, A. and Sanes, J. R. (1997) Lamina-specific connectivity in the brain: regulation by N-cadherin, neurotrophins, and glycoconjugates. *Science* **276,** 1428–1431.

82. Tanaka, H., Shan, W., Phillips, G. R., et al. (2000) Molecular modification of N-cadherin in response to synaptic activity. *Neuron* **25,** 93–107.

83. Fannon, A. M. and Colman, D. R. (1996) A model for central synaptic junctional complex formation based on the differential adhesive specificities of the cadherins. *Neuron* **17,** 423–434.

84. Uchida, N., Honjo, Y., Johnson, K. R., Wheelock, M. J., and Takeichi. M. (1996) The catenin/cadherin adhesion system is localized in synaptic junctions bordering transmitter release zones. *J. Cell Biol.* **135,** 767–779.

85. Zhou, M., Tian, X., and Suszkiw, J. B. (2000) Developmental stage-dependent protective effect of NGF against lead cholinotoxicity in the rat septum. *Brain Res.* **866,** 268–273.

86. Reinhard, E., Nedivi, E., Wegner, J., Skene, J. H. P., and Westerfield, M. (1994) Neural selective activation and temporal regulation of a mammalian GAP-43 promotor in zebrafish. *Development* **120,** 1767–1775.

87. Bernstein, H.-G. and Muller, M. (1999) The cellular localization of the L-ornithine decarboxylase/polyamine sytemin normal and diseased central nervous system. *Prog. Neurobiol.* **57,** 485–505.

88. Klekner, A., Rohn, A. G., Schillinger, G., Schroder, R., Klug, N., and Ernestus, R. I. (2001) ODC mRNA as a prognostic factor for predicting recurrence in meningiomas. *J. Neurooncol.* **53,** 67–75.

89. Hilliard, A., Ramesh, A., and Zawia, N. H. (1999) Correlation between lead-induced changes in cerebral ornithine decarboxylase and protein kinase C activities during development and in cultured PC12 cells. *Int. J. Dev. Neurosci.* **17,** 777–785.

90. Toews, A. D., Krigman, M. R., Thomas, D. J., and Morell, P. (1980) Effect of inorganic lead exposure on myelination in the rat. *Neurochem. Res.* **5,** 605–616.

91. Toews, A. D., Blaker, W. D., Thomas, D. J., et al. (1983) Myelin deficit produced by early postnatal exposure to inorganic lead or triethyltin are persistent. *J. Neurochem.* **41,** 816–822.

92. Harry, G. J., Toews, A. D., Kirgman, M. R., and Morell, P. (1985) The effect of lead toxicity and milk deprivation on myelination in the rat. *Toxicol. Appl. Pharmacol.* **77,** 458–464.

93. Sundstr^m, R. and Karlsson, B. (1987) Myelin basic protein in brains of rats with low dose lead encephalopathy. *Arch. Toxicol.* **59,** 341–345.

94. Seppalainen, A. M., Hernberg, S., Vesanto, R., and Kock, B. (1983) Early neurotoxic effects of occupational lead exposure: a prospective study. *Neurotoxicology* **4(2),** 181–192.

95. Araki, S., Sato, H., Yokoyama, K., and Murata, K. (2000) Subclinical neuro-physiological effects of lead: a review on peripheral, central, and autonomic nervous system effects in lead workers. *Am. J. Ind. Med.* **37,** 193–204.

96. Harry, G. J., Billingsley, M., Bruinink, A., et al. (1998) In vitro techniques for the assessment of neurotoxicity. *Environ. Health Perspect.* **106(Suppl.),** 131–158.

97. Dabrowska-Bouta, B., Sulkowski, G., Bartosz, G., Walski, M., and Rafalowska, U. (1999) Chronic lead intoxication affects the myelin membrane status in the central nervous system of adult rats. *J. Mol. Neurosci.* **13,** 127–139.

98. Wu, J.-N. and Tiffany-Castiglioni, E. (1987) Reduction by lead of hydrocortisone-induced glycerol phosphate dehydrogenase activity in cultured rat oligodendroglia. *In Vitro Dev. Cell. Biol.* **23,** 765–774.

99. Sierra, E. M., Rowles, T. K., Martin, J., Bratton, G. R., Womac, C., and Tiffany-Castiglioni, E. (1989) Low level lead neurotoxicity in a pregnant guinea pig model: Neuroglial enzyme activities and brain trace metal concentrations. *Toxicology* **59,** 81–96.

100. Gordon, M. N., Kumar, S., Espinosa de los Monteros, A., and de Vellis, J. (1992) Ontogeny of glycerol phosphate dehydrogenase-positive oligodendrocytes in rat brain. Impaired differentiation of oligodendrocytes in the myelin deficient mutant rat. *Int. J. Devel. Neurosci.* **10,** 243–253.

101. Deng, W. and Poretz, R. D. (2002) Protein kinase C activation is required for the lead- induced inhibition of proliferation and differentiation of cultured oligodendroglial progenitor cells. *Brain Res.* **929,** 87–95.

102. Yim, S. H., Farrer, R. G., and Quarles, R. H. (1995) Expression of glycolipids and myelin- associated glycoprotein during the differentiation of oligodendrocytes: comparison of the CG-4 glial cell line to primary cultures. *Dev. Neurosci.* **17,** 171–180.

103. Deng, W. and Poretz, R. D. (2001) Lead exposure affects levels of galactolipid metabolic enzymes in the developing rat brain. *Toxicol. Appl. Pharmacol.* **172,** 98–107.

104. Deng, W. and Poretz, R. D. (2001) Lead alters the developmental profile of the galactolipid metabolic enzymes in cultured oligodendrocyte lineage cells. *Neurotoxicology* **22,** 429–437.

105. Poretz, R. D., Yang, A., Deng, W., and Manowitz, P. (2000) The interaction of lead exposure and arylsulfatase A genotype affects sulfatide catabolism in human fibroblasts. *Neurotoxicology* **21,** 379–387.

106. Chen, X. G. and Poretz, R. D. (2001) Lead causes human fibroblasts to mis-sort arylsulfatase A. *Toxicology* **163,** 107–114.

107. S·nchez, I., Hassinger, L., Paskevich, P. A., Shine, H. D., and Nixon, R. A. (1996) Oligodendroglia regulate the regional expansion of axon caliber and local accumulation of neurofilaments during development independently of myelin formation. *J. Neurosci.* **16,** 5095–5105.

108. Sortwell, C. E., Daley, B. F., Pitzer, M. R., McGuire, S. O., Sladek, J. R., and Collier, T. J. (2000) Oligodendrocyte-type 2 astrocyte-derived trophic factors increase survival of developing dopamine neurons through the inhibition of apoptotic cell death. *J. Comp. Neurol.* **426,** 143–153.

109. Kaplan, M. R., Meyer-Franke, A., Lambert, S., et al. (1997) Induction of sodium channel clustering by oligodendrocytes. *Nature* **386,** 724–728.

110. Taniike, M., Mohri, I., Eguchi, N., Beuckmann, C. T., Suzuki, K., and Urade, Y. (2002) Perineuronal oligodendrocytes protect against neuronal apoptosis through the production of lipocalin-type prostaglandin D synthase in a genetic demyelinating model. *J. Neurosci.* **22,** 4885–4896.

111. Zawia, N. H. and Harry, G. J. (1995) Exposure to lead-acetate modulates the developmental expression of myelin genes in the rat frontal lobe. *Int. J. Dev. Neurosci.* **13,** 639–644.

112. Popko, B., Pearl, D. K., Walker, D. M., et al. (2002) Molecular markers that identify human astrocytomas and oligodendrogliomas. *J. Neuropathol. Exp. Neurol.* **61,** 329–338.

113. Anttila A. Heikkila P. Nykyri E. et al. (1996) Risk of nervous system cancer among workers exposed to lead. *J. Occup. Environ. Med.* **38,** 131–136.

114. Cohen, R. D., Bowser, D. H., and Costa, M. (1996) Carcinogenicity and genotoxicity of lead, beryllium, and other metals, in *Toxicology of Metals* (Chang, L. W., Magos, L., and Suzuki, T., eds.), CRC/Lewis, Boca Raton, FL, pp. 253–284.

115. Johnson, F. M. (1998) The genetic effects of environmental lead. *Mutat. Res.* **410,** 123–140.

116. Gencic, S. and Hudson, L. D. (1990) conservative amino acid substitution in the myelin proteolipid protein of jimpymsd mice. *J. Neurosci.* **10,** 117–124.

117. Henson, J., Saffer, J., and Furneaux, H. (1992) The transcription factor Sp1 binds to the JC virus promoter and is selectively expressed in glial cells in human brain. *Ann. Neurol.* **32,** 72–77.

118. Kumar, A. P., Mar, P. K., Zhao, B., Montgomery, R. L., Kang, D. C., and Butler, A. P. (1995) Regulation of rat ornithine decarboxylase promoter activity by binding of transcription factor Sp1. *J. Biol. Chem.* **270,** 4341–4348.

119. Bai, G. and Kusiak, J. W. (1995) Functional analysis of the proximal 5'-flanking region of the *N*-methyl-D-aspartate receptor subunit gene, NMDAR1. *J. Biol. Chem.* **270,** 7737–7744.

120. Saffer, J. D., Jackson, S. P., and Annarella, M. B. (1991) Developmental expression of Sp1 in the mouse. *Mol. Cell Biol.* **11,** 2189–2199.

121. Zawia, N. H., Sharan, R., Brydie, M., Oyama, T., and Crumpton, T. (1998) Sp1 as a target site for metal-induced perturbations of transcriptional regulation of developmental brain gene expression. *Dev. Brain Res.* **107,** 291–298.

122. Razmiafshari, M. and Zawia, N. H. (2000) Utilization of a synthetic peptide as a tool to study the interaction of heavy metals with the zinc finger domain of proteins critical for gene expression in the developing brain. *Toxicol. Appl. Pharmacol.* **166,** 1–12.

123. Razmiafshari, M., Kao, J., d'Avignon, A., and Zawia, N. H. (2001) NMR identification of heavy metal-binding sites in a synthetic zinc finger peptide: toxicological implications for the interactions of xenobiotic metals with zinc finger proteins. *Toxicol. Appl. Pharmacol.* **172,** 1–10.

124. Miskimins, R. and Miskimins, W. K. (2001) A role for an AP-1-like site in the expression of the myelin basic protein gene during differentiation. *Int. J. Dev. Neurosci.* **19,** 85–91.

125. Tiffany-Castiglioni, E., Sierra, E. M., Wu, J.-N., and Rowles, T. K. (1989) Lead toxicity in neuroglia. *Neurotoxicology* **10,** 383–410.

126. Tiffany-Castiglioni, E., Legare, M. E., Schneider, L. A., et al. (1996) Heavy metal effects on glia, in *Methods in Neurosciences, Volume 30* (Regino Perez-Polo, J., ed.) Academic, New York, pp. 135–165.

127. Tiffany-Castiglioni, E. and Qian, Y. (2001) Astroglia as metal depots: molecular mechanisms for metal accumulation, storage and release. *Neurotoxicology* **22,** 577–592.

128. Lidsky, T. I. and Schneider, J. S. (2003) Lead neurotoxicity in children: basic mechanisms and clinical correlates. *Brain* **126,** 5–19.

129. Opanashuk, L. A. and Finkelstein, J. N. (1995) Induction of newly synthesized proteins in astroglial cells exposed to lead. *Toxicol. Appl. Pharmacol.* **131,** 21–30.

130. Opanashuk, L. A. and Finkelstein, J. N. (1995) Relationship of lead-induced proteins to stress response proteins in astroglial cells. *J. Neurosci. Res.* **42,** 623–632.

131. Selvin-Testa, A., Capani, F., Loidl, C. F., Lopez, E. M., and Pecci-Saavedra, J. (1997) Prenatal and postnatal lead exposure induces 70 kDa heat shock protein in young rat brain prior to changes in astrocyte cytoskeleton. *Neurotoxicology* **18,** 805–817.

132. Li, P. and Rossman, T. G. (2001) Genes upregulated in lead-resistant glioma cells reveal possible targets for lead-induced developmental neurotoxicity. *Toxicol. Sci.* **64,** 90–99.

133. Bradbury, M. W. B. and Deane, R. (1993) Permeability of the blood-brain barrier to lead. *Neurotoxicology* **14,** 131–136.

134. Lindahl, L., Bird, L., Legare, M. E., Mikeska, G., Bratton, G. R, and Tiffany-Castiglioni, E. (1999) Differential ability of astroglia and neuronal cells to accumulate lead: dependence on cell type and on degree of differentiation. *Toxicol. Sci.* **50,** 236–243.

135. Thomas, J. A., Dallenbeck, F. D., and Thomas, M. (1973) The distribution of radioactive lead [^{210}Pb] in the cerebellum of developing rats. *J. Pathol.* **109,** 45–50.

136. Shirabe, T. and Hirano, A. (1977) X-ray microanalytical studies of lead-implanted rat brains. *Acta Neuropathol.* **40,** 189–192.

137. Zurich, M. G., Monnet-Tschudi, F., Bérode, M., and Honegger, P. (1998) Lead acetate toxicity in vitro: dependence on the cell composition of the cultures. *Toxicol. In Vitro* **12,** 191–196.

138. Vaguera-Orte, J., Cervos-Navarro, J., Martin-Giron, F., and Becerra-Ratia, J. (1981) Fine structure of the perivascular-limiting membrane, in *Cerebral Microcirculation and Metabolism* (Cervos-Navarro, J. and Fitschka, E., eds.), Raven, New York, pp. 129–138.

139. Young, J. K., Garvey, J. S., and Huang, P. C. (2000) Glial immunoreactivity for metallothionein in the rat brain. *Glia* **4,** 602–620.

140. Penkowa, M., Nielsen, H., Hidalgo, J., Bernth, N., and Moos, T. (1999) Distribution of metallothionein I + II and vesicular zinc in the developing central nervous system: Correlative study in the rat. *J. Comp. Neurol.* **412,** 303–318.

141. Masters, B. A., Quaife, C. J., Erickson, J. C., et al. (1994) Metallothionein III is expressed in neurons that sequester zinc in synaptic vesicles. *J. Neurosci.* **14,** 5844–5857.

142. Erickson, J. C., Hollopeter, G., Thomas, S. A., Froelick, G. J., and Palmiter, R. D. (1997) Disruption of the metallothionein-III gene in mice: analysis of brain zinc, behavior, and neuron vulnerability to metals, aging, and seizures. *J. Neurosci.* **17,** 1271–1281.

143. Carrasco, J., Giralt, M., Molinero, A., Penkowa, M., Moos, T., and Hidalgo, J. (1999) Metallothionein (MT)-III: generation of polyclonal antibodies, comparison with MT-I + II in the freeze lesioned rat brain and in a bioassay with astrocytes, and analysis of Alzheimer's disease brains. *J. Neurotrauma* **16,** 1115–1129.

144. Aschner, M., Conklin, D. R. Yao, C. P., Allen, J. W., and Tan, K. H. (1998) Induction of astrocyte metallothioneins (Mts) by zinc confers resistance against the acute cytotoxic effects of methylmercury on cell swelling, Na$^+$ uptake, and K$^+$ release. *Brain Res.* **813,** 254–261.

145. Kramer, K. K., Zoelle, J. T., and Klaassen, C. D. (1996) Induction of metallothionein mRNA and protein in primary murine neuron cultures. *Toxicol. Appl. Pharmacol.* **141,** 1–7.

146. Raps, S. P., Lai, J. C., Hertz, L., and Cooper, A. J. (1989) Glutathione is present in high concentrations in cultured astrocytes but not in cultured neurons. *Brain Res.* **493,** 398–401.

147. Slivka, A., Mytilineou, C., and Cohen, G. (1987) Histochemical evaluation of glutathione in brain. *Brain Res.* **409,** 275–284.

148. Philbert, M. A., Beiswanger, C. M., Waters, D. K., Reuhl, K. R., and Lowndes, H. E. (1991) Cellular and regional distribution of reduced glutathione in the nervous system of the rat: histochemical localization by mercury orange and *o*-phthaldialdhyde-induced histofluorescence. *Toxicol. Appl. Pharmacol.* **107,** 215–227.

149. Klomp, L., Farhangrazi, Z., Dugan, L., and Gitlin, J. (1996) Ceruloplasmin gene expression in the murine central nervous system. *J. Clin. Invest.* **98,** 207–215.

150. Patel, B. N. and David, S. (1997) A novel glycosylphosphatidylinositol-anchored form of ceruloplasmin is expressed by mammalian astrocytes. *J. Biol. Chem.* **272,** 20,185–20,190.

151. Kaler, S. G. and Schwartz, J. P. (1998) Expression of the menkes disease homolog in rodent neuroglial cells. *Neurosci. Res. Commun.* **23,** 61–66.

152. Qian, Y., Tiffany-Castiglioni, E., and Harris, E. D. (1997) A Menkes P-type ATPase involved in copper homeostasis in the central nervous system of the rat. *Mol. Brain. Res.* **48,** 60–66.

153. Niklowitz, W. J. (1980) Toxicology of lead, in *Advances in Neurotoxicology* (Manso, L., Lory, N., Lacasse, Y., and Roche, L., eds.), Permagon, New York, pp. 27–43.

154. Rehman, S.-U. and Chandra, O. (1984) Regional interrelationships of zinc, copper, and lead in the brain following lead intoxication. *Bull. Environ. Contam. Toxicol.* **32,** 157–165

155. Tiffany-Castiglioni, E., Garcia, D. M., Wu, J. N., Zmudzki, J., and Bratton, G. R. (1988) Effects of lead on viability and intracellular metal content of C6 rat glioma cells. *J. Toxicol. Environ. Health* **23,** 267–279.

156. Wedler, F. C. and Denman, R. B. (1984) Glutamine synthetase: the major Mn(II) enzyme in mammalian brain. *Curr. Topics Cell. Regul.* **24,** 153–169.

157. Norenberg, M. D. and Martinez-Hernandez, A. (1979) Fine structural localization of glutamine synthetase in astrocytes of rat brain. *Brain Res.* **161,** 303–310.

158. Kodama, H., Meguro, Y., Abe, T., et al. (1991) Genetic expression of Menkes disease in cultured astrocytes of the macular mouse. *J. Inherit. Metab. Dis.* **14,** 896–901.

159. Kodama, H. (1993) Recent developments in Menkes disease. *J. Inherit. Metab. Dis.* **16,** 791–799.

160. Hartmann, H. A. and Evenson, M. A. (1992) Deficiency of copper can cause neuronal degeneration. *Med. Hypotheses* **38,** 75–85.

161. Scortegagna, M. and Hanbauer, I. (2000) Increase AP-1 binding activity and nuclear REF-1 accumulation in lead-exposed primary cultures of astroglia. *Neurochem. Res.* **25,** 861–866.

162. Buchner, J. (1999). Hsp90 & Co.—a holding for folding. *Trends Biochem. Sci.* **24,** 36–141.

163. Caplan, A. J. (1999). Hsp90's secrets unfold: new insights from structural and functional studies. *Cell Biol.* **9,** 262–268.

164. Lee, A. S. (1992) Mammalian stress response: induction of the glucose-regulated protein family. *Curr. Opin. Cell Biol.* **4,** 267–273.

165. Gething, M. J. (1997) *Guidebook to Molecular Chaperones and Protein-Folding Catalysts.* Oxford University Press, Oxford.

166. Chapman, R., Sidrauski, C., and Walter, P. (1998) Intracellular signaling from the endoplasmic reticulum to the nucleus. *Annu. Rev. Cell. Dev. Biol.* **14,** 459–485.

167. Kaufman, R. J. (1999) Stress signaling from the lumen of the endoplasmic reticulum: coordination of gene transcriptional and translational controls. *Genes Dev.* **13,** 1211–1233.

168. Kozutsumi, Y., Segal, M., Normington, K., Gething, M. J., and Sambrook, J. (1988) The presence of malfolded proteins in the endoplasmic reticulum signals the induction of glucose-regulated proteins. *Nature* **332,** 462–464.

169. Wooden, S. K., Li, L. J., Navarro, D., Qadri, I., Pereira, L., and Lee, A. S. (1991) Transactivation of the grp78 promoter by malfolded proteins,

glycosylation block, and calcium ionophore is mediated through a proximal region containing a CCAAT motif which interacts with CTF/NF-I. Mol. *Cell. Biol.* **11,** 5612–5623.

170. Miyata, T., Kokame, K., Agarwala, K.L., and Kato, H. (1998) Analysis of gene expression in homocysteine-injured vascular endothelial cells: demonstration of GRP78/BiP expression, cloning and characterization of a novel reducing agent-tunicamycin regulated gene. *Semin. Thromb. Hemost.* **24,** 285–291.

171. Cao, X., Zhou, Y., and Lee, A. S. (1995) Requirement of tyrosine- and serine/ threonine kinases in the transcriptional activation of the mammalian grp78/ BiP promoter by thapsigargin. *J. Biol. Chem.* **270,** 494–502.

172. Tully, D. B., Collins, B. J., Overstreet, J. D., et al. (2000) Effects of arsenic, cadmium, chromium, and lead on gene expression regulated by a battery of 13 different promoters in recombinant HepG2 cells. *Toxicol. Appl. Pharmacol.* **168,** 79–90.

173. Fernandez, P. M., Tabbara, S. O., Jacobs, L. K., et al. (2000) Overexpression of the glucose-regulated stress gene GRP78 in malignant but not benign human breast lesions. *Breast Cancer Res. Treat.* **59,** 15–26.

174. Liu, H., Miller, E., van de Water, B., and Stevens, J. L. (1998) Endoplasmic reticulum stress proteins block oxidant-induced Ca^{2+} increases and cell death. *J. Biol. Chem.* **273,** 12,858–12,862.

175. Norenberg, M. (1996) Reactive astrocytosis, in *The Role of Glia in Neurotoxicity* (Aschner, M. and Kimelberg, H. K., eds.), CRC, Boca Raton, FL, pp. 93–107.

176. Stoltenburg-Didinger, I., Pünder, B., Peters, M., et al. (1996) Glial fibrillary acidic protein and RNA expression in adult rat hippocampus following low-level lead exposure during development. *Histochem. Cell Biol.* **105,** 431–442.

177. Harry, G. J., Schmitt, T. J., Gong, Z., Brown, H., Zawia, N., and Evans, H. L. (1996) Lead- induced alterations of glial fibrillary acidic protein (GFAP) in the developing rat brain. *Toxicol. Appl. Pharmacol.* **139,** 84–93.

178. Selvin-Testa, A., Loidl, C. F., Lopez, E. M., Capani, F., Lopez-Costa, J. J., and Pecci- Saavedra, J. (1995) Prolonged lead exposure modifies astrocyte cytoskeletal proteins in the rat brain. *Neurotoxicology* **16,** 389–401.

179. Struzyñska, L. Bubko, I., Walski, M., and Rafalwska, U. (2001) Astroglial reaction during the early phase of acute lead toxicity in the adult rat brain. *Toxicology* **165,** 121–131.

<h1>8</h1>

Effects of Toxicants on Neural Differentiation

**Stanley Barone, Jr., Prasada R. S. Kodavanti,
and William R. Mundy**

1. INTRODUCTION

1.1. What Is Differentiation and Why Is It an Important Process for Studies of Developmental Neurotoxicology?

Differentiation is a complex process by which a terminal cell phenotype is determined. During neural development, in vivo cells of the nervous system reach this terminal phenotype through both preprogrammed genetic signaling and epigenetic signaling. This genetic program can set up initial organizational planes and an initial temporal sequence of events, but epigenetic signals drive much of the later gene expression and subsequent protein expression that determines different phases of differentiation. This epigenetic signaling can stimulate pluripotent cells to become more restricted in their fate, usually leading to multipotent cells and eventually to a final terminal phenotype. Epigenetic signals include a number of morphogenic and neurotrophic molecules that determine phenotype based on (1) the level of exposure to these endogenous substances, (2) the order of exposure, and (3) the mixture of exposure to these different epigenetic signaling molecules. These complex signaling events are being elucidated with advances in stem cell research in which the signals that stimulate multipotent cells to become neurons, glia, muscle, or bone are starting to be revealed *(1)*. Because of this complexity, it is difficult to tease these different signaling events apart in many in vivo systems and this is why a reductionist approach with in vitro systems is often favored.

From: *Methods in Pharmacology and Toxicology: In Vitro Neurotoxicology: Principles and Challenges*
Edited by: E. Tiffany-Castiglioni © Humana Press Inc., Totowa, NJ

Many subtle but clinically important developmental disorders of the nervous system involve perturbation of neural differentiation at one stage of this process or another (e.g., autism, schizophrenia, Down syndrome; for review, see ref. *2*). These perturbations are believed to be associated with critical windows in the ontogeny of this process. Thus, the question arises: If you are using a reductionist approach; what stages of the process of differentiation are you trying to model in vitro and what epigenetic signaling molecules are pertinent for the experimental system you are studying? Understanding that in vivo differentiation includes the determination of both neuronal and glial lineages and noting that there are different time scales for differentiation of these two cell lineages and differences in time-scales even within the same lineage among different regions of the nervous system is very important *(3)*.

1.2. Perturbation of What Mechanisms Leads to Effects on This Process?

In the case of neuronal development, this process involves the development of specific structures, properties, and connections. This includes differentiation of cell bodies, axons, and dendrites. This differentiation overlaps greatly with other processes of neural development in vivo and these processes are regionally and temporally regulated (*see* Fig. 1). The process of differentiation leads the neuron to a mature state in which neurons can perform normal functions such as neurotransmitter synthesis, neurotransmitter release, synaptic plasticity, synaptic transmission, and electrical excitability.

As the nervous system goes through these critical phases of ontogeny, there are regional and cell-type-specific windows of unique vulnerability ("critical windows of exposure") to toxicants. In contrast, when the process is complete, the window of vulnerability has closed (reviewed in ref. *2*). Injury caused by exposure to toxicants at these critical times can result in transient or permanent changes in the structure and function of the nervous system. The complexity of multiple events occurring sequentially during development also increases the number of targets to be affected by developmental neurotoxicants. This idea is supported by evidence that the initial phase of differentiation likely begins as soon as neuronal precursors complete their last division and are primed for migration to the cortical plate *(4,5)*. Thus, disruption of an early process that causes delays in proliferation and migration theoretically can have downstream effects on cell differentiation because the temporal and regional coordination of neurotrophic signaling molecules of differentiation can be disrupted. Alteration in critical regulatory molecules by toxicants can perturb the growth and development of the nervous system. These critical molecules include morphogenic sig-

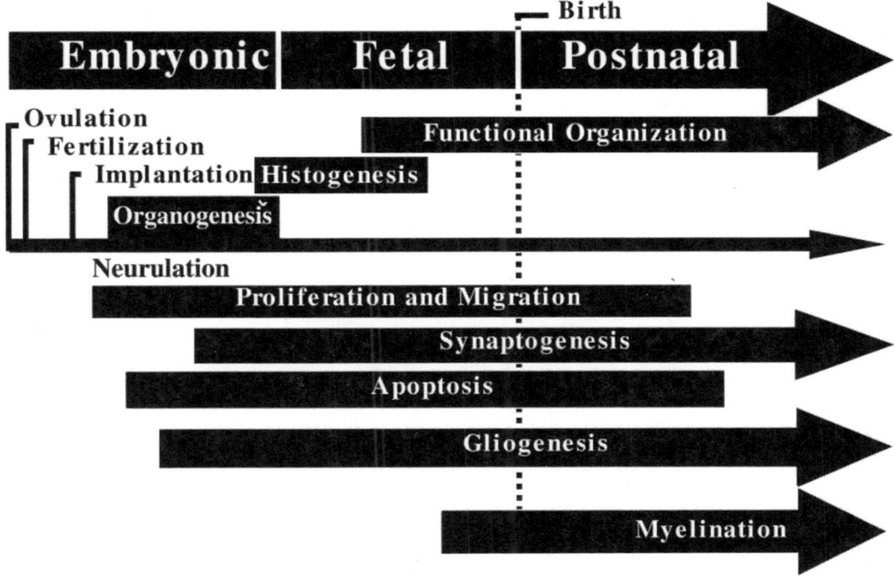

Fig. 1. Critical developmental periods and processes. This illustration depicts developmental periods in the upper portion of the panel and the general timetable of developmental processes that include organogenesis and histogenesis. The bottom two-thirds emphasizes the processes intrinsic to development of the nervous system (i.e., proliferation, migration, synaptogenesis, apoptosis, gliogenesis, and myelination). Note that the time span is not specific for a given regionM9f the nervous system. Each region of the nervous system has its distinct progression through these processes. As result, a punctate exposure to an environmental agent can affect multiple regions and multiple processes that are occurring simultaneously.

naling molecules like neurotransmitters, neurotrophic factors, substrate adhesion molecules, and cell adhesion molecules. Toxicant exposure can interfere with the expression of these gene products, their receptors, or intracellular second-messenger signaling.

During the process of differentiation, neuronal cells go through a number of steps on their way to a mature and stable terminal state. In addition to the visible change in appearance and morphology, typically characterized by an increase in the size of the cell soma and extension of neurites (*see* Fig. 2), there are profound changes in the expression of specific genes that result in the arrest of cell division and increased synthesis of proteins that underlie the unique morphologic, physiologic, and biochemical properties of mature neurons and glia. As well as increasing the expression of potential targets for neurotoxicants, this change in the cellular protein complement can be used as an indication of the state of differentiation.

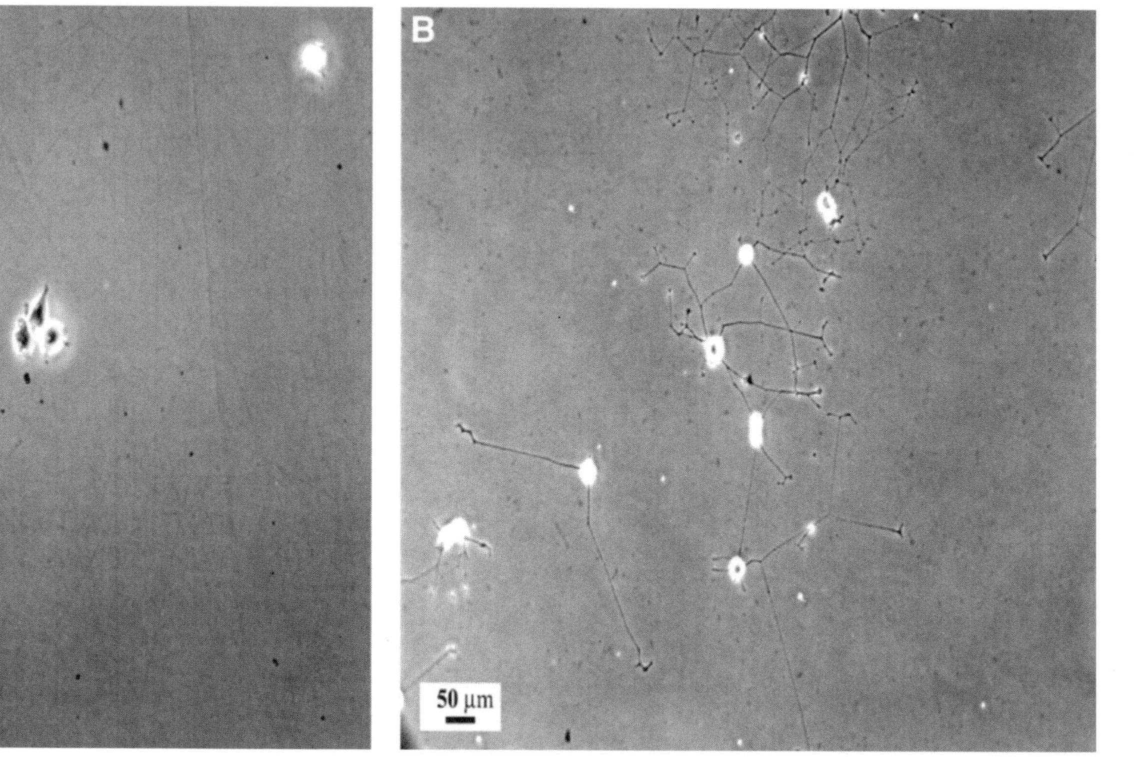

Fig. 2. Initiation *vs* elaboration. PC12 cells can be used to examine differentiation. Key characteristics of unprimed PC12 cells naive to nerve growth factor exposure are the small cell body size and limited neurites. Primed PC12 cells have significant neurite outgrowth and much larger cell bodies.

2. MORPHOLOGICAL INDICES

2.1. What Do You Measure Morphologically and How?

In vivo, morphological assessments of specific changes in differentiation include elaboration of dendritic arbors, axonal growth, and synapse formation and all require the use of advanced techniques, including immunocytochemical staining, microinjection of cell dyes, and/or electron microscopy. These approaches often require specialized equipment and software, can be labor intensive, and require specialized training. The methods used for morphological measurement of differentiation in vitro include assessment of cell size, number of cells exhibiting neurites, extent of neurite outgrowth, and fiber branching. These measurements of differentiation can be simpler and more efficient than similar correlate measures made in vivo, particularly in cell lines or primary cultures plated at low densities.

Many in vitro studies have used neurite outgrowth as a measure of differentiation after trophic factor stimulation *(6–10)* or to investigate the effects of drug or chemical exposure on this process in cell lines *(11–15)* and primary *(16–19)* or slice cultures *(20,21)*. Although many studies use measures of neurite outgrowth, most of these methods are semiquantitative at best. Most of these studies employ some criteria of measurement of processes that cross circular annulae that exceed two times the cell body diameter (e.g., ref. *22*). This approach is rapid and simple but is limited in dose–response analysis and focuses on neurite elaboration and not neurite initiation. Other, more quantitative approaches to measuring neurite outgrowth are applicable for use in measuring neurite initiation and elaboration *(8)*. This approach has been used to measure neurite initiation in PC12 cells that have no history of exposure to nerve growth factor (NGF) but receive acute exposure to this differentiating agent and coexposure to test chemicals. This approach can also reveal alterations in elaboration of neurite outgrowth in primed PC12 cells. Primed cells have had a history of NGF exposure and are differentiated to a point where they have a significant neurite network but then are replated. These primed cells are genetically identical to unprimed cells but are different in that they have reached the cell size of a differentiated neuronal phenotype. These primed cells will rapidly elaborate neurites over a 24-h period and recapitulate what would take approx 7 d of NGF stimulation to achieve in this same cell line without a history of NGF exposure (*see* Fig. 3). The methodological approach for measuring neurite outgrowth can utilize sophisticated image analysis software to objectively quantify cell size, neurite out growth, number of branch points, and branch segment length. This approach employs utilizing differential thresholds in a way that does not require drawing of the entire neurite network (*see* Fig. 4).

 Barone, Kodavanti, and Mundy

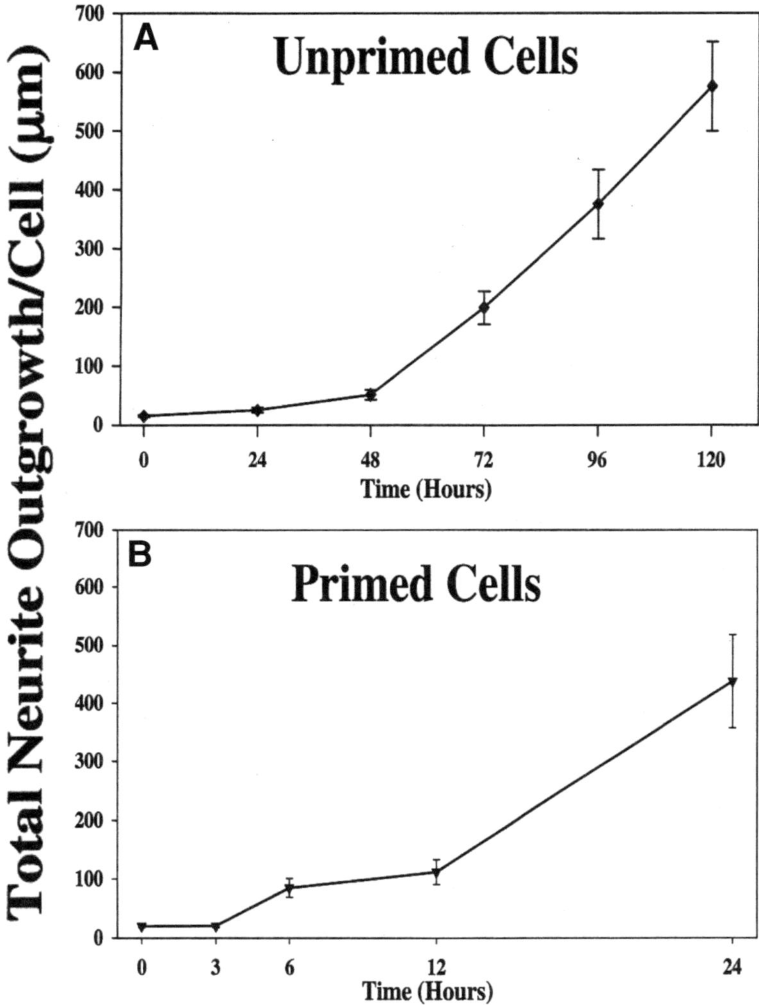

Fig. 3. Time-course and NGF concentration study of neurite outgrowth in PC12 cells. (**A**) Unprimed PC12 cells were cultured for different periods of time (24, 48, 72, 96, 120 h), during the priming period, in the presence of NGF (50 ng/mL) and resulted in a time-dependent increase in neurite outgrowth. (**B**) Primed PC12 cells were cultured for different periods of time (3, 6, 12, 24 h), during the exposure period, in the presence of NGF (50 ng/mL) and resulted in a time- dependent increase in neurite outgrowth. Note that it takes almost 24 h for primed cells to elaborate as much neurite outgrowth unprimed cells. The results depicted are representative of at least six independent measures and are expressed as mean ± SE.

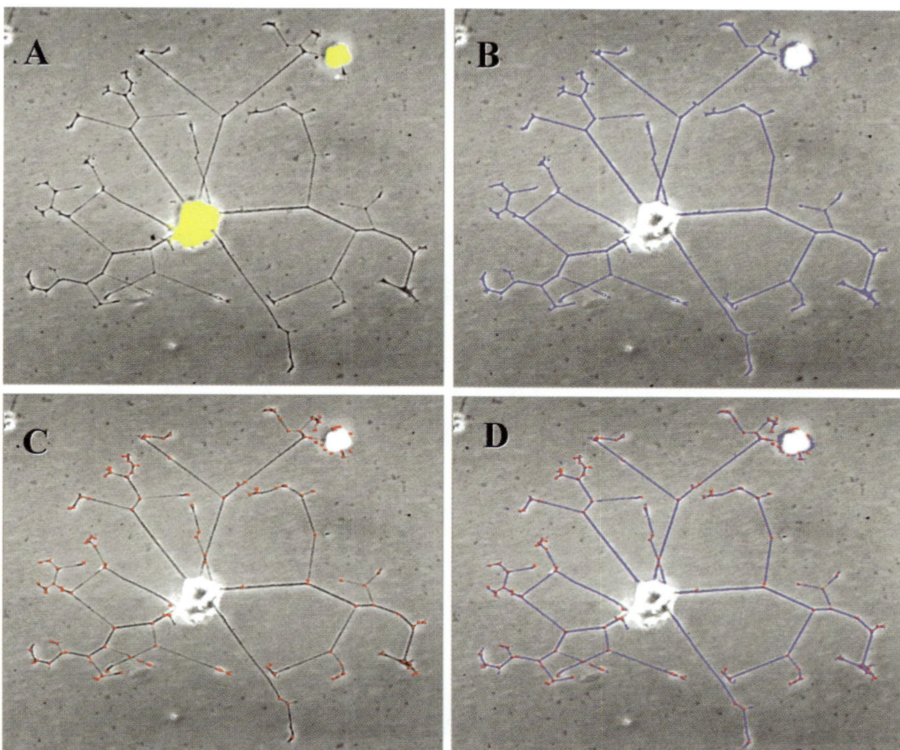

Fig. 4. Image analysis can be used to quantify neurite outgrowth. (**A**) The cell bodies of neurons can be discerned from the background by differential thresholds in digital images and mean cell body area can be determined (yellow). (**B**) The total neurite network can be discerned from the background by differential thresholds in digital images and digitally processes (skeletonized) to one pixel width to determine the mean total neurite outgrowth per cell (blue). (**C**) The skeletonized image of the total neurite network can be processed to determine where more than three pixels come into contact (triple point) to quantify fiber branching and crossing. (**D**) Subtraction of triple points from skeletonized total neurite network can provide the fiber segments that can then be uniquely labeled to provide a mean fiber branch segment length.

2.2. Case Studies of In Vitro and In Vivo Lead and Methylmercury

Examination of results of numerous studies of neurite outgrowth data by means of the same analysis system with PC12 cells can be used to draw some conclusions about relative potency of neurotoxicants on different aspects of differentiation (*see* Table 1). Even within a single class of toxicants

Table 1
Neurite Outgrowth in Rat Pheochromocytoma (PC12) Cells

Class	Agent	Unprimed (LOEL)	Primed (LOEL)
Positive control	Nerve growth factor (8)	⇑	⇑
	Fibroblast growth factor (8)	Not tested	⇑
Control inhibitors	K252A (8,23) inhibits trk autophosphorylation	Not tested	⇓
	U0126 (23) inhibits MAPK phosphorylation	Not tested	⇓
	NGF antibody (8)	Not tested	⇓
	FGF antibody (8)	Not tested	⇓
Neurotoxicants metals	Lead acetate (12)	⇑(0.025 μM) ⇓(1 μM) biphasic	⇑(0.025 μM) ⇓(1 μM) biphasic
	Methylmercury (13)	⇓(0.3 μM)	⇓(0.01 μM)
	Mercury chloride (13)	⇑(0.1 μM)	⇓(0.01 μM)
	Trimethyltin[a]	Not tested	⇓(4 μM)
	Monomethyltin[a]	Not tested	⇔[b]
	Dimethyltin[a]	Not tested	⇓(2 μM)
	Dibutyltin[a]	Not tested	⇓(0.1 μM)
Cholinesterase inhibitors and metabolites	Chlorpyrifos (11)	⇔	⇓(1 μM)
	Chlorpyrifos-oxon (11)	⇔	⇓(1 nM)
	Trichlorpyridinol (11)	⇔	⇓(1 μM)
	Burroughs Welcome compound (11)	Not tested	⇓(1 μM)

Note: All effects on neurite outgrowth were seen at concentrations did not produce changes in cell viability at LOELs (lowest effective levels).

[a]Unpublished data from Jenkins and Barone.

[b]No effect seen at any concentrations tested.

such as metals, the effects on initiation and elaboration can be qualitatively different. For example, low levels of lead can actually stimulate molecular and morphological characteristics of differentiation in both unprimed and primed PC12 cells at relatively similar potencies *(12)*. On the other hand, methylmercury exposure inhibits differentiation but with much greater potency on elaboration versus initiation *(13)*. The effect of low level lead or mercury chloride exposure to accelerate initiation might be related to potentiation of calcium-mediated signaling of differentiation *(12)*. Accelerated differentiation should not be viewed uniformly as a good thing, but must be considered in the context of the full concentration–response curve. A deviation from normal timing of differentiation might be indicative of altered cell determination. In addition, this premature differentiation can have secondary consequences on pattern formation. Timing of differentiation has dramatic effects on downstream and upstream synaptic targets.

The relevance of in vitro findings to in vivo effects can be demonstrated qualitatively with two prototypical developmental neurotoxicants that affect differentiation: lead and methylmercury. In the case of lead, numerous investigators have shown that in vitro lead exposure can have a wide range of effects on differentiation depending on the exposure *(23)*. In our in vitro assay system, lead appears to have stimulatory effects at lower concentrations and inhibitory effects at higher concentrations *(12)*. Recent evidence from our lab would also suggest that in vivo perinatal exposure to lead in rats also has a stimulatory effect on the differentiation of specific neurotransmitter systems during postnatal development. The transmitter systems examined were the catacholaminegic and sertonergic systems that have been shown to be affected by postnatal lead exposure using functional and biochemical analyses *(25–27)*. The in vivo effects of perinatal lead exposure are consistent with premature differentiation, but it appears that this effect can come with a cost, because markers of later dendritic and synaptic elaboration appear to be stunted when compared to controls *(27)*. In the case of methylmercury, differentiation is inhibited at low concentrations in vitro and this inhibition might involve changes in neurotrophic factor signaling *(13,28)*, tubulin polymerization *(29)*, and cell adhesion molecule expression *(30,31)*. In vivo, the effects of low-dose gestational exposure to methylmercury in rats also results in the inhibition of what is believed to be dendritic elaboration *(32)*. Although these are studies of developmental neurotoxicity of two heavy metals, their proposed mechanisms of action are very different. Furthermore, the key point made here is that the in vitro effects can be used to design in vivo studies and can be useful in determining the mechanism(s) by which a toxicant might be affecting a specific developmental process.

3. NEUROCHEMICAL INDICES

The use of neurochemical methods to monitor differentiation and maturation of neuronal cells in culture is not a new concept. In the development of cell culture systems for use in neuroscience, biochemical measurements have been used to characterize the differentiation and maturation of primary neuronal cells *(33)* and neuronal cell lines *(34)*. However, although the assessment of specific proteins associated with developmental processes has been used successfully to detect chemical-induced injury in the developing nervous system in vivo *(35,36)*, it is only recently that neurochemical measurement of proteins associated with cellular differentiation was recognized for its potential as a marker of neurotoxicity in cell culture test systems *(37,38)*. Although not widely applied to date, the use of neurochemical measures of differentiation for in vitro neurotoxicity testing has the potential to add to and improve upon the data obtained from traditional morphologic measures of differentiation. Neurochemical methods for assessing differentiation, including radioligand binding, immunoblotting, and ELISA (enzyme-linked immunosorbent assay) might prove to be more efficient and are potentially amenable to high-throughput screening. A change in a particular neurochemical marker can also provide information regarding the site or mechanism of action of a neurotoxicant. The sensitivity of neurochemical markers compared to morphologic assessment of neuronal differentiation is a critical issue that remains to be determined.

The process of differentiation results in mature neurons with unique properties that subserve their ultimate function: the transfer of information both intercellularly from one cell to another and intracellularly within cells. These properties include the elaboration of dendrites and axons (which contain specific neuronal cytoskeletal elements), electrical excitability (which depends on the presence of ion channels), synthesis and release of neurotransmitters (based on the expression of particular neurotransmitter-metabolizing enzymes), the expression of neurotransmitter receptors, and formation of the synaptic terminal. In many cases, the process of differentiation results in an increase in expression over time in the culture of the proteins that underlie these functions. Thus, by critically evaluating the relationship between expression of these cell-specific proteins and the state of morphological or functional maturity within a particular cell culture model, a subset of proteins can be identified that can serve as neurochemical markers of differentiation. Although it is clear that the synthesis of many proteins is increased in differentiating cells, it should be noted that the number is fewer than may be expected from the dramatic change in structure and function that is observed. For example, in PC12 cells differentiated with NGF, examination of 700–800 individual proteins by one- or two-dimensional gel electrophoresis showed that a quantitative change was apparent in only 5% of the proteins *(39–41)*.

Appropriate growth of axons underlies the development of connections in the nervous system. Molecules that promote axon growth comprise very different classes of protein acting on distinct sets of neuronal receptors. Soluble growth factors such as neurotrophins and fibroblast growth factors (FGF) act mostly on receptor-type protein tyrosine kinases, whereas extracellular matrix (ECM) proteins such as laminin and fibronectin act on heterodimeric integrins and cell adhesion molecules. Although the proteins involved in the stimulation of axon growth are varied, both tyrosine phosphorylation and calcium mobilization are components of many pathways activated by axonal growth-promoting molecules. The onset of critical protein expression determines whether the developing neurite becomes a dendrite or an axon *(42)*. The initial process is short and contains both microtubule-associated protein 2 (MAP2) and growth- associated protein-43 (GAP-43) proteins. The critical step in axonal differentiation is the restriction of GAP-43 and the appearance of tau protein in one neurite, and all the rest become dendrites. After differentiation of the axon, other processes begin to extend and take on the branching appearance of dendrites. New proteins, such as phosphokinase A and calcium/calmodulin kinase, appear differentially in the dendrites. Neurofilaments are present both in dendrites and axons. They are much more numerous and more heavily phosphorylated in axons.

There are numerous examples of in vitro studies examining the expression of neuron- specific cytoskeletal proteins, ion channels, neurotransmitter-metabolizing enzymes, and neurotransmitter receptors in primary neuronal cultures or neuronal cell lines. However, the number of studies in which a correlation is made between the ontogeny of these proteins and a morphological or functional measure of differentiation are far fewer. The following subsections will focus on those neurochemical parameters that are clearly associated with an independent measure of neuronal differentiation.

3.1. Neurotransmitter-Metabolizing Enzymes

Increases in various neurotransmitter-metabolizing enzymes are observed in both clonal cell lines and primary neuronal cultures. The identity and final levels of these enzymes in vitro will depend on the cell type, developmental stage of the starting material, and culture conditions. The PC12 cell clone is probably the most widely used model for the study of neuronal differentiation. When cultured in the presence of NGF, PC12 cells stop dividing, extend neuronal processes, and become electrically excitable *(6)*. These changes are accompanied by increases in enzymes involved in acetylcholine and catecholamine synthesis and degradation. The acetylcholine-metabolizing enzymes choline acetyltransferase (ChAT) and acetylcholinesterase (AChE) are increased twofold to threefold upon treatment with NGF *(43–47)*, whereas the catecholamine-synthesizing enzyme tyrosine hydroxylase (TH) is increased twofold *(48)*. Increases in metabolizing enzymes are also observed in primary neuronal cultures. For example, in primary cultures from fetal rat telencephalon, increases in ChAT, AChE, and glutamic acid decarboxylase (GAD) increase over time in culture and are accompanied by an increase in cell size, neurite outgrowth, and the appearance of mature synapses *(33)*.

Recently, there has been much interest in the idea that AChE has a morphogenic role during neuronal development distinct from its enzymatic ability to break down acetylcholine *(49,50)*. Thus, even in cells that are noncholinergic, AChE is expressed at high levels during periods of neurite outgrowth. In cultured dorsal root ganglion neurons prepared from rat embryos, the level of AChE expression correlates with neurite outgrowth, whereas pharmacologic inhibition of AChE or treatment with an anti-AChE antibody reduces neurite outgrowth *(51–53)*.

3.2. Receptors and Ion Channels

The depolarization of PC12 cells in response to application of acetylcholine is increased by NGF-induced differentiation *(54,55)*. This response is a result of the presence of nicotinic cholinergic receptors in the PC12 cell membrane *(43,56)*, which show a sixfold increase with time in culture after differentiation with NGF, as assessed by binding of a monoclonal antibody *(57)*. PC12 cells also express muscarinic cholinergic receptors in the cell membrane *(58,59)*. In addition, muscarinic cholinergic receptors show a progressive increase (twofold to fourfold) over time after differentiation when measured by the specific binding of the antagonists quinuclidinyl benzilate *(58)* or *N*-methylscopolamine *(60)*.

The *N*-methyl-D-aspartate (NMDA) subtype of glutamate receptor is widely distributed in the central nervous system and increases with development in vivo *(61)*. Several NMDA receptor subunits have been cloned, including the NR1 subunit and four NR2 (A–D) subunits *(62,63)*. The coexpression of the NR1 subunit with one or more of the NR2 subunits is required for the generation of a functional receptor. In primary neurons from fetal rat or mouse brain, the expression of the NMDA receptor subunits increases over time in culture as measured by expression of NMDA receptor subunit mRNA or binding of the NMDA antagonist MK-801 *(64–66)*. This increase follows the morphologic maturation of neurons in culture and is thought to be related to the emergence of glutamate-stimulated calcium flux and excitotoxicity in mature cultures *(67)*.

Electrical excitability and the release of a neurotransmitter from presynaptic stores generally increase with differentiation and maturation of neurons in culture largely resulting from the increased expression of voltage-gated ion channels. In PC12 cells, NGF-induced differentiation results in a 10- to 20-fold increase in the density of Na^{2+} channels *(68)*, and the cells acquire electrical excitability. The expression of voltage-gated Ca^{2+} channels is also changed with differentiation and maturation in vitro. The influx of Ca^{2+} through voltage-gated Ca^{2+} channels plays an important role in neurotransmitter release during synaptic transmission. In neurons, a number of different Ca^{2+} channel subtypes have been identified, including the N type, L type, P type, and Q type *(69,70)*. Three of these subtypes, the N-, P-, and Q-type Ca^{2+} channels, are involved in evoking fast neurotransmitter release *(71,72)*. PC12 cells express at least two of these Ca^{2+} channel subtypes *(73)*. Differentiation of PC12 cells results in both an increase in Ca^{2+} channel expression and a change in the predominant subtype. As measured by electrophysiologic recordings and channel-type-selective inhibitors, differentiation of PC12 cells with NGF results in a shift from predominantly L-type Ca^{2+} channels to predominantly N-type channels *(74–76)*. This change in the predominant Ca^{2+} channel subtype is accompanied by an increase in Ca^{2+} channel expression of twofold to fourfold as determined by measuring Ca^{2+} current *(76–79)* or ligand binding to the Ca^{2+} channel *(76,79)*. The effect of methylmercury on Ca^{2+} channels was examined in differentiating PC12 cells. Cells exposed to 10 n*M* methylmercury during 7 d of differentiation with NGF showed a 36% decrease in Ca^{2+} current on DIV 7 (80). However, a similar exposure resulted no change in ligand binding to Ca^{2+} channels and no change in neurite outgrowth *(80)*, suggesting the effects of methylmercury were the result of the direct inhibition of ion channel function. These results indicate that measurement of changes in ion channel function may not be a good measure of differentiation in cases where a toxicant can directly block the channel. A more limited set of studies has examined the changes in Ca^{2+} channels during differentiation and maturation of primary neuronal cultures. Porter et al. *(81)* examined Ca^{2+} channels in fetal hippocampal neurons in culture. Morphologically, an increase in the size of the cell soma and elongation of neurites was noted at 3 d in vitro (DIV), with more extensive networks formed by DIV 6. Ca^{2+} channel currents increased rapidly during the first 7 d in culture, then continued to rise more slowly up to DIV 28. Further studies from the same laboratory showed that the initial increase was the result of Ca^{2+} flux through L-, N-, and P/Q- type channels, whereas increases after DIV 7 were the result of L-type channels *(82)*.

3.3. Cytoskeletal Proteins

There are several cytoskeletal proteins that increase with neurite growth that can be useful as markers of differentiation and growth as well as for visualization of axons and dendrites. These include neurofilament proteins, MAPs, GAP-43, and proteins associated with the synaptic terminal (synapsin, synaptophysin, synuclein). The involvement of these proteins in the formation of neuronal processes and synaptic maturation have made them particularly well suited for the study of developing cultures (*see* Fig. 5). Neurofilaments that belong to the class of intermediate filaments are among the most phosphorylated proteins in the cytoskeleton and are prominent in large axons playing a role in the maintenance of cell shape and axonal transport. They are composed of light (68 kDa), medium (160 kDa) and heavy (200 kDa) subunits.

Inhibition of neurite outgrowth assessed by an ELISA for the light and medium neurofilament subunits has been examined in two cell lines. In the mouse NB41A3 neuroblastoma cell line, treatment of the cells for 6 d with the excitatory amino acid analogs β-*N*-methyl-1 amino alanine or kainate decreased neurofilament proteins with a corresponding decrease in neurite outgrowth *(38)*. Similar results were observed in human SK- N-SH neuroblastoma cells exposed to mercuric chloride for 6 d *(83)*.

Although both microfilaments and intermediate filaments are involved in neuronal development and are possible sites for toxicants *(84)*, much of the focus has been given to microtubules. Microtubules are long polymers composed of longitudinally aligned tubulin dimers (α and β monomers). Microtubule-associated proteins (MAPs) are high-molecular-weight structural proteins (>200 kDa) that are associated with and stabilize the microtubules. Microtubules exist in a number of isoforms that differ in the content of α- and β-tubulins and decoration by MAPs *(85)*. There are several subtypes of MAP that occur at high levels in neurons, including MAP2a and MAP2b (288 and 280 kDa, respectively; expressed mainly in nerve cell bodies and dendrites) and MAP2c (70 kDa; expressed transiently in developing axons). The developmental regulation of MAPs suggests that they are involved in neuronal morphogenesis *(86,87)*. PC12 cells contain several MAP subtypes, including MAP5/1b, MAP1, MAP2, and MAP3 *(88)*. As assessed by immunobloting, at least one of these subtypes (MAP5/1b) shows a large (10- to 15-fold) and progressive increase after differentiation of PC12 cells with NGF *(88,89)*. In primary neuronal cultures, MAP2 is a developmentally regulated subtype that is generally restricted to the cell soma and dendrites. It is useful for staining and identifying dendritic processes, although it can be found in all the minor processes early in differentiation *(51,86)*.

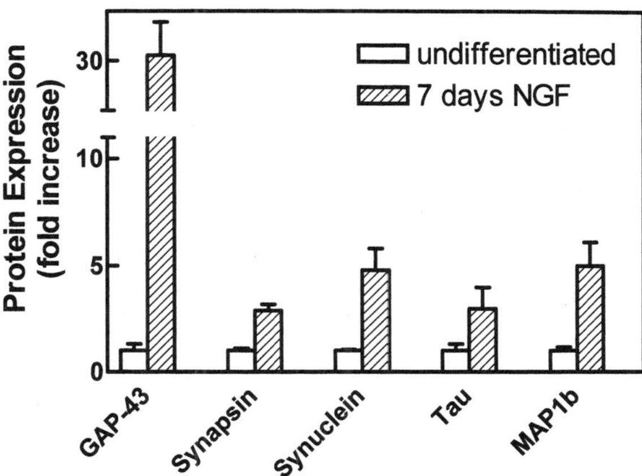

Fig. 5. Changes in protein levels for cytoskeletal and synaptic proteins upon differentiation of PC12 cells. The elaboration of neurites and formation of synapses results in the upregulation of a number cytoskeletal and synaptic proteins. Unprimed (undifferentiated) PC12 cells were treated with 50 ng/mL NGF for 7 d. On d 7, cell lysates were prepared and proteins separated using sodium dodecyl sulfate–polyaerylamide gel electrophoresis. Protein levels were determined using commercially available antibodies by Western blot analysis. The results depicted are representative of at least three independent experiments and are expressed as mean ± SE.

MAP2 staining and MAP2 protein levels in primary neuronal cultures increase in association with increasing dendritic length *(90–92)*. Several neurotoxicants have been shown to affect the microtubule system. Methylmercury has been shown to interfere with maturation of microtubules in cultured cells *(29,93,94)*. 2,4-Dichlorophenoxyacetic acid (2,4-D), a potent neurotoxic herbicide, has been shown to inhibit microtubule assembly and decrease neurite outgrowth in a dose-dependent manner *(95)*. Dichlorvos, an organophosphorous insecticide, induced hyperphosphorylation of tubulin and MAP2 which, in turn, destabilizes microtubule assembly *(96)*.

A related protein, tau, is a microtubule-associated protein that appears to play a major role in the polymerization and stabilization of microtubules during neuronal differentiation and axon elongation *(97)*. In primary cells developing in culture, tau is found in neurons but not in glia, and it is initially present in both dendrites and axons *(98)*. However, as the neurons mature in vitro, tau can become segregated to the axon *(99)*. A number of studies in both PC12 cells *(10,100,101)* and primary neuronal cultures *(101)* indicate that a dramatic increase in tau protein levels is coincidental with neurite outgrowth.

3.4. Synapses

GAP-43 is a growth-associated phosphoprotein that has long been known for its role in growth cone function and axonal elongation, regeneration after axonal damage, and synaptic plasticity in the mature nervous system *(102)*. Neurons growing either in vivo or in vitro express high levels of GAP-43 coincident with the beginning of neurite outgrowth *(103–106)*. It is preferentially distributed in the growth cone and elongating axon of developing neurons *(104,107,108)*. In PC12 cells, differentiation with NGF results in a 5- to 10-fold increase in GAP-43 levels that correlates with the increase in neurite outgrowth *(109–111)*. Inhibition of NGF-induced neurite outgrowth with dexamethasone *(110)* or the MAP kinase inhibitor U0126 *(111)* produced a corresponding decrease in GAP-43 expression. GAP-43 levels can also be correlated with axonal outgrowth in primary neuronal cultures *(112)*.

There are a number of proteins that are preferentially distributed to the synapse. The best characterized of these are synapsin and synaptophysin, proteins that are localized to the presynaptic membrane and involved in synaptic vesicle fusion resulting in neurotransmitter release *(113)*. Synaptobrevin is a small protein that is anchored to the vesicle membrane and plays a key role in exocytosis. Synaptotagmin is an integral membrane protein and also plays a key role in calcium-dependent exocytosis *(113)*. These protein levels increase with the active formation of synapses in the developing rat brain *(36,114)*. The time-course of this in vivo increase parallels that of synaptogenesis and suggests that these proteins can be used as markers of nerve terminal maturation. In addition, the study of O'Callaghan and Miller *(36)* examined the effect of developmental exposure in vivo to organotins on the levels of synapsin and synaptophysin. Both proteins were decreased in brain regions previously shown to be damaged by the organotins, suggesting that synapsin and synaptophysin can be used as markers of nerotoxicant-induced damage to developing nerve terminals. The levels of synapsin and synaptophysin also increase in neuronal cultures. In PC12 cells, differentiation with NGF results in a threefold increase in synapsin which correlates with the appearance of synaptic vesicles in mature nerve terminals *(115)*. In primary neurons, both synapsin and synaptophysin increase with time in culture, coincident with extent of synapse formation *(116)* and the ability to evoke neurotransmitter release *(117)*. Less well studied are the synucleins, another family of proteins expressed predominantly in the brain and enriched in presynaptic terminals. Although their normal physiologic functions are not entirely known, they can act to regulate membrane stability and/or turnover *(118)*. Unlike synapsin and synaptophysin, α-synuclein does not appear in synaptic terminals in cultured neurons until several days after functional synapses begin to form *(119)* and thus do not appear to be a constitutive component of synapses. α-Synuclein is upregulated in areas of the brain where synaptic architecture is undergoing rearrangements associated with learning and memory *(120–122)*. Thus, α-synuclein can be a marker for mature synapses, and levels correlate with the degree of functional plasticity in the synapse. In the rodent brain, α-synuclein levels undergo a large increase during the brain growth spurt and remain high in adulthood *(123)*. In both PC12 cells *(124)* and primary hippocampal neurons *(119)*, α-synuclein levels increase during the later stages of differentiation, after synapses have formed.

3.5. Cell Adhesion Molecules

Cell adhesion and substrate adhesion are extremely important to differentiation. Neural cell adhesion molecules (NCAMs) are the most widely studied and well characterized of the adhesion molecules involved in neurogenesis. NCAM is a surface glycoprotein whose structure is highly conserved across species. There are three isoforms that are temporally and spatially regulated during development. The 120- and 140-kDa isoforms appear early in neural development and the 180-kDa isoform appears first in postmitotic, postmigratory neurons *(125)*. Although NCAM plays a central role in brain morphogenesis *(126,127)*, little is known about its role in developmental neurotoxicity. Of the various classes of toxicants, heavy metals such as lead and methylmercury have been shown to clearly affect NCAM in developing animals *(128,129)*, which might be related to defective arborization and synaptogenesis reported in brains of treated animals *(129,130)*.

4. MOLECULAR METHODS FOR DETECTING DIFFERENTIATION

Measurements of steady-state mRNA levels for developmentally regulated proteins are often useful as markers for their function. In addition, toxic insults that target a given cell type or function might be expected to result in somewhat specific alterations in mRNA expression of proteins involved in those functions. Alterations in mRNA levels depend on the extent of toxicity caused by the chemical (i.e., mRNA expression might be repressed or be upregulated in some conditions by a mechanism compensating for toxicant exposure). Thus, measurements of steady-state mRNA levels for selected proteins can serve as molecular markers for altered nervous system function consequent to exposure to a toxicant. There are several probes available for specific proteins in neurons and axons. These include neurofilament proteins, which are the sites of action of a number of neurotoxicants *(131)*. Changes in mRNA levels for synapsin I have been noted during brain development *(132)* in a number of neurological disorders *(133)* and following exposure to various pharmaceutical agents *(86)*. Expression of both GAP-43 and its mRNA is upregulated in neurons during axonal regeneration following injury *(134)*. Measurement of mRNA levels for this protein can be useful as a general marker of axonal regeneration. Several neurotoxicants including lead have been shown to stimulate GAP-43 mRNA expression *(135,136)*, suggesting that perturbations in levels of this growth-associated protein might play a role in the retarded nervous system development. In addition, mRNAs of the microtubule associated proteins tau and MAP-2 are also modulated during brain development *(137)*.

There are several experimental approaches to measure mRNA. Advantages of using this measurement are that it is a uniform, relatively simple, rapid, and usually inexpensive approach. This contrasts with direct assays of a protein of interest, which requires at the very least a good antibody for the protein being examined. These are very expensive to generate or purchase, and assays are complicated and time-consuming. On the other hand, many RNA species can be measured simultaneously with relatively simple techniques. Northern blot analysis is the most commonly used technique for mRNA quantitation where RNA (total or mRNA) is electrophoretically separated on denaturing agarose gels according to molecular size, transferred to a nylon or similar membrane, and then hybridized with labeled DNA probes complimentary to the mRNA species being examined *(138)*. After unbound probe is rinsed from these membranes, the amount of the label in each sample can be determined either autoradiographically or with electronic imaging systems. The Northern blot analysis has an advantage over the quicker "dot-blot" or "slot-blot" analysis, where RNA is directly immobilized on the membrane without any size fractionation, because the specificity of probe hybridization can be confirmed by examining the sizes of mRNA species that bind the labeled cDNA probe. A further advantage is that if multiple mRNA transcripts are present (alternative splicing of RNA), levels of each individual transcript can be quantified. Another approach, roughly an order of magnitude more sensitive than Northern, is the ribonuclease (RNase) protection assay *(139)*. In this assay, RNA prepared from the tissue is hybridized within solution with a labeled antisense RNA probe. After hybridization, samples will be subjected to ribonuclease digestion, which removes all RNA except double-stranded RNA formed when target mRNA binds the labeled probe. These fragments will be separated electrophoretically and the label in appropriate bands will be quantified. This assay allows the determination of a number of different messages at the same time. Another procedure that is a more sensitive, but less quantitative strategy is reverse transcriptase–polymerase chain reaction (RT-PCR). This methodology is very useful for examining genes that are expressed at very low levels, at or below the limits of detection of Northern analysis or RNase protection assay. The new technology in this area is DNA microarray. In this procedure, differential expression of a large number of genes can be monitored quickly and at high levels of sensitivity.

5. SUMMARY, CONCLUSIONS, AND FUTURE DIRECTIONS

5.1. Summary and Conclusions

Morphological indices of differentiation can provide qualitative and quantitative information about concentration responses in vitro depending on the test system used. This chapter provides some review of methods but also provides examples with numerous positive controls and test chemicals in the same cell line with the same quantitative approach. The current morphological approaches for examining differentiation can be associated with effects on differentiation at relatively low-level exposures in vivo of two reference compounds (lead and methylmercury) that produce developmental neurotoxicity leading to functional deficits.

Biochemical measures of differentiation can provide quantitative information that recapitulates in vitro differentiation under defined conditions. Although some data exist for selected regions for biochemical markers of differentiation, additional data are needed to show the sensitivity of regional and temporal profiles to developmental neurological disorders and developmental neurotoxicants.

Molecular methods can provide qualitative evidence for mechanism of action on the process of differentiation; however, more data are needed on toxicant-induced changes and dose–response assessment.

For all three approaches for examining differentiation, further evaluation is required to determine the reliability, sensitivity, and predictive validity of assays to detect toxicant-induced changes in these markers of differentiation.

5.2. Future Directions

Future research should address in vitro to in vivo extrapolation of the markers and methods for determining the differentiation state of multiple neural cell types. More attention needs to be given to evaluating the relationship between in vitro concentration responses and to in vivo target-tissue doses. This would greatly enhance the predictive validity of these in vitro assays. Molecular indices of differentiation could be useful for elucidating mechanism(s) of action for drugs and toxicants but more work is required to provide proof of principle of a multitude of molecular approaches. One of the most promising areas where this in vitro research could have an impact is in the arena of screening mixtures of toxicants found in the environment. If these approaches have predictive validity, then for in vivo effects on the same processes regardless of their mechanism of action, one might determine that effects on this developmental process could serve as a mode of action for developmental neurotoxicity. Moreover, this approach could provide more rapid screening of very complex environmental mixtures and constituents of mixtures for cumulative dose–response assessment.

ACKNOWLEDGMENTS

The authors are grateful for the technical assistance of Lori White, Scott Jenkins, Connie Meacham, and Theresa Freudenrich. The authors are also grateful for the photographic assistance of Mr. Keith Tarpley and for the editorial comments of Dr. Tim Shafer, Dr. Stephanie Padilla, and Dr. Evelyn Tiffany-Castiglioni on an earlier draft of this manuscript.

This manuscript was reviewed by the NHEERL, US Environmental Protection Agency, and approved for publication. Mention of trade names or commercial products does not constitute endorsement or recommendation for use. The opinions expressed by the authors are not to be misconstrued as US Environmental Protection Agency policy.

REFERENCES

1. Panchision, D. M. and McKay, R. D. (2002) The control of neural stem cells by morphogenic signals. *Curr. Opin. Genet. Dev.* **12,** 478–487.
2. Rice, D. C. and Barone, S. J. (2000) Critical Periods of vulnerability for the developing nervous system: evidence from humans and animal models. *Environ. Health Perspect.* **108(Suppl. 3),** 511–533.
3. Edenfeld, G., Pielage, J., and Klambt, C. (2002) Cell lineage specification in the nervous system. *Curr. Opin. Genet. Dev.* **12,** 473–477.
4. McConnell, S. K. (1990) The specification of neuronal identity in the mammalian cerebral cortex. *Experientia* **46,** 922–929.
5. Eagleson, K. L., Lillien, L., Chan, A. V., and Levitt, P. (1997) Mechanisms specifying area fate in cortex include cell-cycle-dependent decisions and the capacity of progenitors to express phenotype memory. *Development* **124,** 1623–1630.
6. Greene, L. A. and Tischler, A. S. (1976) Establishment of a noradrenergic clonal line of rat adrenal pheochromocytoma cells which respond to nerve growth factor. *Proc. Natl. Acad. Sci. USA* **73,** 2424–2428.
7. Greene, L. A., Bernd, P., Black, M. M., et al. (1983) Genomic and non-genomic actions of nerve growth factor in development. *Prog. Brain Res.* **58,** 347–357.

8. Shaughnessy, L. W. and Barone, S. J. (1997) Damage to the NBM leads to a sustained lesion-induced increase in functional NGF in the cortex. *NeuroReport* **8,** 2767–2774.

9. Bosco, A. and Linden, R. (1999) BDNF and NT-4 differentially modulate neurite outgrowth in developing retinal ganglion cells. *J. Neurosci. Res.* **57,** 759–769.

10. Drubin, D. G., Feinstein, S. C., Shooter, E. M., and Kirschner, M. W. (1985) Nerve growth factor-induced neurite outgrowth in PC12 cells involves the coordinate induction of microtubule assembly and assembly-promoting factors. *J. Cell Biol.* **101,** 1799–1807.

11. Das, K. D. and Barone, S. J. (1999) Neuronal differentiation in PC12 cells is inhibited by chlorpyrifos and its metabolites: is acetylcholinesterase inhibition the site of action? *Toxicol. Appl. Pharmacol.* **160,** 217–230.

12. Crumpton, T. L., Atkins, D., Zawia, N., and Barone, S., Jr. (2001) Lead exposure in pheochromocytoma (PC12) cells alters neural differentiation and Sp1 DNA-binding. *Neurotoxicology* **22,** 49–62.

13. Parran, D. K., Mundy, W. R., and Barone, S. J. (2001) Effects of methylmercury and mercuric chloride on differentiation and cell viability in PC12 cells. *Toxicol. Sci.* **59,** 278–290.

14. Smith, S. L., Sadler, C. J., Dodd, C. C., et al. (2001) The role of glutathione in the neurotoxicity of artemisinin derivatives in vitro. *Biochem. Pharmacol.* **61,** 409–416.

15. Brat, D. J. and Brimijoin, S. (1992) A paradigm for examining toxicant effects on viability, structure, and axonal transport of neurons in culture. *Mol. Neurobiol.* **6,** 125–135.

16. Audesirk, T. and Cabell, L. (1999) Nanomolar concentrations of nicotine and cotinine alter the development of cultured hippocampal neurons via non-acetylcholine receptor-mediated mechanisms. *Neurotoxicology* **20,** 639–646.

17. Mariussen, E., Myhre, O., Reistad, T., and Fonnum, F. (2002) The polychlorinated biphenyl mixture aroclor 1254 induces death of rat cerebellar granule cells: the involvement of the *N*- methyl-D-aspartate receptor and reactive oxygen species. *Toxicol. Appl. Pharmacol.* **179,** 137–144.

18. Layer, P. G. (1991) Cholinesterases during development of the avian nervous system. *Cell Mol. Neurobiol.* **11,** 7–33.

19. Layer, P. G., Weikert, T., and Alber, R. (1993) Cholinesterases regulate neurite growth of chick nerve cells in vitro by means of a non-enzymatic mechanism. *Cell Tissue Res.* **273,** 219–226.

20. Bywood, P. T. and Johnson, S. M. (2000) Dendrite loss is a characteristic early indicator of toxin-induced neurodegeneration in rat midbrain slices. *Exp. Neurol.* **161,** 306–316.

21. Lotto, R. B. and Price, D. J. (1996) Effects of subcortical structures on the growth of cortical neurites in vitro. *NeuroReport* **7,** 1185–1188.

22. Bilsland, J., Rigby, M., Young, L., and Harper, S. (1999) A rapid method for semi- quantitative analysis of neurite outgrowth from chick DRG explants using image analysis. *J. Neurosci. Methods* **92,** 75–85.

23. Audesirk, G. and Audesirk, T. (1998) Neurite development, in *Handbook of Developmental Neurotoxicology* (Slikker, W. J. and Chang, L. W., eds.), Academic, San Diego, pp. 61–86.

24. Cory-Slechta, D. A. (1995) Relationships between lead-induced learning impairments and changes in dopaminerigic, cholinerigic, and glutamatergic neurotransmitter system functions. *Annu. Rev. Pharmacol. Toxicol.* **35,** 391–415.

25. Lasley, S. M. and Lane, J. D. (1988). Diminished regulation of mesolimbic dopaminergic activity in rat after chronic inorganic lead exposure. *Toxicol. Appl. Pharmacol.* **95,** 474–483.

26. Lasley, S. M., Greenland, R. D., Minnema, D. J., and Michaelson, I. A. (1984) Influence of chronic inorganic lead exposure on regional dopamine and 5-HT turnover in rat brain. *Neurochem. Res.* **9,** 1675–1688.

27. Moreira, E. G., Vassilieff, V. S., Vassilieff, I., et al. (2002) Developmental lead exposure: neurochemical and neuroanatomical effects in the rat. *Toxicologist* **66,** 125.

28. Parran, D. K., Barone, S., Jr., and Mundy, W. R. (2003) Methylmercury inhibits NGF-induced TrkA autophosphorylation and neurite outgrowth in PC12 cells. *Dev. Brain Res.* **141(1-2),** 71–81.

29. Graff, R. D., Falconer, M. M., Brown, D. L., and Reuhl, K. R. (1997) Altered sensitivity of posttranslationally modified microtubules to methylmercury in differentiating embryonal carcinoma-derived neurons. *Toxicol. Appl. Pharmacol.* **144,** 215–224.

30. Lagunowich, L. A., Bhambhani, S., Graff, R. D., and Reuhl, K. (1991) Cell adhesion molecules in the cerebellum: Targets of methylmercury toxicity? *Soc. Neurosci.* **17,** 515.

31. Dey, P. M., Gochfeld, M., and Reuhl, K. R. (1999) Developmental methylmercury administration alters cerebellar PSA-NCAM expression and Golgi sialyltransferase activity. *Brain Res.* **845,** 139–151.

32. Barone, S. J., Haykal-Coates, N., Parran, D. K., and Tilson, H. A. (1998) Gestational exposure to methylmercury alters the developmental pattern of trk-like immunoreactivity in the rat brain and results in cortical dysmorphology. *Dev. Brain Res.* **109,** 13–31.

33. Honegger, P. (1985) Biochemical differentiation in serum-free aggregating brain cell cultures, in *Cell Culture in the Neurosciences* (Bottenstein, J. E. and Sato, G., eds.), Plenum, New York, pp. 223–243.

34. Guroff, G. (1985) PC12 cells as a model of neuronal differentiation, in *Cell Culture in the Neurosciences* (Bottenstein, J. and Sato, G., eds.), Plenum, New York, pp. 245–272.

35. O'Callaghan, J. P. (1988) Neurotypic and gliotypic proteins as biochemical markers of neurotoxicity. *Neurotoxicol. Teratol.* **10,** 445–452.

36. O'Callaghan, J. P. and Miller, D. B. (1989) Assessment of chemically-induced alterations in brain development using assays of neuron- and glia-localized proteins. *Neurotoxicology* **10,** 393–406.

37. Reinhardt, C. A. (1993) Neurodevelopmental toxicity in vitro: primary cell culture models for screening and risk assessment. *Reprod. Toxicol.* **7(Suppl. 1),** 165–170.

38. Abdulla, E. M. and Campbell, I. C. (1993) L-BMAA and kainate-induced modulation of neurofilament concentrations as a measure of neurite outgrowth: implications for an in vitro test of neurotoxicity. *Toxicol. In Vitro* **7,** 341–344.
39. Garrels, J. I. and Schubert, D. (1979) Modulation of protein synthesis by nerve growth factor. *J. Biol. Chem.* **254,** 7978–7985.
40. McGuire, J. C., Greene, L. A., and Furano, A. V. (1978) NGF stimulates incorporation of fucose or glucosamine into an external glycoprotein in cultured rat PC12 pheochromocytoma cells. *Cell* **15,** 357–365.
41. McGuire, J. C. and Greene, L. A. (1980) Stimulation by nerve growth factor of specific protein synthesis in rat PC12 pheochromocytoma cells. *Neuroscience* **5,** 179–189.
42. Goslin, K. and Banker, G. (1989) Experimental observations on the development of polarity by hippocampal neurons in culture. *J. Cell Biol.* **108,** 1507–1516.
43. Greene, L. A. and Rein, G. (1977) Synthesis, storage and release of acetylcholine by a noradrenergic pheochromocytoma cell line. *Nature* **268,** 349–351.
44. Edgar, D. H. and Thoenen, H. (1978) Selective enzyme induction in a nerve growth factor- responsive pheochromocytoma cell line (PC 12). *Brain Res.* **154,** 186–190.
45. Lucas, C. A., Czlonkowska, A., and Kreutzberg, G. W. (1980) Regulation of acetylcholinesterase by nerve growth factor in the pheochromocytoma PC12 cell line. *Neurosci. Lett.* **18,** 333–337.
46. Rieger, F., Shelanski, M. L., and Greene, L. A. (1980) The effects of nerve growth factor on acetylcholinesterase and its multiple forms in cultures of rat PC12 pheochromocytoma cells: increased total specific activity and appearance of the 16 S molecular form. *Dev. Biol.* **76,** 238–243.
47. Greene, L. A. and Rukenstein, A. (1981) Regulation of acetylcholinesterase activity by nerve growth factor. Role of transcription and dissociation from effects on proliferation and neurite outgrowth. *J. Biol. Chem.* **256,** 6363–6367.
48. Hatanaka, H. (1981) Nerve growth factor-mediated stimulation of tyrosine hydroxylase activity in a clonal rat pheochromocytoma cell line. *Brain Res.* **222,** 225–233.
49. Layer, P. G. and Willbold, E. (1995) Novel functions of cholinesterases in development, physiology and disease. *Prog. Histochem. Cytochem.* **29,** 1–94.
50. Bigbee, J. W., Sharma, K. V., Gupta, J. J., and Dupree, J. L. (1999) Morphogenic role for acetylcholinesterase in axonal outgrowth during neural development. *Environ. Health Perspect.* **107(Suppl. 1),** 81–87.
51. Caceres, A., Banker, G., Steward, O., Binder, L., and Payne, M. (1984) MAP2 is localized to the dendrites of hippocampal neurons which develop in culture. *Brain Res.* **315,** 314–318.
52. Dupree, J. L. and Bigbee, J. W. (1994) Retardation of neuritic outgrowth and cytoskeletal changes accompany acetylcholinesterase inhibitor treatment in cultured rat dorsal root ganglion neurons. *J. Neurosci. Res.* **39,** 567–575.
53. Sharma, K. V. and Bigbee, J. W. (1998) Acetylcholinesterase antibody treatment results in neurite detachment and reduced outgrowth from cultured neu-

rons: further evidence for a cell adhesive role for neuronal acetylcholinesterase. *J. Neurosci. Res.* **53,** 454–464.

54. Dichter, M. A., Tischler, A. S., and Greene, L. A. (1977) Nerve growth factor-induced increase in electrical excitability and acetylcholine sensitivity of a rat pheochromocytoma cell line. *Nature* **268,** 501–504.
55. Ifune, C. K. and Steinbach, J. H. (1990) Regulation of sodium currents and acetylcholine responses in PC12 cells. *Brain Res.* **506,** 243–248.
56. Boyd, N. D. (1987) Two distinct kinetic phases of desensitization of acetylcholine receptors of clonal rat PC12 cells. *J. Physiol.* **389,** 45–67.
57. Whiting, P. J., Schoepfer, R., Swanson, L. W., Simmons, D. M., and Lindstrom, J. M. (1987) Functional acetylcholine receptor in PC12 cells reacts with a monoclonal antibody to brain nicotinic receptors. *Nature* **327,** 515–518.
58. Jumblatt, J. E. and Tischler, A. S. (1982) Regulation of muscarinic ligand binding sites by nerve growth factor in PC12 phaeochromocytoma cells. *Nature* **297,** 152–154.
59. Cross, A. J., Johnson, J. A., Frith, C., and Taylor, G. R. (1984) Muscarinic cholinergic receptors in a rat pheochromocytoma cell line. *Biochem. Biophys. Res. Commun.* **119,** 163–167.
60. Viana, G. B., Davis, L. H., and Kauffman, F. C. (1988) Effects of organophosphates and nerve growth factor on muscarinic receptor binding number in rat pheochromocytoma PC12 cells. *Toxicol. Appl. Pharmacol.* **93,** 257–266.
61. McDonald, J. W., Johnston, M. V., and Young, A. B. (1990) Differential ontogenic development of three receptors comprising the NMDA receptor/channel complex in the rat hippocampus. *Exp. Neurol.* **110,** 237–247.
62. Ishii, T., Moriyoshi, K., Sugihara, H., et al. (1993) Molecular characterization of the family of the N-methyl-D-aspartate receptor subunits. *J. Biol. Chem.* **268,** 2836–2843.
63. Monyer, H., Sprengel, R., Schoepfer, R., et al. (1992) Heteromeric NMDA receptors: molecular and functional distinction of subtypes. *Science* **256,** 1217–1221.
64. Williams, K., Russell, S. L., Shen, Y. M., and Molinoff, P. B. (1993) Developmental switch in the expression of NMDA receptors occurs in vivo and in vitro. *Neuron* **10,** 267–278.
65. Zhong, J., Russell, S. L., Pritchett, D. B., Molinoff, P. B., and Williams, K. (1994) Expression of mRNAs encoding subunits of the N-methyl-D-aspartate receptor in cultured cortical neurons. *Mol. Pharmacol.* **45,** 846–853.
66. Mizuta, I., Katayama, M., Watanabe, M., Mishina, M., and Ishii, K. (1998) Developmental expression of NMDA receptor subunits and the emergence of glutamate neurotoxicity in primary cultures of murine cerebral cortical neurons. *Cell. Mol. Life Sci.* **54,** 721–725.
67. Cheng, C., Fass, D. M., and Reynolds, I. J. (1999) Emergence of excitotoxicity in cultured forebrain neurons coincides with larger glutamate-stimulated [Ca(2+)](i) increases and NMDA receptor mRNA levels. *Brain Res.* **849,** 97–108.

68. Rudy, B., Kirschenbaum, B., Rukenstein, A., and Greene, L. A. (1987) Nerve growth factor increases the number of functional Na channels and induces TTX-resistant Na channels in PC12 pheochromocytoma cells. *J. Neurosci.* **7,** 1613–1625.

69. Nowycky, M. C., Fox, A. P., and Tsien, R. W. (1985) Three types of neuronal calcium channels with different calcium agonist sensitivity. *Nature* **316,** 440–443.

70. Tsien, R. W., Lipscombe, D., Madison, D. V., Bley, K. R., and Fox, A. P. (1988) Multiple types of neuronal calcium channels and their selective modulation. *Trends Neurosci.* **11,** 431–438.

71. Takahashi, T. and Momiyama, A. (1993) Different types of calcium channels mediate central synaptic transmission. *Nature* **366,** 156–158.

72. Wheeler, D. B., Randall, A., and Tsien, R. W. (1994) Roles of N-type and Q-type Ca^{2+} channels in supporting hippocampal synaptic transmission. *Science* **264,** 107–111.

73. Shafer, T. J. and Atchison, W. D. (1991) Methylmercury blocks N- and L-type Ca++ channels in nerve growth factor-differentiated pheochromocytoma (PC12) cells. *J. Pharmacol. Exp. Ther.* **258,** 149–157.

74. Streit, J. and Lux, H. D. (1987) Voltage dependent calcium currents in PC12 growth cones and cells during NGF-induced cell growth. *Pflugers Arch.* **408,** 634–641.

75. Plummer, M. R., Logothetis, D. E., and Hess, P. (1989) Elementary properties and pharmacological sensitivities of calcium channels in mammalian peripheral neurons. *Neuron* **2,** 1453–1463.

76. Usowicz, M. M., Porzig, H., Becker, C., and Reuter, H. (1990) Differential expression by nerve growth factor of two types of Ca^{2+} channels in rat pheochromocytoma cell lines. *J. Physiol.* **426,** 95–116.

77. Furukawa, K., Onodera, H., Kogure, K., and Akaike, N. (1993) Time-dependent expression of Na and Ca channels in PC12 cells by nerve growth factor and cAMP. *Neurosci. Res.* **16,** 143–147.

78. Lewis, D. L., De Aizpurua, H. J., and Rausch, D. M. (1993) Enhanced expression of Ca^{2+} channels by nerve growth factor and the v-src oncogene in rat pheochromocytoma cells. *J. Physiol.* **465,** 325–342.

79. Bouron, A., Becker, C., and Porzig, H. (1999) Functional expression of voltage-gated Na+ and Ca^{2+} channels during neuronal differentiation of PC12 cells with nerve growth factor or forskolin. *Naunyn Schmiedebergs Arch. Pharmacol.* **359,** 370–377.

80. Shafer, T. J., Meacham, C. A., and Barone, S. (2002) Effects of prolonged exposure to nanomolar concentrations of methylmercury on voltage-sensitive sodium and calcium currents in PC12 cells. *Dev. Brain Res.* **136,** 151–164.

81. Porter, N. M., Thibault, O., Thibault, V., Chen, K. C., and Landfield, P. W. (1997) Calcium channel density and hippocampal cell death with age in long-term culture. *J. Neurosci.* **17,** 5629–5639.

82. Blalock, E. M., Porter, N. M., and Landfield, P. W. (1999) Decreased G-protein-mediated regulation and shift in calcium channel types with age in hippocampal cultures. *J. Neurosci.* **19,** 8674–8684.

83. Abdulla, E. M., Calaminici, M., and Campbell, I. C. (1995) Comparison of neurite outgrowth with neurofilament protein subunit levels in neuroblastoma cells following mercuric oxide exposure. *Clin. Exp. Pharmacol. Physiol.* **22,** 362–363.

84. Clarkson, T. W., Sager, P. R., and Syversen, T. L. (1986) *The Cytoskeleton. A Target for Toxic Agents*, Plenum, New York.

85. Nunez, J. (1986) Differential expression of microtubule components during brain development. *Dev. Neurosci.* **8,** 125–141.

86. Matus, A., Bernhardt, R., Bodmer, R., and Alaimo, D. (1986) Microtubule-associated protein 2 and tubulin are differently distributed in the dendrites of developing neurons. *Neuroscience* **17,** 371–389.

87. Kobayashi, N. and Mundel, P. (1998) A role of microtubules during the formation of cell processes in neuronal and non-neuronal cells. *Cell Tissue Res.* **291,** 163–174.

88. Brugg, B. and Matus, A. (1988) PC12 cells express juvenile microtubule-associated proteins during nerve growth factor-induced neurite outgrowth. *J. Cell Biol.* **107,** 643–650.

89. Greene, L. A., Liem, R. K., and Shelanski, M. L. (1983) Regulation of a high molecular weight microtubule-associated protein in PC12 cells by nerve growth factor. *J. Cell Biol.* **96,** 76–83.

90. Caceres, A., Banker, G. A., and Binder, L. (1986) Immunocytochemical localization of tubulin and microtubule-associated protein 2 during the development of hippocampal neurons in culture. *J. Neurosci.* **6,** 714–722.

91. Fletcher, T. L., De Camilli, P., and Banker, G. (1994) Synaptogenesis in hippocampal cultures: evidence indicating that axons and dendrites become competent to form synapses at different stages of neuronal development. *J. Neurosci.* **14,** 6695–6706.

92. Guo, X., Chandrasekaran, V., Lein, P., Kaplan, P. L., and Higgins, D. (1999) Leukemia inhibitory factor and ciliary neurotrophic factor cause dendritic retraction in cultured rat sympathetic neurons. *J. Neurosci.* **19,** 2113–2121.

93. Sager, P. R. and Matheson, D. W. (1988) Mechanisms of neurotoxicity related to selective disruption of microtubules and intermediate filaments. *Toxicology* **49,** 479–492.

94. Hunter, A. M. and Brown, D. L. (2000) Effects of microtubule-associated protein (MAP) expression on methylmercury-induced microtubule disassembly. *Toxicol. Appl. Pharmacol.* **166,** 203–213.

95. Rosso, S. B., Caceres, A. O., de Duffard, A. M., Duffard, R. O., and Quiroga, S. (2000) 2,4- Dichlorophenoxyacetic acid disrupts the cytoskeleton and disorganizes the Golgi apparatus of cultured neurons. *Toxicol. Sci.* **56,** 133–140.

96. Choudhary, S., Joshi, K., and Gill, K. D. (2001) Possible role of enhanced microtubule phosphorylation in dichlorvos induced delayed neurotoxicity in rat. *Brain Res.* **897,** 60–70.

97. Paglini, G., Peris, L., Mascotti, F., Quiroga, S., and Caceres, A. (2000) Tau protein function in axonal formation. *Neurochem. Res.* **25,** 37–42.

98. Dotti, C. G., Banker, G. A., and Binder, L. I. (1987) The expression and distribution of the microtubule-associated proteins tau and microtubule-associated protein 2 in hippocampal neurons in the rat in situ and in cell culture. *Neuroscience* **23,** 121–130.

99. Litman, P., Barg, J., Rindzoonski, L., and Ginzburg, I. (1993) Subcellular localization of tau mRNA in differentiating neuronal cell culture: implications for neuronal polarity. *Neuron* **10,** 627–638.

100. Rasouly, D., Rahamim, E., Ringel, I., et al. (1994) Neurites induced by staurosporine in PC12 cells are resistant to colchicine and express high levels of tau proteins. *Mol. Pharmacol.* **45,** 29–35.

101. Smith, C. J., Anderton, B. H., Davis, D. R., and Gallo, J. M. (1995) Tau isoform expression and phosphorylation state during differentiation of cultured neuronal cells. *FEBS Lett.* **375,** 243–248.

102. Benowitz, L. I. and Routtenberg, A. (1997) GAP-43: an intrinsic determinant of neuronal development and plasticity. *Trends Neurosci.* **20,** 84–91.

103. Perrone-Bizzozero, N. I., Finklestein, S. P., and Benowitz, L. I. (1986) Synthesis of a growth-associated protein by embryonic rat cerebrocortical neurons in vitro. *J. Neurosci.* **6,** 3721–3730.

104. Meiri, K. F., Willard, M., and Johnson, M. I. (1988) Distribution and phosphorylation of the growth-associated protein GAP-43 in regenerating sympathetic neurons in culture. *J. Neurosci.* **8,** 2571–2581.

105. Costello, B., Meymandi, A., and Freeman, J. A. (1990) Factors influencing GAP-43 gene expression in PC12 pheochromocytoma cells. *J. Neurosci.* **10,** 1398–1406.

106. Dani, J. W., Armstrong, D. M., and Benowitz, L. I. (1991) Mapping the development of the rat brain by GAP-43 immunocytochemistry. *Neuroscience* **40,** 277–287.

107. McGuire, C. B., Snipes, G. J., and Norden, J. J. (1988) Light-microscopic immunolocalization of the growth- and plasticity-associated protein GAP-43 in the developing rat brain. *Brain Res.* **469,** 277–291.

108. Goslin, K., Schreyer, D. J., Skene, J. H., and Banker, G. (1990) Changes in the distribution of GAP-43 during the development of neuronal polarity. *J. Neurosci.* **10,** 588–602.

109. Jap Tjoen, S. E., Schmidt-Michels, M. H., Spruijt, B. M., Oestreicher, A. B., Schotman, P., and Gispen, W. H. (1991) Quantitation of the growth-associated protein B-50/GAP-43 and neurite outgrowth in PC12 cells. *J. Neurosci. Res.* **29,** 149–154.

110. Jap Tjoen, S. E., Schmidt-Michels, M., Oestreicher, A. B., Schotman, P., and Gispen, W. H. (1992) Dexamethasone-induced effects on B-50/GAP-43 expression and neurite outgrowth in PC12 cells. *J. Mol. Neurosci.* **3,** 189–195.

111. Das, K. P., Freudenrich, T. M., and Mundy, W. R. (2001) Evaluation of protein markers for neuronal differentiation in PC12 cells. *Toxicologist* **61,** 373.

112. Przyborski, S. A. and Cambray-Deakin, M. A. (1994) Developmental changes in GAP-43 expression in primary cultures of rat cerebellar granule cells. *Mol. Brain Res.* **25,** 273–285.

113. Thiel, G. (1993) Synapsin I, synapsin II, and synaptophysin: marker proteins of synaptic vesicles. *Brain Pathol.* **3,** 87–95.
114. Knaus, P., Betz, H., and Rehm, H. (1986) Expression of synaptophysin during postnatal development of the mouse brain. *J. Neurochem.* **47,** 1302–1304.
115. Romano, C., Nichols, R. A., Greengard, P., and Greene, L. A. (1987) Synapsin I in PC12 cells. I. Characterization of the phosphoprotein and effect of chronic NGF treatment. *J. Neurosci.* **7,** 1294–1299.
116. Ferreira, A., Kao, H. T., Feng, J., Rapoport, M., and Greengard, P. (2000) Synapsin III: developmental expression, subcellular localization, and role in axon formation. *J. Neurosci.* **20,** 3736–3744.
117. Ehrhart-Bornstein, M., Treiman, M., Hansen, G. H., Schousboe, A., Thorn, N. A., and Frandsen, A. (1991) Parallel expression of synaptophysin and evoked neurotransmitter release during development of cultured neurons. *Int. J. Dev. Neurosci.* **9,** 463–471.
118. George, J. M. (2002) The synucleins. Genome Biol. 3, REVIEWS3002.
119. Withers, G. S., George, J. M., Banker, G. A., and Clayton, D. F. (1997) Delayed localization of synelfin (synuclein, NACP) to presynaptic terminals in cultured rat hippocampal neurons. *Dev. Brain Res.* **99,** 87–94.
120. George, J. M., Jin, H., Woods, W. S., and Clayton, D. F. (1995) Characterization of a novel protein regulated during the critical period for song learning in the zebra finch. *Neuron* **15,** 361–372.
121. Maroteaux, L. and Scheller, R. H. (1991) The rat brain synucleins; family of proteins transiently associated with neuronal membrane. *Mol. Brain Res.* **11,** 335–343.
122. Shibayama-Imazu, T., Okahashi, I., Omata, K., et al. (1993) Cell and tissue distribution and developmental change of neuron specific 14 kDa protein (phosphoneuroprotein 14). *Brain Res.* **622,** 17–25.
123. Hsu, L. J., Mallory, M., Xia, Y., et al. (1998) Expression pattern of synucleins (non-Abeta component of Alzheimer's disease amyloid precursor protein/alpha-synuclein) during murine brain development. *J. Neurochem.* **71,** 338–344.
124. Stefanis, L., Kholodilov, N., Rideout, H. J., Burke, R. E., and Greene, L. A. (2001) Synuclein-1 is selectively up-regulated in response to nerve growth factor treatment in PC12 cells. *J. Neurochem.* **76,** 1165–1176.
125. Pollerberg, G. E., Burridge, K., Krebs, K. E., Goodman, S. R., and Schachner, M. (1987) The 180-kD component of the neural cell adhesion molecule N-CAM is involved in a cell–cell contacts and cytoskeleton-membrane interactions. *Cell Tissue Res.* **250,** 227–236.
126. Edelman, G. M. (1986) Cell adhesion molecules in the regulation of animal form and tissue pattern. *Annu. Rev. Cell Biol.* **2,** 81–116.
127. Brackenbury, R., Sorkin, B. C., and Cunningham, B. A. (1987) Molecular features of cell adhesion molecules involved in neural development. *Res. Publ. Assoc. Res. Nerv. Ment. Dis.* **65,** 155–167.
128. Cookman, G. R., King, W., and Regan, C. M. (1987) Chronic low-level lead exposure impairs embryonic to adult conversion of the neural cell adhesion molecule. *J. Neurochem.* **49,** 399–403.

129. Regan, C. M. (1993) Neural cell adhesion molecules, neuronal development and lead toxicity. *Neurotoxicology* **14,** 69–74.

130. Reuhl, K. R., Rice, D. C., Gilbert, S. G., and Mallett, J. (1989) Effects of chronic developmental lead exposure on monkey neuroanatomy: visual system. *Toxicol. Appl. Pharmacol.* **99,** 501–509.

131. Pyle, S. J. and Reuhl, K. R. (1997) Cytoskeletal elements in neurotoxicity, in *Nervous System and Behavioral Toxicology* (Lowndes, H. E. and Reuhl, K. R., eds.), Elsevier, New York, Vol. II, pp. 79–97.

132. Zurmohle, U. M., Herms, J., Schlingensiepen, R., Schlingensiepen, K. H., and Brysch, W. (1994) Changes of synapsin I messenger RNA expression during rat brain development. *Exp. Brain Res.* **99,** 17–24.

133. Tcherepanov, A. A. and Sokolov, B. P. (1997) Age-related abnormalities in expression of mRNAs encoding synapsin 1A, synapsin 1B, and synaptophysin in the temporal cortex of schizophrenics. *J. Neurosci. Res.* **49,** 639–644.

134. Curtis, R., Green, D., Lindsay, R. M., and Wilkin, G. P. (1993) Up-regulation of GAP-43 and growth of axons in rat spinal cord after compression injury. *J. Neurocytol.* **22,** 51–64.

135. Schmitt, T. J., Zawia, N., and Harry, G. J. (1996) GAP-43 mRNA expression in the developing rat brain: alterations following lead-acetate exposure. *Neurotoxicology* **17,** 407–414.

136. Zawia, N. H. and Harry, G. J. (1996) Developmental exposure to lead interferes with glial and neuronal differential gene expression in the rat cerebellum. *Toxicol. Appl. Pharmacol.* **138,** 43–47.

137. Ginzburg, I., Scherson, T., Giveon, D., Behar, L., and Littauer, U. Z. (1982) Modulation of mRNA for microtubule-associated proteins during brain development. *Proc. Natl. Acad. Sci. USA* **79,** 4892–4896.

138. Thomas, P. S. (1980) Hybridization of denatured RNA and small DNA fragments transferred to nitrocellulose. *Proc. Natl. Acad. Sci. USA* **77,** 5201–5205.

139. Berk, A. J. and Sharp, P. A. (1977) Sizing and mapping of early adenovirus mRNAs by gel electrophoresis of S1 endonuclease-digested hybrids. *Cell* **12,** 721–732.

9

Impairment of Synaptic Function by Exposure to Lead

Stephen M. Lasley and Mary E. Gilbert

1. INTRODUCTION

Of all known neurotoxicants, lead (Pb) has received by far the most research attention. Because of increasing awareness of its untoward effects, investigation of the metal's central nervous system (CNS) actions has extended over several decades and across multiple experimental species, methods, and approaches. As a result, numerous actions of lead on the brain have been uncovered at the cellular and systems levels (e.g., ref. *1*). Nonetheless, progress toward defining the specific bases of the neurotoxicity observed in exposed young children has been slow and inefficient and has not been commensurate with the magnitude of effort invested. Multiple factors have limited the development of this new information, but one of the most prominent has been the difficulty in linking findings obtained with in vitro approaches to neurotoxicity present in vivo.

Cellular mechanisms of toxicity are most readily examined employing in vitro systems, and in recent years many neurotoxicologists have come to recognize that in vitro approaches and lead exposure parameters must better relate to exposure in the intact animal for the results to have meaningful significance. In this chapter we will examine two methodological approaches that have been successful in meeting these criteria. Studies utilizing acute exposure to Pb^{2+} in vitro and expressing the effects of the metal in terms of *free* Pb^{2+} concentrations have produced results on retinal and synaptic activity corresponding well to independent measures of function in exposed intact animals. In addition, experiments utilizing hippocampal slices harvested from

From: *Apoptosis Methods in Pharmacology and Toxicology: In Vitro Neurotoxicology: Principles and Challenges*
Edited by: Evelyn Tiffany-Castiglioni © Humana Press Inc., Totowa, NJ

chronically exposed animals have generated similarly valuable findings on synaptic physiology, suggesting that these slices constitute a valid model of hippocampal function in the whole animal when studied ex vivo. We will review results generated in investigations of lead neurotoxicity utilizing each of these approaches, compare the findings to those from analogous studies conducted in vivo, and evaluate each methodology for its ability to elucidate neurotoxic mechanisms in the intact animal. It is our belief that more focused use of specific in vitro methodologies such as these will permit progress in this research area to proceed at a greater pace.

2. UTILIZATION OF FREE ION CONCENTRATIONS IN IN VITRO SYSTEMS

Studies utilizing acute exposure to Pb^{2+} in vitro have most often employed nominal metal ion concentrations, thereby ignoring the affinity of Pb^{2+} to form complexes with other ions in physiological buffer systems. Because of the complexity of metal–ligand equilibria in these solutions, control of *free* Pb^{2+}-ion speciation is necessary to ensure the reliability of data concerning the actions of this metal ion. Furthermore, this approach provides a common basis for comparison of results across studies or laboratories investigating Pb^{2+} effects and establishes a potential basis for linking data from in vitro and in vivo systems once metal speciation in vivo is known. This methodology has been employed in several studies of the actions of metal ions on cellular processes *(2–6)*.

The desired concentrations of free Pb^{2+} are set by use of a chelating agent present in excess, metal–ligand stability constants, and computer software. A number of chelators have been utilized including citrate, nitrilotriacetate, EDTA, and EGTA; the choice is based on their affinity for Pb^{2+} and on the desired range of free ion concentrations. These compounds also serve to buffer physiological media against any contaminant sources of Pb^{2+} in tissue or reagents.

Stability constants are obtained from reference compilations or from the original research reports (e.g., refs. *7,8*). Figure 1 shows the relationship among a chelating agent, stability constant, and nominal and free metal ion concentrations. Because ions such as Pb^{2+} can form complexes with several components of physiological buffer systems, equations such as that in Fig. 1 must be expressed for each Pb^{2+}–ligand combination. Computer software is generally required to calculate the Pb^{2+} and ligand concentrations necessary to simultaneously solve all of the stability relationships. The software utilized for this purpose has included Chelator *(9)*, a program provided by Fabiato *(10)*, and commercially available products *(11)*.

$$M(CH_3COO)_2 + \text{citrate} \xrightarrow{\;K_{citrate}\;} [\, M^{2+} \,] + M(\text{citrate})$$

nominal metal concentration	chelating agent	stability constant	*free* metal ion	chelated metal

Fig. 1. Chemical equation expressing a metal–ligand equilibrium utilizing a chelating agent and resulting in a free metal ion concentration. In this manner a nominal metal concentration is converted to a free ion concentration. Stability constants (e.g., $K_{citrate}$) are found in reference compilations and in original research publications. M and M^{2+} are a metal and its divalent cation, such as lead, zinc, or calcium; CH_3COO- is an acetate ion.

There is little direct evidence that the biologically active moiety of lead is the free ion, as some other positively charged complexed form of Pb^{2+} could behave similarly. However, the ability to describe the actions of free Pb^{2+} utilizing classical modeling approaches (e.g., sigmoidal concentration–effect curves as opposed to multiphasic curves) suggests that the free ion is the active form. In addition, results obtained with free ion concentrations computed by use of Pb^{2+}–ligand stability constants agree well with findings based on concentrations determined by other means (*see* refs. *2* and *4*), and free Pb^{2+} levels have also been verified by independent analytical methods (e.g., ref. *11*).

3. CANDIDATE MECHANISMS OF Pb NEUROTOXICITY DERIVED FROM IN VITRO SYSTEMS

3.1. Neurotransmitter Release

It has long been known that acute addition of Pb^{2+} to incubation media containing nerve synapse preparations inhibits Ca^{2+}-dependent neurotransmission by decreasing depolarization-evoked acetylcholine release (e.g., refs. *12,13*). Subsequent work demonstrated that Pb^{2+} added in vitro competitively inhibits Ca^{2+} influx through voltage-sensitive channels in rat brain synaptosomes (nominal K_i ~1 μM) and diminishes the associated acetylcholine release *(14)*. A generalized action of Pb^{2+} on neuronal function is indicated by extension of these findings to synaptosomal preparations in which dopamine *(15)* and GABA *(16)* release are reduced with nominal concentrations of 1–10 μM Pb^{2+}. In contrast, nominal concentrations of 1–30 μM Pb^{2+} increase spontaneous release in a concentration-dependent manner, a phenomenon that persists in the presence of Ca^{2+} channel blockers or absence of Ca^{2+} in the perfusion medium *(14–17)*. Pb^{2+} added to Ca^{2+}-deficient medium has also been shown to directly trigger exocytosis of acetylcholine with potency much greater than that of Ca^{2+} *(18)*, indicative of a Ca^{2+}-mimetic action of Pb^{2+}.

The above studies largely preceded the use of free Pb^{2+} concentrations to study the actions of the metal on transmitter release. It was left to these latter efforts to identify the sensitivity of various synaptic mechanisms to the actions of Pb^{2+} and thereby implicate those effects associated with environmentally relevant exposures. Multiple laboratories have investigated the inhibition of depolarization-induced Ca^{2+} currents produced by acute exposure of cultured cells, resulting in free Pb^{2+} IC_{50} values in the range of 0.3–1.3 μM (e.g., refs. *19,20*). Other workers examined the stimulation of spontaneous transmitter release by acute exposure of permeabilized synaptosomes or cultured cells *(18,21)* and reported a free Pb^{2+} EC_{50} of 4 nM. Westerink and Vijverberg *(22)* addressed this same question using fluorescent dyes and confocal laser scanning microscopy of permeabilized PC12 cells, an independent approach also based on the determination of free Pb^{2+} concentrations. They observed a threshold for acute Pb^{2+} to induce exocytosis of between 10 and 20 nM. It has been proposed that the synaptic concentrations of free Pb^{2+} in experimental animals chronically exposed to environmentally relevant levels of the metal are in the low nanomolar range *(23)*, indicating the importance of the mechanism of Pb^{2+}-induced transmitter release.

Recent studies utilizing nominal Pb^{2+} concentrations and patch clamping of cultured hippocampal cells identified these same mechanisms as underlying the metal's actions on GABA and glutamate release *(24,25)*. Braga et al. *(24)* reported a nominal Pb^{2+} IC_{50} of 68 nM to block the evoked release of these transmitters. Somewhat higher Pb^{2+} concentrations (≥ 100 nM) were required to increase tetrodotoxin-insensitive spontaneous glutamate and GABA release *(25)*. The patch clamp technique is sensitive to much lower nominal Pb^{2+} levels than the older literature cited earlier.

Analogous studies conducted in intact animals employing intracerebral microdialysis have identified the same release components as being affected as a result of chronic lead exposure. Lasley and co-workers have established that environmentally relevant exposure diminishes K^+-stimulated hippocampal glutamate and GABA release, an effect that can be traced to the actions of exposure on the Ca^{2+}-dependent component *(26–28)*. On the other hand, these investigators have also discerned an increase in K^+-stimulated glutamate and GABA release when extracellular Ca^{2+} levels and Ca^{2+} influx are minimized (i.e., the Ca^{2+}-independent release component), although this effect is observable only at higher exposure levels [blood lead ≥ 62 μg/100 mL *[28]).* Clearly, there is good agreement between the synaptic mechanisms identified utilizing chronically exposed animals and acutely exposed in vitro preparations.

In summary, the historical interest in the actions of Pb^{2+} on transmitter release resulted in some elucidation of the mechanisms involved prior to the emergence of investigative approaches utilizing free ion concentrations. Thus, these latter studies have focused more on refining the observations reported earlier and delineating the sensitivity of various synaptic processes to the actions of Pb^{2+}. Although experiments performed in the context of free Pb^{2+} levels have precisely defined the transmitter release components affected by exposure, they have had little opportunity to extend what is known of the actions of the metal on this synaptic process.

3.2. NMDA Receptors

Because of the importance of the NMDA receptor channel in cognitive function and synaptic plasticity, the effect of Pb^{2+} on this receptor has been one focus of attempts to define the bases of lead-induced cognitive impairments. In general, these studies have addressed the issue of whether environmental exposure can be mediated through direct effects of this ion on channel function. Most investigators have approached this question by employing brief exposure to nominal concentrations of Pb^{2+} in vitro. Alkondon et al. *(29)* reported that this form of Pb^{2+} exposure produced decreases in NMDA receptor-mediated currents in patch-clamped fetal hippocampal cells by decreasing the frequency of NMDA-activated channel openings. Decreases in the use-dependent binding of the noncompetitive NMDA antagonist MK-801 to its receptor channel site have been noted *(29–31).* IC_{50} values determined in rat hippocampal *(29,30)* or mouse forebrain preparations *(31)* ranged from 7 to 10 μM Pb^{2+} based on nominal metal concentrations.

Similarities in the inhibitory effects of Pb^{2+} and Zn^{2+} on access to the NMDA receptor channel have also been found *(29,32).* An increase in the IC_{50} of Pb^{2+} to inhibit MK-801 binding has been observed in the presence of Zn^{2+} *(31,33),* suggesting competition for the same binding site. Consistent with this proposal, Pb^{2+} has been reported to decrease the rate of dissociation of MK-801 binding similarly to Zn^{2+} *(32).* However, using nominal metal concentrations in forebrain membranes from adult animals, the presence of Pb^{2+} has also been reported not to affect the Zn^{2+} IC_{50} for MK-801 binding *(32).* Control of *free* metal ion speciation is necessary to ensure the reliability of data concerning Pb^{2+}–Zn^{2+} interactions and has clarified some of the findings of these studies. This approach assumes free Pb^{2+} is the active form of the ion and there is some evidence to support this assumption (*see* Subheading 2.), although the actual speciation in vivo is unknown.

Lasley and Gilbert *(34)* addressed these issues through experiments to identify the effects of acute exposure in vitro to free Pb^{2+} and/or Zn^{2+} on access to the NMDA receptor channel. Their results indicated that the properties of these free metal ions in adult rat cortical membranes are similar in inhibiting channel access to MK-801, but Pb^{2+} is more potent, exhibiting an IC_{50} of 0.55 μM versus 1.30 μM for Zn^{2+}. Moreover, interaction studies clearly demonstrated that these metal ions have independent sites of action on the receptor channel and indicated a combined inhibitory effect when both Pb^{2+} and Zn^{2+} are present. As noted earlier, the synaptic concentrations of free Pb^{2+} in experimental animals chronically exposed to environmentally relevant levels of the metal are thought to be in the low nanomolar range *(23)*. The fact that the Pb^{2+} IC_{50} for access to the NMDA receptor channel is in the low micromolar range indicates that the effect on the receptor of chronic environmental exposure to this metal is most likely mediated via an indirect mechanism.

Studies examining the actions of chronic exposure on NMDA receptor function have also been performed. The majority of these efforts have utilized continuous lead administration throughout development with testing conducted in adult animals. Ma et al. *(35)* continuously exposed female rats from just after conception to adulthood and found 15–41% increases compared to controls in NMDA receptor numbers in cortical and hippocampal areas. This increase in receptor number was determined by MK-801 autoradiography in the presence of blood lead values of 39 μg/100 mL. Guilarte et al. *(36)* also reported a 31% increase in forebrain NMDA receptors in animals exposed continuously from conception until sacrifice as adults employing Scatchard analyses of MK-801 binding. These increases were observed at blood lead concentrations of 14 μg/100 mL. Lasley et al. *(37)* examined hippocampal tissue and also performed Scatchard analyses of MK-801 binding. These workers observed 30–38% increases in NMDA receptor density in groups with blood lead values of 39 and 62 μg/100 mL, findings consistent with Ma et al. *(35)*. In addition, Chen et al. *(38)* utilized autoradiography and reported 19% increases in NMDA receptor number in hippocampal CA1 in animals exhibiting blood lead values of 30 μg/100 mL.

Whereas exposure-induced alterations of NMDA receptors have been observed in multiple laboratories, there has not been uniform agreement as to the direction of this change. Cory-Slechta et al. *(39,40)* employed autoradiography to investigate NMDA receptors in adult rats and found 15–30% decreases in MK-801 binding in several brain areas in exposed groups exhibiting blood lead values of 16–74 μg/100 mL. A plausible basis for these discrepancies is not evident, as Ma et al. *(35)* and Chen et al. *(38)* utilized similar methodology. Of course, it is possible that the distinction is based on the use of a postweaning exposure protocol as opposed to continual exposure initiated during gestation or at birth. However, it is worth noting that behavioral findings of enhanced responsiveness to NMDA *(41,42)* and diminished sensitivity to MK-801 *(43,44)* are consistent with increases in receptor density. Thus, the weight of the evidence appears to indicate that chronic exposure increases NMDA receptor numbers.

In comparing results on NMDA receptor function obtained employing acute exposure to free Pb^{2+} in vitro with those produced utilizing chronic exposure, some conclusions are apparent. It is clear that the increase in NMDA receptor density observed in the majority of reports involving chronic exposure is not a direct effect of Pb^{2+} on access to the receptor channel, but must be the result of some other cellular mechanism. As these changes induced by chronic lead are an opposite reflection of those found in evoked glutamate release, a link between these two observations has been proposed *(37,45)*. Furthermore, the evidence suggests that direct inhibition of the receptor channel does not occur with typical environmental exposures. Thus, although alterations induced by acute exposure in terms of free Pb^{2+} concentrations elucidate the changes seen after chronic exposure, they do not parallel them.

3.3. Protein Kinase C

The ability of Pb^{2+} to stimulate protein kinase C (PKC) activity with high potency has received substantial research interest because of its potential implications for cellular and synaptic toxicity and because of its apparent importance at environmental exposure levels. Using nominal metal concentrations Markovac and Goldstein *(46)* found that Pb^{2+} could selectively stimulate PKC activity at picomolar levels in partially purified enzyme from rat brain compared to the micromolar levels of Ca^{2+} required to elicit the same effect. Studies conducted in immature rat brain microvessels also employed nominal concentrations to demonstrate that micromolar Pb^{2+} stimulates PKC activity and causes translocation of the kinase from the soluble to the particulate fraction *(47)*. This potency was equivalent to that of Ca^{2+} and suggested that Pb^{2+} activated PKC in a Ca^{2+}-mimetic fashion.

Subsequently, Long et al. *(2)* quantified the properties of Pb^{2+} activation by utilizing a chelating agent to buffer free Pb^{2+} and Ca^{2+} in the PKC assay mixture and then measuring free ion concentrations by fluorine-19 nuclear magnetic resonance spectroscopy. These workers found the K_m for free Pb^{2+} stimulation of PKC in rat brain cortical extracts to be 55 pM, whereas the analogous value for Ca^{2+} was 0.26 µM. These mechanisms were further elucidated by Tomsig and Suszkiw *(4)* employing chelating agents to set free Pb^{2+}/Ca^{2+} concentrations in permeabilized adrenal chromaffin cells. Three

Pb^{2+} interaction sites with PKC were discriminated: an activation site with a K_m of 2.4 pM (compared to 1.0 μM for Ca^{2+}) and competitive and noncompetitive inhibitory sites with K_m's of 7.1 nM and 0.28 μM, respectively. The opposing actions at these interactive sites resulted in a maximal efficacy for Pb^{2+} activation of PKC that was less than half that of Ca^{2+}, in agreement with Long et al. *(2)*, leading to the proposal that Pb^{2+} was a partial agonist of the kinase *(4)*. Further work utilizing free ion concentrations and recombinant human PKC isozymes demonstrated that the picomolar potency of Pb^{2+} to activate the kinase resided in the Ca^{2+}-dependent or conventional isoforms *(48)*, whereas the inhibitory micromolar affinity interactions were evident in all of the Ca^{2+}-dependent and Ca^{2+}-independent isozymes examined. The data indicated that the picomolar affinity activation of PKC by Pb^{2+} occurred at the Ca^{2+}-binding sites, and thus these observations underscored the importance of the C2 domain of the enzyme as a molecular target of the metal ion.

Attempts have been made to build on the observed effects of Pb^{2+} on PKC in vitro by obtaining more functional measures of the induced changes in kinase activity. Capillary-like structure formation within astroglial–endothelial cell cocultures was inhibited with a nominal K_i of 0.5 μM Pb^{2+}, whereas the metal was found to increase membrane-associated PKC *(49)*. These effects mimicked the actions of phorbol esters in activating PKC, suggesting a stimulation of kinase activity by Pb^{2+}. Similarly, Lu et al. *(50)* found in human astrocytoma cells that Pb^{2+} induced a concentration-dependent increase in DNA synthesis that was mediated by activation of the α-isoform of PKC. Ca^{2+}-independent isozymes of the kinase were not involved. On the other hand, Kim et al. *(51)* demonstrated that exposure of PC12 cells to Pb^{2+} induced the expression of immediate early genes such as *c-fos* by a PKC-dependent mechanism. This induction was associated with activation of PKC δ- and ε-isoforms (Ca^{2+}-independent), but not the α- and β-isoforms (Ca^{2+}-dependent).

The effects of chronic lead exposure on PKC signaling have been more difficult to discriminate. Most investigators have utilized broken cell preparations and measures of either kinase translocation or enzyme activity. There is no basis on which to simulate in a broken cell preparation the intracellular milieu that existed in a chronically exposed intact animal. In the preparation of a tissue extract for determination of kinase activity, the unbound Pb^{2+} is removed or greatly diluted, so that the resulting activity measure largely reflects changes in total PKC expression resulting from the exposure; that is, this measure does not identify a synaptic pool of PKC or necessarily represent the pool of kinase involved in signal transduction. Alternatively, the translocation of kinase from a cytosolic to membrane cellular fraction is a somewhat nonspecific measure and observed changes should be independently confirmed. For example, chronic exposure has been reported to reduce expression of the γ-isozyme of PKC in rat hippocampal cytosolic and membrane fractions, but this change was not manifested in phorbol ester binding in tissue slices from these animals or in measures of Ca^{2+}-dependent or Ca^{2+}-independent PKC activity *(52)*. In other work, phorbol ester-stimulated PKC translocation was assessed in hippocampal slices and found to be enhanced in chronically exposed animals *(53)*, suggesting a lead-induced activation of the kinase. However, the number of phorbol ester binding sites in the membrane fraction was decreased as was expression of the PKC γ-isoform, leading the authors to suggest the presence of a downregulation of the enzyme. Reinholz et al. *(54)* reported decreased PKC activity in chronically exposed neonatal rats at postnatal day 8, but found enhanced expression of the γ-isozyme at this same time point.

From the effects of acute Pb^{2+} exposure in vitro, it is abundantly clear that PKC is a toxicologically significant intracellular target for the metal ion. However, various investigators have been unable to define how this acute effect translates, if at all, to chronic exposure in the intact animal. Neither is it evident how one could discriminate inhibition of PKC activity (e.g., resulting from decreased efficacy relative to that associated with Ca^{2+}) from a downregulated enzyme from prolonged stimulation. Judgment as to whether in vitro approaches employing free Pb^{2+} concentrations have the ability to elucidate neurotoxic mechanisms involving PKC in intact chronically exposed animals awaits the results of future experiments.

3.4. Neurite Initiation

Neurite initiation is known to be highly sensitive to neurotoxic compounds and has been the focus of studies examining morphological alterations caused by exposure to Pb^{2+} in vitro. Kern and Audesirk *(3)* assessed this endpoint in cultured rat hippocampal neurons exposed acutely to nominal 100 n*M* Pb^{2+} in combination with kinase or calmodulin inhibitors. They found that Pb^{2+} inhibited neurite initiation, and on the basis of the results with inhibitors concluded that this occurred by inappropriate stimulation of protein phosphorylation by Ca^{2+}-calmodulin-dependent (CaMKII) or cyclic AMP-dependent (PKA) protein kinases, possibly through stimulation of calmodulin. Intracellular free Ca^{2+} concentrations were measured in these neurons by fura-2 spectrofluorometry and were not altered by up to 48 h exposure to nominal 100 n*M* Pb^{2+}, leading these workers to propose that the stimulation of CaMKII, PKA, or calmodulin was not via increased Ca^{2+} but attributable to intracellular Pb^{2+} concentrations.

In contrast, Crumpton et al. *(55)* have observed a biphasic potentiation of neurite outgrowth in PC12 cells after exposure for up to 72 h to nominal 0.025–10 μM Pb^{2+}. These workers found that Pb^{2+} stimulated differentiation, but produced an effect of greater magnitude when the cells had been primed by nerve growth factor. Also, 1 and 10 μM Pb^{2+} were not as effective as lower concentrations. These investigators proposed that Pb^{2+} initiates neuronal differentiation via exposure-induced increases observed in binding of the zinc-finger protein Sp1 to DNA.

Subsequent work demonstrated that concentrations of free Pb^{2+} as low as 100–300 pM activates calmodulin and that in the presence of physiological concentrations of free Ca^{2+}, free Pb^{2+} stimulates calmodulin at levels below 50 pM *(56)*. In agreement with these observations, Pb^{2+} was also shown to activate the Ca^{2+}-calmodulin-dependent phosphatase, calcineurin, with a threshold of approx 100 pM free ion, although concentrations >200 pM reduced activity *(57)*. Combined with subsaturating Ca^{2+} concentrations, as little as 20 pM free Pb^{2+} enhanced activity of this phosphatase. Furthermore, exposure of cultured hippocampal neurons to nominal 100 nM Pb^{2+} resulted in 9–16% decreases in the free Ca^{2+}/fura-2 signal at periods up to 2 d of exposure, indicating that Pb^{2+} decreased intracellular free Ca^{2+} levels *(58)*. Other experiments on these cells demonstrated a transient calmodulin-dependent increase in Ca^{2+} efflux, probably through stimulation of Ca^{2+} extrusion by plasma membrane Ca^{2+}-ATPase.

Other reported actions of Pb^{2+} related to neurite initiation have been associated with Ca^{2+}-activated enzymes, but do not involve calmodulin. Audesirk et al. *(59)* demonstrated that Pb^{2+} inhibited the Ca^{2+}-dependent cysteine protease μ-calpain, which is thought to be important in neuronal differentiation. Free Pb^{2+} alone did not affect calpain activity, but it competed with Ca^{2+} for the binding sites on the enzyme and exhibited the properties of a noncompetitive inhibitor. Potential mechanisms underlying the inhibition of neurite initiation by free Pb^{2+} are summarized in Table 1.

Evidence of Pb^{2+}-induced inhibition of neurite outgrowth is in general agreement with observations made after chronic exposure to lead employing in vivo models. Cline et al. *(60)* employed an exposure protocol of 0.1 nM to 100 μM nominal Pb^{2+} for 6 wk localized to the retinotectal system of frog tadpoles and observed a severely reduced area and branch tip number of retinal ganglion cell axon arborizations within the optic tectum at nanomolar Pb^{2+} concentrations. Reuhl et al. *(61)* exposed primates to 2 mg lead/kg/d from infancy to 6 yr of age and found that neuronal volume density was reduced in primary visual area V1 and in visual projection area V2 compared to a group exposed to 25 μg lead/kg/d. Moreover, a relative

Table 1
**Potential Mechanisms Underlying Lead-Induced Inhibition
of Neuronal Development**

Mechanism	Source
Inappropriate stimulation of CaMKII, PKA activity	Kern and Audesirk, *(3)*
Pb^{2+}-induced activation of calmodulin	Kern et al. *(56)*
Activation of calcineurin at low $[Pb^{2+}]$	Kern and Audesirk *(57)*
Stimulation of Ca^{2+} efflux via Ca^{2+}-ATPase	Ferguson et al. *(58)*
Noncompetitive inhibition of μ-calpain	Audesirk et al. (59)

decrease in the number of arborizations among pyramidal neurons in both areas V1 and V2 was observed in the higher dose group.

Thus, there is good correspondence between reports that acute Pb^{2+} exposure in vitro and extended exposure in animal models in vivo results in diminished neuronal growth and differentiation at Pb^{2+} concentrations of apparent environmental relevance. Although studies employing intact animals have not progressed to the investigation of specific cellular mechanisms underlying these effects, it is apparent that the use of in vitro systems has identified the level of detail needed. Moreover, the use of free Pb^{2+} levels has specified a set of actions of the metal that could readily account for the changes observed in neuronal development after chronic exposure. It is left to future studies in intact animals to verify the accuracy of the cellular effects determined by in vitro work, but certainly there are well-defined points at which to begin.

3.5. Rod Photoreceptors

The actions of lead on retinal cells have been a focus of research investigation for over two decades. It has long been recognized that Pb^{2+} exhibits a selective effect on rod cells *(62)* and, more recently, that the associated loss of rod and bipolar cells was the result of exposure-induced apoptotic changes (e.g., ref. *63*). These observations have been linked with exposure-related alterations in rod-mediated visual function, and in vitro studies utilizing free ion concentrations have done much to elucidate the mechanistic bases of these observations.

These latter efforts have established the concentration-dependent inhibition of cyclic GMP (cGMP) hydrolysis by free Pb^{2+}, in addition to increases in retinal cGMP and rod Ca^{2+} levels (e.g., ref. *11*). Kinetic studies utilizing purified rod cGMP phosphodiesterase have shown that picomolar free Pb^{2+} concentrations competitively inhibit the enzyme relative to millimolar concentrations that are required for Mg^{2+} cofactor activity, thus binding with 10^4 to 10^6-fold higher affinity than Mg^{2+} and preventing cGMP hydrolysis *(11,64)*. When retinas are incubated in free Ca^{2+} and/or Pb^{2+} in vitro, the rods selectively die by apoptosis associated with mitochondrial depolarization, release of mitochondrial cytochrome-*c*, and increased caspase activity *(65,66)*. Fox et al. *(65)* have proposed that apoptosis is triggered by Ca^{2+} and Pb^{2+} overload as a result of altered cGMP phosphodiesterase activity. Subsequent work found the elevations in free Ca^{2+} and Pb^{2+} to be localized to photoreceptors and determined that the effects of the two ions were additive and blocked by a mitochondrial permeability transition pore inhibitor *(66)*. This suggested that the two ions bind to the internal metal binding site of this pore and thereby initiate the apoptosis cascade.

These mechanisms are entirely consistent with electroretinogram (ERG) changes observed in animals chronically exposed during early development: decreases in maximal ERG amplitude, decreases in absolute ERG sensitivity, and increases in mean ERG latency that were selective for rod photoreceptors *(67,68)*. Also in agreement with these mechanisms are observed elevations in retinal cGMP levels and reductions in light-activated cGMP phosphodiesterase activity. Moreover, the exposure level-dependent degeneration of rod and bipolar cells exhibited the classical morphological features of apoptotic cell death *(63)*. Other measures of visual function in chronically exposed animals also have been found to be consistent with the mechanistic data. Long-term dose-dependent elevations in response thresholds are present but only at scotopic (i.e., rod-mediated) backgrounds, and dark adaptation is delayed *(69)*. In addition, exposure-induced decreases in rhodopsin content that were proportional to the loss of rod cells have been reported *(63)* as well as dose-dependent decreases in retinal Na^+, K^+-ATPase activity *(70)*.

These studies investigating rod photoreceptors are perhaps the best examples of the ability to correlate data obtained in vitro in terms of free Pb^{2+}/Ca^{2+} concentrations with findings derived from in vivo exposure and with changes in visual physiology. In multiple instances the same cellular mechanisms are affected with each approach and are consistent with ERG and rod-mediated functional measures. The use of free ion concentrations has thus contributed greatly to our understanding of the effects of chronic Pb exposure on visual function. These relationships are summarized in Table 2.

4. THE HIPPOCAMPAL SLICE AND Pb-INDUCED ALTERATIONS IN SYNAPTIC PLASTICITY

The hippocampal slice has been widely used throughout neuroscience research in studies measuring biochemical activity or physiological function. In particular, field potential recordings made in these slices have proven to be a valuable model system for identifying mechanisms of toxicity that are present in vivo, when the tissue is taken from chronically exposed animals, i.e., when the tissue is examined ex vivo (*see* Fig. 2). These slices retain components of local neuronal circuitry as well as much of the extracellular and intracellular milieu present in vivo. Thus, the hippocampal slice constitutes a capable *in situ* model of tissue in exposed intact animals, and valuable findings on synaptic physiology have resulted. The use of these slices to generate the observations described in Subheading 4.1. is based on these principles.

4.1. Long-Term Potentiation

Hippocampal long-term potentiation (LTP) is a widely accepted cellular model of learning and memory that is characterized by a persistent increase

Table 2
Mechanisms of Pb-Induced Impairment of Retinal Function

In vitro evidence	In vivo evidence	Physiological changes
Competitive inhibition of cGMP PDE → increased retinal cGMP	Increased retinal cGMP	
	Decreased stimulated cGMP PDE activity	Decreased maximal ERG amplitude
		Decreased absolute ERG sensitivity
Increased rod $[Ca^{2+}]$		Increased mean ERG latency
Apoptosis from increased photoreceptor Ca^{2+}/Pb^{2+} via binding to mitochondrial permeability transition pore	Morphological features of apoptotic rod, bipolar cell death	Increased response thresholds at scotopic backgrounds
	Decreased rhodopsin proportional to cell loss	Delayed dark adaptation
Decreased retinal Na^+,K^+-ATPase activity	Decreased retinal Na^+,K^+-ATPase activity	

Abbreviations: PDE, phosphodiesterase; ERG, electroretinogram.

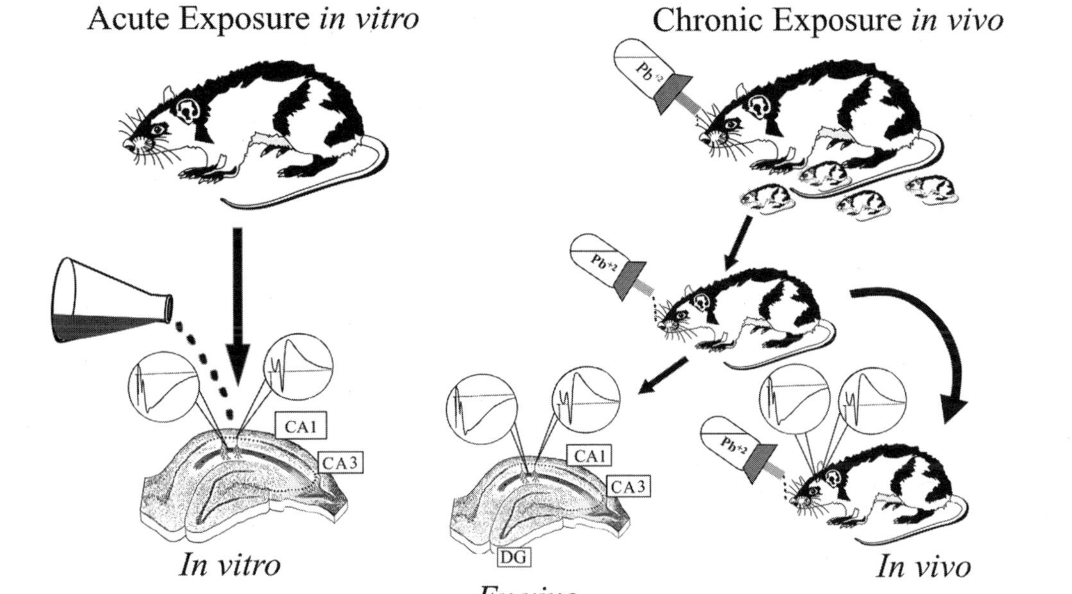

Fig. 2. Diagram depicting the distinctions between acute Pb^{2+} exposure in vitro and chronic lead exposure in vivo in the conduct of neurophysiological studies in hippocampus. For acute exposure in vitro, slices are harvested from control animals and Pb^{2+} is applied in perfusing solutions such as shown in the flask. For chronic developmental exposure in vivo, lead is administered to the dam through the drinking water prior to weaning of the pups, and testing is performed at some later time point on individual offspring maintained on lead water. Ex vivo studies utilize in vitro systems to examine tissue (such as hippocampal slices) from these chronically exposed offspring, whereas in vivo studies employ measurements made directly in intact animals. The waveforms display typical excitatory postsynaptic potentials and population spikes and the indicated recording locations. The CA1, CA3, and dentate gyrus (DG) subregions are also indicated.

in synaptic efficacy following delivery of brief tetanic stimulation *(71,72)*. Several lines of evidence support the hypothesis that the processes of LTP provide a neurophysiological substrate for learning and information storage. Although the link between this increase in synaptic efficacy and learning is far from conclusive (*see* e.g., refs. *73–75*), LTP is thought to utilize the same synaptic mechanisms as the learning process.

Findings from studies investigating the neurophysiological effects of chronic lead exposure have been remarkably consistent, whether utilizing chronically exposed intact animals or hippocampal slices examined ex vivo. No changes in baseline field potential measures (i.e., excitatory postsynaptic potential [EPSP] or population spike [PS]) evoked by single pulse stimulation have been observed (e.g., refs. *76–78*). On the other hand, LTP requires more complex patterns of stimulation for initiation. In studies focused on the effects on LTP in hippocampal subregions CA1 and dentate gyrus, whether in intact animals or tissue slices studied ex vivo, there has been 100% concordance that exposure diminishes potentiation. A summary of these reports organized by hippocampal subregion is provided in Table 3.

Three distinct actions of chronic lead exposure on measures of LTP have been identified. It is evident from the studies listed in Table 3 that exposure increases the threshold for induction and reduces the magnitude of potentiation, but exposure has also been shown to shorten LTP duration by accelerating its rate of decay *(82)*. Clearly, diminished LTP magnitude is commonly observed whether using in vivo or ex vivo preparations. Although an elevation in the threshold for induction of potentiation has been evaluated only in whole animal studies (Table 3), a decreased incidence of LTP induction has been reported in tissue slices also *(91)*, suggesting an impairment of induction processes. On the other hand, a meaningful comparison of decay of long-lasting LTP in intact animals and hippocampal slices is not possible: investigation of the decay of potentiation required a period of weeks *(82)*, whereas tissue slices are only viable for periods up to 6–8 h. Nonetheless, it is apparent that there is a good correspondence between the effects of chronic lead exposure on LTP when actions of the metal are studied in vivo and ex vivo. Tissue slices from chronically exposed animals therefore present an effective means to further investigate the cellular and/or biochemical bases of the actions of lead on LTP.

Moreover, measures of hippocampal LTP obtained from chronically exposed animals as a function of developmental period and exposure level *(76,81)* have exhibited striking similarities to data collected in parallel studies which quantified hippocampal glutamate release. These observations have suggested that lead-induced changes in stimulated glutamate release

Table 3
Hippocampal LTP and Chronic Lead Exposure

Exposure Duration[a]	Blood Pb[b]	Brain Pb[c]	Model	Effect of exposure on LTP	Ref.
Dentate gyrus					
PN0—PN85–105	37.5	378	In vivo	Impaired induction	Lasley et al. *(79)*
PN0—PN90–120	37.2	ND	In vivo	Elevated induction threshold	Gilbert et al. *(77)*
PN0—PN90–115	30.1	180	In vivo	Diminished magnitude	Ruan et al. *(80)*
G16—PN130–210	40.2	378	In vivo	Elevated induction threshold	Gilbert et al. *(76)*
PN30—PN130–210	38.7	350		and diminished magnitude	
G16—PN120–180	26.8[d]	220	in vivo	Elevated induction threshold	Gilbert et al. *(81)*
	40.2	378		and diminished magnitude	
	61.8	670			
G16—PN210–540	ND	ND	In vivo	Accelerated decay	Gilbert and Mack *(82)*
G0—PN50	31.9	587	In vivo	Diminished magnitude	Nihei et al. *(83)*
CA1					
G0—PN70–210	14.3	160	Slices	Blocked, required exposure during early development	Altmann et al. *(84)*
56–70 d[e]	24.1	ND	Slices	Blocked in presence of strong tetanus	Grover and Frye *(78)*
G16—PN91	31.5	ND	In vivo	Diminished magnitude	Zaiser and Miletic *(85)*
PN0—PN21	30.1[f]	333	Slices	Diminished magnitude	Xu et al. *(86)*
G0—PN90–130	16.0	135	Slices	Diminished magnitude	Gutowski et al. *(87)*
PN0—PN21	30.1	776	Slices	Diminished magnitude	Zhao et al. *(88)*
G16—PN28	23[d]	ND	In vivo	Diminished magnitude	Zaiser and Miletic *(89)*
	50				
PN0–PN21	33	364	Slices	Diminished magnitude	Cai et al. *(90)*

[a]Exposure duration in terms of gestational (G) or postnatal (PN) days of age; PN0 = day of birth.
[b]Values expressed as μg/deciliter.
[c]Values expressed as ng/g tissue.
[d]Different blood Pb values generated by differing levels of exposure.
[e]Duration of exposure in young adult rats, ages not reported.
[f]Blood and brain Pb values determined at weaning; all others determined at the age of testing.

(such as the diminished Ca^{2+}-dependent responses) are an important factor in the exposure-related alterations seen in LTP *(28,45)*. Moreover, these effects on glutamate release are intuitively consistent with the observed decreases in LTP magnitude and elevations in induction threshold *(76,77,81)*. These lead actions could also relate to impairments in ontogenesis of the barrel field cortex in rats (a model of developmental plasticity) resulting from exposure during early development *(92)*, as the mechanisms involved in barrel field plasticity have been closely linked to those underlying LTP *(93)*. Other workers have also drawn parallels between the plasticity that guides establishment and maintenance of synaptic connections in cortical structures during brain ontogeny and the induction and maintenance of LTP in mature organisms *(94)*.

5. SUMMARY

In this chapter, we have demonstrated the value of two methodological approaches that better relate in vitro exposure parameters to those present in a chronically exposed intact animal, thus producing in vitro results of more meaningful significance. Investigations utilizing acute exposure to Pb^{2+} in vitro and expressing the effects of the metal in terms of *free* Pb^{2+} concentrations have clarified several aspects of lead effects on synaptic function. This approach has contributed greatly to our understanding of the effects of chronic exposure on visual function by uncovering evidence of the cellular actions of Pb^{2+} on rod photoreceptors that correspond to analogous findings derived from in vivo exposure and with changes in visual physiology. It is apparent that acute Pb^{2+} exposure in vitro and extended exposure in vivo results in diminished neuronal growth and differentiation at Pb^{2+} concentrations of environmental relevance, and the use of in vitro systems and free Pb^{2+} levels have identified mechanisms that could account for these alterations. This approach has resulted in refinement of earlier observations of Pb^{2+}-induced changes in transmitter release and in definition of the release components that are affected. Furthermore, the alterations in NMDA receptor function induced by acute exposure in terms of free Pb^{2+} concentrations have significantly clarified the changes seen after chronic lead administration. Although it is quite clear from in vitro studies that PKC is a toxicologically significant intracellular target for Pb^{2+}, judgment as to the validity of these observations awaits scientifically sound future experiments.

In addition, experiments utilizing hippocampal slices harvested from chronically exposed animals to investigate changes in LTP have produced findings on synaptic physiology that have corresponded well to observations made in vivo, suggesting that these slices constitute a valid model of hippocampal function in the whole animal when studied ex vivo. As such, they represent untapped potential to further investigate the cellular and/or biochemical bases of the actions of lead on LTP.

ACKNOWLEDGMENT

This document has been subjected to review by the National Health and Environmental Effects Research Laboratory and approved for publication. Approval does not signify that the contents reflect the views of the Agency, nor does mention of trade names or commercial products constitute endorsement or recommendation for use.

REFERENCES

1. Cory-Slechta, D. A. (1995) Relationships between lead-induced learning impairments and changes in dopaminergic, cholinergic, and glutamatergic neurotransmitter system functions. *Annu. Rev. Pharmacol. Toxicol.* **35,** 391–415.
2. Long, G. J., Rosen, J. F., and Schanne, F. A. X. (1994) Lead activation of protein kinase C from rat brain. *J. Biol. Chem.* **269,** 834–837.
3. Kern, M. and Audesirk, G. (1995) Inorganic lead may inhibit neurite development in cultured rat hippocampal neurons through hyperphosphorylation. *Toxicol. Appl. Pharmacol.* **134,** 111–123.
4. Tomsig, J. L. and Suszkiw, J. B. (1995) Multisite interactions between Pb^{2+} and protein kinase C and its role in norepinephrine release from bovine adrenal chromaffin cells. *J. Neurochem.* **64,** 2667–2773.
5. Paoletti, P., Ascher, P., and Neyton, J. (1997) High-affinity zinc inhibition of NMDA NR1-NR2A receptors. *J. Neurosci.* **17,** 5711–5725.
6. Traynelis, S. F., Burgess, M. F., Zheng, F., Lyuboslavsky, P., and Powers, J. L. (1998) Control of voltage-independent zinc inhibition of NMDA receptors by the NR1 subunit. *J. Neurosci.* **18,** 6163–6175.
7. Smith, R. M. and Martell, A. E. (1976) Critical Stability Constants, Plenum, New York.
8. Simons, T. J. B. (1985) Influence of lead ions on cation permeability in human red cell ghosts. *J. Membr. Biol.* **84,** 61–71.
9. Schoenmakers, T. J. M., Visser, G. J., Flik, G., and Theuvenet, A. P. R. (1992) Chelator: an improved method for computing metal ion concentrations in physiological solutions. *BioTechniques* **12,** 870–879.
10. Fabiato, A. (1988) Computer programs for calculating total from specified free or free from specified total ionic concentrations in aqueous solutions containing multiple metals and ligands. *Methods Enzymol.* **157,** 378–417.
11. Srivastava, D., Hurwitz, R. L., and Fox, D. A. (1995) Lead- and calcium-mediated inhibition of bovine rod cGMP phosphodiesterase: interactions with magnesium. *Toxicol. Appl. Pharmacol.* **134,** 43–52.
12. Kober, T. E. and Cooper, G. P. (1976) Lead competitively inhibits calcium-dependent synaptic transmission in the bullfrog sympathetic ganglion. *Nature* **262,** 704–705.
13. Manalis, R. S., Cooper, G. P., and Pomeroy, S. L. (1984) Effects of lead on neuromuscular transmission in the bullfrog. *Brain Res.* **294,** 95–109.
14. Suszkiw, J., Toth, G., Murawsky, M., and Cooper, G. P. (1984) Effects of Pb^{2+} and Cd^{2+} on acetylcholine release and Ca^{2+} movements in synaptosomes and subcellular fractions from rat brain and *Torpedo* electric organ. *Brain Res.* **323,** 31–46.
15. Minnema, D. J., Greenland, R. D., and Michaelson, I. A. (1986) Effect of *in vitro* inorganic lead on dopamine release from superfused rat striatal synaptosomes. *Toxicol. Appl. Pharmacol.* **84,** 400–411.

16. Minnema, D. J. and Michaelson, I. A. (1986) Differential effects of inorganic lead and delta-aminolevulinic acid *in vitro* on synaptosomal gamma-aminobutyric acid release. *Toxicol. Appl. Pharmacol.* **86,** 437–447.
17. Minnema, D. J., Michaelson, I. A., and Cooper, G. P. (1988) Calcium efflux and neurotransmitter release from rat hippocampal synaptosomes exposed to lead. *Toxicol. Appl. Pharmacol.* **92,** 351–357.
18. Shao, Z. and Suszkiw, J. B. (1991) Ca^{2+} surrogate action of Pb^{2+} on acetylcholine release from rat brain synaptosomes. *J. Neurochem.* **56,** 568–574.
19. Audesirk, G. and Audesirk, T. (1991) Effects of inorganic lead on voltage-sensitive calcium channels in N1E-115 neuroblastoma cells. *NeuroToxicology* **12,** 519–528.
20. Sun, L. R. and Suszkiw, J. B. (1995) Extracellular inhibition and intracellular enhancement of Ca^{2+} currents by Pb^{2+} in bovine adrenal chromaffin cells. *J. Neurophysiol.* **74,** 574–581.
21. Tomsig, J. L. and Suszkiw, J. B. (1996) Metal selectivity of exocytosis in α-toxin-permeabilized bovine chromaffin cells. *J. Neurochem.* **66,** 644–650.
22. Westerink, R. H. S. and Vijverberg, H. P. M. (2002) Ca^{2+}-independent vesicular catecholamine release in PC12 cells by nanomolar concentrations of Pb^{2+}. *J. Neurochem.* **80,** 861–873.
23. Goldstein, G. W. (1993) Evidence that lead acts as a calcium substitute in second messenger metabolism. *NeuroToxicology* **14,** 97–102.
24. Braga, M. F. M., Pereira, E. F. R., and Albuquerque, E. X. (1999) Nanomolar concentrations of lead inhibit glutamatergic and GABAergic transmission in hippocampal neurons. *Brain Res.* **826,** 22–34.
25. Braga, M. F. M., Pereira, E. F. R., Marchioro, M., and Albuquerque, E. X. (1999) Lead increases tetrodotoxin-insensitive spontaneous release of glutamate and GABA from hippocampal neurons. *Brain Res.* **826,** 10–21.
26. Lasley, S. M. and Gilbert, M. E. (1996) Presynaptic glutamatergic function in dentate gyrus in vivo is diminished by chronic exposure to inorganic lead. *Brain Res.* **736,** 125–134.
27. Lasley, S. M., Green, M. C., and Gilbert, M. E. (1999) Influence of exposure period on *in vivo* hippocampal glutamate and GABA release in rats chronically exposed to lead. *NeuroToxicology* **20,** 619–630.
28. Lasley, S. M. and Gilbert, M. E. (2002) Rat hippocampal glutamate and GABA release exhibit biphasic effects as a function of chronic lead exposure level. *Toxicol. Sci.* **66,** 139–147.
29. Alkondon, M., Costa, A. C. S., Radhakrishnan, V., Aronstam, R. S., and Albuquerque, E. X. (1990) Selective blockade of NMDA-activated channel currents may be implicated in learning deficits caused by lead. *FEBS Lett.* **261,** 124–130.
30. Guilarte, T. R. and Miceli, R. C. (1992) Age-dependent effects of lead on [3H]MK-801 binding to the NMDA receptor-gated ionophore: in vitro and in vivo studies. *Neurosci. Lett.* **148,** 27–30.

31. Schulte, S., Muller, W. E., and Friedberg, K. D. (1995) *In vitro* and *in vivo* effects of lead on specific ^{3}H-MK-801 binding to NMDA receptors in the brain of mice. *NeuroToxicology* **16,** 309–318.

32. Guilarte, T. R., Miceli, R. C., and Jett, D. A. (1995) Biochemical evidence of an interaction of lead at the zinc allosteric sites of the NMDA receptor complex: effects of neuronal development. *NeuroToxicology* **16,** 63–72.

33. Guilarte, T. R., Miceli, R. C., and Jett, D. A. (1994) Neurochemical aspects of hippocampal and cortical Pb^{2+} neurotoxicity. *NeuroToxicology* **15,** 459–466.

34. Lasley, S. M. and Gilbert, M. E. (1999) Lead inhibits the rat *N*-methyl-D-aspartate receptor channel by binding to a site distinct from the zinc allosteric site. *Toxicol. Appl. Pharmacol.* **159,** 224–233.

35. Ma, T., Chen, H-H., Chang, H. L., Hume, A. S., and Ho, I. K. (1997) Effects of chronic lead exposure on [^{3}H]MK-801 binding in the brain of rat. *Toxicol. Lett.* **92,** 59–66.

36. Guilarte, T. R., Miceli, R. C., Altmann, L., Weinsberg, F., Winneke, G., and Wiegand, H. (1993) Chronic prenatal and postnatal Pb^{2+} exposure increases [^{3}H]MK-801 binding sites in adult rat forebrain. *Eur. J. Pharmacol.* **248,** 273–275.

37. Lasley, S. M., Green, M. C., and Gilbert, M. E. (2001) Rat hippocampal NMDA receptor binding as a function of chronic lead exposure level. *Neurotoxicol. Teratol.* **23,** 185–189.

38. Chen, H-H., Ma, T., and Ho, I. K. (2001) Effects of developmental lead exposure on inhibitory avoidance learning and glutamate receptors in rats. *Environ. Toxicol. Pharmacol.* **9,** 185–191.

39. Cory-Slechta, D. A., Garcia-Osuna, M., and Greenamyre, J. T. (1997) Lead-induced changes in NMDA receptor complex binding: correlations with learning accuracy and with sensitivity to learning impairments caused by MK-801 and NMDA administration. *Behav. Brain Res.* **85,** 161–174.

40. Cory-Slechta, D. A., McCoy, L., and Richfield, E. K. (1997) Time course and regional basis of Pb-induced changes in MK-801 binding: Reversal by chronic treatment with the dopamine agonist apomorphine but not the D_1 agonist SKF-82958. *J. Neurochem.* **68,** 2012–2023.

41. Cohn, J. and Cory-Slechta, D. A. (1994) Lead exposure potentiates the effects of NMDA on repeated learning. *Neurotoxicol. Teratol.* **16,** 455–465.

42. Cory-Slechta, D. A., Pokora, M. J., and Johnson, J. L. (1996) Postweaning lead exposure enhances the stimulus properties of *N*-methyl-D-aspartate: Possible dopaminergic involvement? *NeuroToxicology* **17,** 509–522.

43. Cohn, J. and Cory-Slechta, D. A. (1993) Subsensitivity of lead-exposed rats to the accuracy-impairing and rate-altering effects of MK-801 on a multiple schedule of repeated learning and performance. *Brain Res.* **600,** 208–218.

44. Cory-Slechta, D. A. (1995) MK-801 subsensitivity following postweaning lead exposure. *NeuroToxicology* **16,** 83–96.

45. Lasley, S. M. and Gilbert, M. E. (2000) Glutamatergic components underlying lead-induced impairments in hippocampal synaptic plasticity. *NeuroToxicology* **21,** 1057–1068.

46. Markovac, J. and Goldstein, G. W. (1988) Picomolar concentrations of lead stimulate brain protein kinase C. *Nature* **334,** 71–73.

47. Markovac, J. and Goldstein, G. W. (1988) Lead activates protein kinase C in immature rat brain microvessels. *Toxicol. Appl. Pharmacol.* **96,** 14–23.

48. Sun, X., Tian, X., Tomsig, J. L., and Suszkiw, J. B. (1999) Analysis of differential effects of Pb^{2+} on protein kinase C isozymes. *Toxicol. Appl. Pharmacol.* **156,** 40–45.

49. Laterra, J., Bressler, J. P., Indurti, R. R., Belloni-Olivi, L., and Goldstein, G. W. (1992) Inhibition of astroglia-induced endothelial differentiation by inorganic lead: a role for protein kinase C. *Proc. Natl. Acad. Sci. USA* **89,** 10,748–10,752.

50. Lu, H., Guizzetti, M., and Costa, L. G. (2001) Inorganic lead stimulates DNA synthesis in human astrocytoma cells: role of protein kinase C. *J. Neurochem.* **78,** 590–599.

51. Kim, K-A., Chakraborti, T., Goldstein, G. W., and Bressler, J. P. (2000) Immediate early gene expression in PC12 cells exposed to lead: requirement for protein kinase C. *J. Neurochem.* **74,** 1140–1146.

52. Nihei, M. K., McGlothan, J. L., Toscano, C. D., and Guilarte, T. R. (2001) Low level Pb^{2+} exposure affects hippocampal protein kinase Cγ gene and protein expression in rats. *Neurosci. Lett.* **298,** 212–216.

53. Chen, H-H., Ma, T., and Ho, I. K. (1999) Protein kinase C in rat brain is altered by developmental lead exposure. *Neurochem. Res.* **24,** 415–421.

54. Reinholz, M. M., Bertics, P. J., and Miletic, V. (1999) Chronic exposure to lead acetate affects the development of protein kinase C activity and the distribution of the PKCγ isozyme in the rat hippocampus. *NeuroToxicology* **20,** 609–618.

55. Crumpton, T., Atkins, D. S., Zawia, N. H., and Barone, S. (2001) Lead exposure in pheochromocytoma (PC12) cells alters neural differentiation and Sp1 DNA-binding. *NeuroToxicology* **22,** 49–62.

56. Kern, M., Wisniewski, M., Cabell, L., and Audesirk, G. (2000) Inorganic lead and calcium interact positively in activation of calmodulin. *NeuroToxicology* **21,** 353–364.

57. Kern, M. and Audesirk, G. (2000) Stimulatory and inhibitory effects of inorganic lead on calcineurin. *Toxicology* **150,** 171–178.

58. Ferguson, C., Kern, M., and Audesirk, G. (2000) Nanomolar concentrations of inorganic lead increase Ca^{2+} efflux and decrease intracellular free Ca^{2+} ion concentrations in cultured rat hippocampal neurons by a calmodulin-dependent mechanism. *NeuroToxicology* **21,** 365–378.

59. Audesirk, T., Pedersen, C., Audesirk, G., and Kern, M. (1998) Low levels of inorganic lead noncompetitively inhibit μ-calpain. *Toxicology* **131,** 169–174.

60. Cline, H. T., Witte, S., and Jones, K. W. (1996) Low lead levels stunt neuronal growth in a reversible manner. *Proc. Natl. Acad. Sci. USA* **93,** 9915–9920.

61. Reuhl, K. R., Rice, D. C., Gilbert, S. G., and Mallett, J. (1989) Effects of chronic developmental lead exposure on monkey neuroanatomy: visual system. *Toxicol. Appl. Pharmacol.* **99,** 501–509.

62. Fox, D. A. and Sillman, A. J. (1979) Heavy metals affect rod, but not cone, photoreceptors. *Science* **206,** 78–80.

63. Fox, D. A., Campbell, M. L., and Blocker, Y. S. (1997) Functional alterations and apoptotic cell death in the retina following developmental or adult lead exposure. *NeuroToxicology* **18,** 645–664.

64. Fox, D. A. and Srivastava, D. (1995) Molecular mechanism of the lead-induced inhibition of rod cGMP phosphodiesterase. *Toxicol. Lett.* **82-83,** 263–270.

65. Fox, D. A., He, L., Poblenz, A. T., Medrano, C. J., Blocker, Y. S., and Srivastava, D. (1998) Lead-induced alterations in retinal cGMP phosphodiesterase trigger calcium overload, mitochondrial dysfunction and rod photoreceptor apoptosis. *Toxicol. Lett.* **102-103,** 359–361.

66. He, L., Poblenz, A. T., Medrano, C. J., and Fox, D. A. (2000) Lead and calcium produce rod photoreceptor cell apoptosis by opening the mitochondrial permeability transition pore. *J. Biol. Chem.* **275,** 12,175–12,184.

67. Fox, D. A. and Farber, D. B. (1988) Rods are selectively altered by lead: I. Electrophysiology and biochemistry. *Exp. Eye Res.* **46,** 597–611.

68. Lilienthal, H., Lenaerts, C., Winneke, G., and Hennekes, R. (1988) Alteration of the visual evoked potential and the electroretinogram in lead-treated monkeys. *Neurotoxicol. Teratol.* **10,** 417–422.

69. Fox, D. A., Srivastava, D., and Hurwitz, R. L. (1994) Lead-induced alterations in rod-mediated visual functions and cGMP metabolism: new insights. *NeuroToxicology* **15,** 503–512.

70. Fox, D. A., Rubinstein, S. D., and Hsu, P. (1991) Developmental lead exposure inhibits adult rat retinal, but not kidney, Na^+,K^+-ATPase. *Toxicol. Appl. Pharmacol.* **109,** 482–493.

71. Barnes, C. (1995) Involvement of LTP in memory: are we "searching under the street light?" *Neuron* **15,** 751–754.

72. Bliss, T. V. P. and Collingridge, G. L. (1993) A synaptic model of memory: long-term potentiation in the hippocampus. *Nature* **361,** 31–39.

73. Cain, D. P., Hargreaves, E. L., Boon, F., and Dennison, Z. (1993) An examination of the relations between hippocampal long-term potentiation, kindling, afterdischarge, and place learning in the water maze. *Hippocampus* **5,** 153–163.

74. Sutherland, R. J., Dringenberg, H. C., and Hoesing, J. M. (1993) Induction of long-term potentiation at perforant path dentate synapses does not affect place learning or memory. *Hippocampus* **3,** 141–148.

75. Hargreaves, E. L., Cain, D. P., and Vanderwolf, C H. (1990) Learning and behavioral long-term potentiation: importance of controlling for motor activity. *J. Neurosci.* **10,** 1472–1478.

76. Gilbert, M. E., Mack, C. M., and Lasley, S. M. (1999) The influence of developmental period of lead exposure on long-term potentiation in the adult rat dentate gyrus *in vivo*. *NeuroToxicology* **20,** 57–70.

77. Gilbert, M. E., Mack, C. M., and Lasley, S. M. (1996) Chronic developmental lead exposure increases threshold for long-term potentiation in the rat dentate gyrus in vivo. *Brain Res.* **736,** 118–124.

78. Grover, C. A. and Frye, G. D. (1996) Ethanol effects on synaptic neurotransmission and tetanus-induced synaptic plasticity in hippocampal slices of chronic in vivo lead-exposed adult rats. *Brain Res.* **734,** 61–71.

79. Lasley, S. M., Polan-Curtain, J., and Armstrong, D. L. (1993) Chronic exposure to environmental levels of lead impairs *in vivo* induction of long-term potentiation in rat hippocampal dentate. *Brain Res.* **614,** 347–351.

80. Ruan, D., Chen, J., Zhao, C., Xu, Y., Wang, M., and Zhao, W. (1998) Impairment of long-term potentiation and paired-pulse facilitation in rat hippocampal dentate gyrus following developmental lead exposure *in vivo*. *Brain Res.* **806,** 196–201.

81. Gilbert, M. E., Mack, C. M., and Lasley, S. M. (1999) Chronic developmental lead exposure and hippocampal long-term potentiation: biphasic dose-response relationship. *NeuroToxicology* **20,** 71–82.

82. Gilbert, M. E. and Mack, C. M. (1998) Chronic developmental lead exposure accelerates decay of long-term potentiation in rat dentate gyrus in vivo. *Brain Res.* **789,** 139–149.

83. Nihei, M. K., Desmond, N. L., McGlothan, J. L., Kuhlmann, A. C., and Guilarte, T. R. (2000) *N*-Methyl-D-aspartate receptor subunit changes are associated with lead-induced deficits of long-term potentiation and spatial learning. *Neuroscience* **99,** 233–242.

84. Altmann, L., Weinsberg, F., Sveinsson, K., Lilienthal, H., Wiegand, H., and Winneke, G. (1993) Impairment of long-term potentiation and learning following chronic lead exposure. *Toxicol. Lett.* **66,** 105–112.

85. Zaiser, A. E. and Miletic, V. (1997) Prenatal and postnatal chronic exposure to low levels of inorganic lead attenuates long-term potentiation in the adult rat hippocampus *in vivo*. *Neurosci. Lett.* **239,** 128–130.

86. Xu, Y., Ruan, D., Wu, Y., et al. (1998) Nitric oxide affects LTP in area CA1 and CA3 of hippocampus in low-level lead-exposed rat. *Neurotoxicol. Teratol.* **20,** 69–73.

87. Gutowski, M., Altmann, L., Sveinsson, K., and Wiegand, H. (1998) Synaptic plasticity in the CA1 and CA3 hippocampal region of pre- and postnatally lead-exposed rats. *Toxicol. Lett.* **95,** 195–203.

88. Zhao, W., Ruan, D., Xu, Y., Chen, J., Wang, M., and Ge, S. (1999) The effects of chronic lead exposure on long-term depression in area CA1 and dentate gyrus of rat hippocampus *in vitro*. *Brain Res.* **818,** 153–159.

89. Zaiser, A. E. and Miletic, V. (2000) Differential effects of inorganic lead on hippocampal long-term potentiation in young rats *in vivo*. *Brain Res.* **876,** 201–204.

90. Cai, L., Ruan, D-Y., Xu, Y-Z., Liu, Z., Meng, X-M., and Dai, X-Q. (2001) Effects of lead exposure on long-term potentiation induced by 2-deoxy-*D*-glucose in area CA1 of rat hippocampus in vitro. *Neurotoxicol. Teratol.* **23,** 481–487.

91. Altmann, L., Gutowski, M., and Wiegand, H. (1994) Effects of maternal lead exposure on functional plasticity in the visual cortex and hippocampus of immature rats. *Dev. Brain Res.* **81,** 50–56.

92. Wilson, M. A., Johnston, M. V., Goldstein, G. W., and Blue, M. E. (2000) Neonatal lead exposure impairs development of rodent barrel field cortex. *Proc. Natl. Acad. Sci. USA* **97,** 5540–5545.

93. Rema, V. and Ebner, F. F. (1999) Effect of enriched environment rearing on impairments in cortical excitability and plasticity after prenatal alcohol exposure. *J. Neurosci.* **19,** 10,993–11,006.

94. Gilbert, M. E. and Lasley, S. M. (2002) Long-term consequences of developmental exposure to lead or polychlorinated biphenyls: synaptic transmission and plasticity in the rodent CNS. *Environ. Toxicol. Pharmacol.* **12,** 105–117.

10

Aggregating Brain Cell Cultures for Neurotoxicological Studies

Marie-Gabrielle Zurich, Florianne Monnet-Tschudi, Lucio G. Costa, Benoît Schilter, and Paul Honegger

1. INTRODUCTION

Because of the limited accessibility of the brain for experimentation, but also for ethical and economical reasons, there is considerable interest in culture models suitable for neurotoxicological research. Although it is generally accepted that in vitro models cannot cover the entire spectrum of brain functions, they have proven to be indispensable for investigations in the life sciences since the early work of Harrison *(1)*. To date, many in vitro models of various complexity are available, ranging from monolayer cultures of immortalized cell lines to organotypic cultures. Each of these culture systems has its particularities, therefore, it is of great importance to select the model that is most appropriate for the question to be solved.

Although many biological problems can be addressed by the use of simple cell culture systems, neurotoxicological research often requires more complex models that allow for interactions between the different cell types present in the nervous system. In addition to the synaptic interactions among neurons, cell-to-cell signaling and metabolic interactions have been observed also between neurons and glial cells, as well as between the different types of glial cell (i.e., astrocytes, oligodendrocytes, and microglial cells). When studying the effect of a potential neurotoxicant in the brain, it is necessary to consider secondary effects that ensue from the primary impact of this toxicant on a given cell type. Such secondary reactions can attenuate neurotoxicity, for example, through the activation of neurotrophic systems, but in most cases they

From: *Methods in Pharmacology and Toxicology: In Vitro Neurotoxicology: Principles and Challenges*
Edited by: E. Tiffany-Castiglioni © Humana Press Inc., Totowa, NJ

will exacerbate neurotoxicity. Both cases are often observed as a consequence of the reactivity of astrocytes and/or microglial cells.

For many neurotoxicological investigations, it appears therefore of interest to make use of in vitro models that offer maximal cell-to-cell interactions, as well as easy handling and high reproducibility. These characteristics are typical for rotation-mediated aggregating brain cell cultures. We have adopted and refined the methodology of this culture system introduced by Moscona *(2)* and we have subsequently applied it for neurotoxicological investigations. Aggregating brain cell cultures are primary, three-dimensional cell cultures consisting of even-sized, spherical structures that are maintained in suspension by constant gyratory agitation. Because of the avidity of freshly dissociated fetal cells to attach to their counterparts, cell aggregates form spontaneously and rapidly under appropriate culture conditions. The cells are able to migrate within the formed aggregates and to interact with each other by direct cell–cell contact, as well as through exchange of nutritional and signaling factors. This tissue-specific environment enables aggregating neural cells to differentiate and to develop specialized structures, such as synapses and compact myelin, resembling those of brain tissue *in situ*. This maturation process makes the aggregates a valuable model for studying the interferences of potential neurotoxicants with critical developmental stages that might cause irreversible structural and functional alterations. The ability of the cells to synthetize and compact myelin around axons also permits one to investigate the potential demyelinating effects of toxicants and to study the power of regeneration of the cells after the insult. The fact that the aggregates can be maintained for long periods of time in culture allows one to study not only acute toxicity at relatively high toxicant concentrations but also chronic exposure to low toxicant concentrations, as well as delayed toxic processes.

The assessment of human health risks from chemical exposure is an important aspect in neurotoxicology. In most cases, the risks for humans are evaluated from biological responses found in experimental animals, based on the assumption that the mechanism of action is similar in all species regardless the doses of exposure. Aggregating brain cell cultures might be of great help in that matter, because mechanisms of action can be studied in such cultures prepared from several species, including man.

2. AGGREGATING BRAIN CELL CULTURES

2.1. Preparation and Maintenance of Serum-Free Aggregating Brain Cell Cultures

Aggregating brain cell cultures can be prepared routinely from 16-d-old embryonic rat telencephalon *(3,4)*. The entire dissection and dissociation procedure is performed in ice-cold, sterile, modified Puck's salt solution D (137 m*M* NaCl, 5.4 m*M* KCl, 0.2 m*M* Na_2HPO_4, 0.2 m*M* KH_2PO_4, 5.6 m*M* D-glucose, 58.4 m*M* sucrose, pH 7.4, 340 mOsm). The excised telencephalons are pooled and dissociated in a two-step process. First, the tissue is forced with a glass rod through a nylon mesh bag with 200-μm pores. The dispersed tissue is then gently triturated with a plastic pipet and filtered by gravity flow through a nylon mesh bag with 115-μm pores. The resulting suspension is sedimented by centrifugation (300*g*, 15 min at 4°C) and washed twice in solution D. After the last centrifugation, the cells are resuspended in cold serum-free culture medium to obtain a cell density of 7.5 × 10^6 cells/mL. Aliquots (4 mL) of this suspension are transferred to 25-mL Erlenmeyer flasks. The chemically defined medium is prepared from Dulbecco's modified Eagle's medium (DMEM) powder, containing high glucose (4.5 g/L) and L-glutamine, but no pyruvate. It is supplemented with insuline, triiodothyronine, transferrine, hydrocortisone-21-phosphate, trace elements, and vitamins. The flasks are placed onto a rotating gyratory shaker, in an atmosphere of 10% CO_2 and 90% humidified air, at 37°C. The initial frequency of agitation (68 rpm) is progressively increased to reach 77 rpm after the transfer of the cultures at day in vitro 2 (DIV 2) to 50-mL Erlenmeyer flasks and the addition of 4 mL of fresh prewarmed culture medium. The final frequency of agitation (80 rpm) is reached at DIV 5.

With the telencephalon of 16-d-old rat embryos as a source, as many as 100 flasks of aggregating brain cell cultures can be prepared from the litters of 12 pregnant rats, each flask containing more than 1000 individual aggregates with a final diameter of 300–400 μm. After DIV 5, the aggregates of several flasks can be pooled and aliquoted so that for each initial flask, six replicate cultures can be obtained. This means that starting with 12 pregnant rats, up to 600 cultures can be generated in one batch. In addition to the mixed brain cell aggregates, cultures highly enriched either in neurons or in glial cells can be prepared, through an easy treatment with either arabino–furanosil–cytosine (Ara-C) or cholera toxin, respectively *(5)*.

2.2. Characteristics of Serum-Free Aggregating Brain Cell Cultures

Mechanically dissociated embryonic brain cells appear to reaggregate in a random fashion, whereas once the three-dimensional structures are formed, the cells undergo migration and they reorganize in a tissue-specific way. The final aggregates contain all types of brain cell (i.e., neurons, astrocytes, oligodendrocytes, and microglia) (*see* Fig. 1), whereas they are devoid of fibroblasts (Monnet-Tschudi and Honegger, unpublished observation) and of blood-borne macrophages *(6)*.

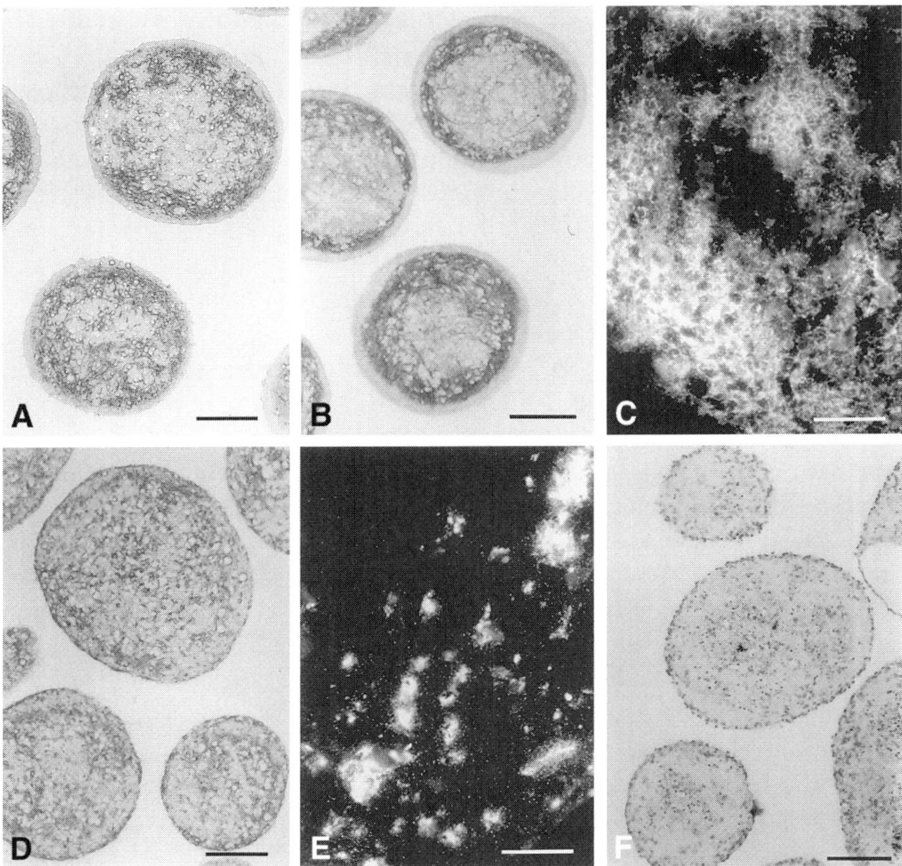

Fig. 1. Aggregate sections immunolabeled with cell-type specific markers illustrating the histotypic organization. (**A**) Neuronal cell bodies, immunostained for MAP-2, are often arranged in patches and are localized throughout the aggregates, except in the periphery and in the center; DIV 21, bar = 150 μm; bright field. (**B**) Neuronal processes, immunolabeled for NF-H, are densely packed in an external ring; DIV 35, bar = 150 μm; bright field. (**C**) Synapses, immnunolabeled with synaptophysin, are superimposed on the neuronal patches seen in (a); DIV 21, bar = 50 μm; fluorescence. (**D**) Astrocytes, immunolabeled with GFAP, are found throughout the aggregates. Moreover, the external surface of the aggregates is formed by a layer of astrocytes. DIV 15, bar = 150 μm; bright field. (**E**) Oligodendrocytes, labeled with MBP, are found in the same regions as neurons. Larger fluorescent areas show sites of myelin synthesis in oligodendrocyte cell bodies, whereas small fluorescent dots represent myelin around neuronal processes. DIV 35, bar = 50 μm; fluorescence. (**F**) Microglia, labeled with the isolectin B4 of *Griffonia simplicifolia*, are found scattered troughout the aggregates; DIV 15, bar = 150 μm; bright field.

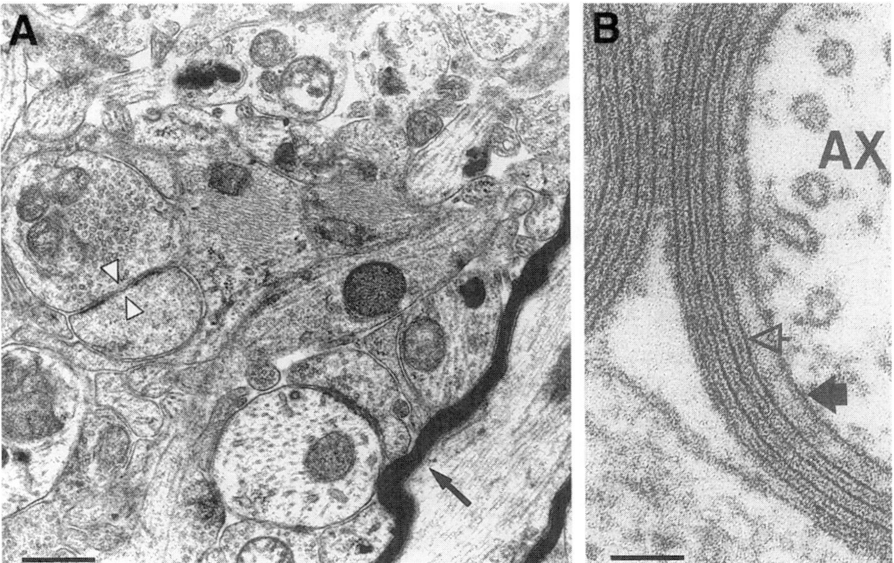

Fig. 2. Electron micrographs showing the histotypic appearance of the aggregates. (**A**) Presence of synapses (arrowheads on each side of synaptic cleft) and of compact myelin sheaths (arrow); bar = 120 nm. (**B**) Myelin fine structure. The preparation shows normal compaction of the myelin membranes around the axon (AX) with formation of major dense lines (open arrows) and intraperiod lines. Filled arrow shows the axolemma. Bar = 40 nm.

Many neuronal cell bodies tend to be localized more toward the center of the aggregate (Fig. 1A) and their processes are more oriented toward the periphery, forming an external layer of fibers (Fig. 1B). The cell bodies of oligodendrocytes are found intermingled with neuronal bodies, with their process-forming myelin sheaths around axons (Figs. 1E and 2), whereas astrocytes occur throughout the three-dimensional structure (Fig. 1D). A small population of microglial cells is found scattered throughout the aggregates (Fig. 1F). Most of the glial cells arise from the proliferation of glioblasts during the first 2 wk in vitro, with a maximal mitotic activity around DIV 5. This proliferative period has been characterized by measuring total protein and total DNA content, as well as by the incorporation of [^{3}H] thymidine *(7)*. Neurons are mostly postmitotic, although autoradiographic examinations at the electron microscopic level showed that some of them are able to incorporate radiolabeled thymidine into their DNA (Honegger and Favrod, unpublished observation). The expression of differentiated characteristics progresses for several weeks, as illustrated by the gradual increase in cell-type-specific enzyme activities *(7)*, cytoskeletal and synaptic proteins *(8)*, and Na⁺,K⁺-ATPase subtypes expression *(9,10)* similar to that observed in vivo. In parallel, extensive morphological maturation is also observed: growth of neuropil and appearance of mature synapses (Figs. 1C and 2A), as well as the accumulation of myelin basic protein and the formation of myelin lamellae around axons (Figs. 1E and 2). Myelination starts in the third week and attains a maximum after 4 wk of culture. With the progression of maturation, the metabolic rate increases substantially and the neurons exhibit spontaneous electrical activity *(4,7,11)*.

2.3. Choice of End Points

Aggregating brain cell cultures can be employed for a large range of applications in neurotoxicology, ranging from routine screening to mechanistic studies. Therefore, the criteria (end points) to be used for analysis need to be in accord with the aim of the study. To keep time-consuming analyses to a strict minimum, a strategy was adopted by which the toxic effects of chemicals is analyzed in sequential steps, starting out with the establishment of a dose–response test with a restricted set of criteria for general cytotoxicity and then proceeding to criteria specific for cell types and for subcellular components. The nature of aggregate cultures, free-floating in the culture medium, greatly facilitates reproducible sampling. Furthermore, the high amount of material permits multidisciplinary analyses of toxicant effects, as well as repetitive sampling for time-course analyses. Biochemical and morphological methods, as well as techniques of molecular biology, such as Western blot, Northern blot, and *in situ* hybridization, are currently used to analyze the effects of neurotoxicants.

General cytotoxicity, or unspecific toxicity, is evaluated by measuring lactate dehydrogenase (LDH) release in culture medium and the remaining intracellular LDH content, as well as total protein content. Increase in LDH release as well as decrease in LDH and protein content may indicate basal cytotoxicity, originally defined as toxicity to common cellular functions and structures, assuming that all types of cells are similarly affected. However, the selective loss of one particular cell type cannot be excluded. Therefore, additional parameters are applied to detect differences in susceptibility between the diverse cell types and to distinguish between the cell-type-specific effects.

Neuron-specific effects are assessed by measuring the activities of neuronal enzymes such as choline acetyl transferase (ChAT), specific for cholinergic neurons, and glutamic acid decarboxylase (GAD), specific for GABAergic neurons. The levels of activity of these enzymes give indications of the maturational state of the different neuronal subtypes, as well as of possible cell-type-specific structural and/or functional changes or cell loss. Because these enzymes are mainly located in synapses, decreases in their activity in the absence of clues suggesting general cytotoxicity might indicate a selective loss of synapses. In that case, structural effects on synapses can be further evaluated by assaying for synapse-specific components such as synapsin or synaptophysin on whole aggregates and, if indicated, on synaptical fractions, by means of immunohistochemistry and Western blotting. Furthermore, structural effects on neuronal processes can be assessed by immunohistochemistry and Western blotting of microtubule-associated protein (MAP2) and neurofilaments (NF-M, NF-H). These parameters give indications of morphological changes and/or changes in the density of processes. The reversibility of decreases in such structural parameters can then be examined by analyzing the same structural parameters 1 and 2 wk later. If type-specific cell loss is observed, follow-up investigations could be conducted in order to determine whether the apoptotic processes are implicated in the neuronal cell death. In that case, soluble nucleosome content and DNA fragmentation assessed by the Tdt-mediated dUPT Nick End Labeling (TUNEL) technique are quantified. In addition to structural changes, neurotoxicants could also induce specific functional changes in neurons. They can be evaluated for example, by measuring 2-deoxyglucose uptake *(10)*, the liberation of neurotransmitters or the modulation of neuronal cytoskeletal protein phosphorylation induced by stimulation, or depolarization *(12,13)*. Intracellular and extracellular recordings of neuronal electrical activity is currently under examination and may eventually become a sensitive endpoint for future studies.

Oligodendrocyte-specific effects are evaluated by measuring the activity of 2',3'-cyclic nucleotide 3'-phosphohydrolase (CNP) or by immunohistochemistry for galactocerebroside, myelin/oligodendrocyte glycoprotein (MOG), or myelin basic protein (MBP), as well as by radioimmunoassay of MBP. These markers allow monitoring of oligodendrocyte maturation, myelination, demyelination, and remyelination processes. Parallel decreases of CNP activity and MBP content in the absence of significant cell death strongly indicates demyelination. In this case, myelin can be extracted from the cultures, quantified, and further analyzed. The reversibility of demyelination can be tested by further sampling and analysis of the same parameters one and 2 wk later, after the end of treatment with the neurotoxicant.

Compared to neurons and oligodendrocytes, astrocytes and microglial cells display a high sensitivity and reactivity to brain injury and neurotoxic insults. Both of these glial cell types are well known to undergo morphological changes corresponding to their process of activation and to synthesize and release numerous signaling molecules in response to a great variety of stimuli. Such reactions can occur at concentrations of neurotoxicants for which no direct effect can be observed on neurons or oligodendrocytes. For this reason, these two types of glial cell are recognized as sensitive indicators of toxicity.

Astrocyte-specific effects are routinely evaluated by measuring the activity of glutamine synthetase (GS). Follow-up analyses include immunohistochemistry for vimentin, GS, and the glial fibrillary acidic protein (GFAP), and quantification of GFAP by enzyme-linked immunosorbent assay (ELISA). All of these criteria are useful markers of the maturational state, whereas GFAP, in addition, is taken as a marker of astrocyte reactivity. Injury to the brain causes the transformation of resting to reactive astrocytes *(14)*, the hallmark of which is an increase in GFAP, the major intermediate filament protein of this cell type. GFAP has been proposed by O'Callaghan *(15)* as a biomarker of neurotoxicity. This implies that a sensitive in vitro model for neurotoxicity should enable the detection of reactive gliosis in response to a chemical insult. Astrocytes in monolayer cultures express abnormally high levels of GFAP, presumably resulting from spontaneous activation *(16,17)*, whereas the presence of neurons on the confluent glial monolayers attenuates the high expression of GFAP *(16,18)*. Aggregating brain cell cultures contain all types of neuron and glial cell present in the original tissue. These cells interact by direct cell–cell contact as well as through the exchange of nutritional and signaling factors. This could explain why chemically induced astrogliosis can be observed in this culture system. A number of examples of chemically induced reactive astrogliosis have already been reported in this model [e.g., after treatment with trimethyltin *(19)* (Fig. 3), mercuric chloride, monomethylmercury chloride *(20)* and parathion *(21)*]. In this context, it is worth noting that in our hands, the immunocytochemical analysis of GFAP is a more sensitive marker of toxicity than the measure of the GFAP content by ELISA. Generally, we observed that the increase in GFAP immunostaining was detectable at concentrations 100 times lower than changes in total GFAP content measured by ELISA. Aquino et al. *(22)* using both monoclonal and polyclonal antibodies reported a temporal delay between the increase in GFAP observed by immunocytochemistry and changes in the content by Western blot analysis in vivo. They attributed the rapid increase in GFAP immunostaining to increased availability of epitopes, perhaps resulting to physical changes in the filament bundles following astrocytic swelling.

Microglial-cell-specific effects are best analyzed by taking advantage of the specific binding of isolectin B4 of *Griffonia simplicifolia (23)*. Microglial cells, also termed resident macrophages, are recognized for their participation in numerous pathological processes of the brain *(24,25)*, and they

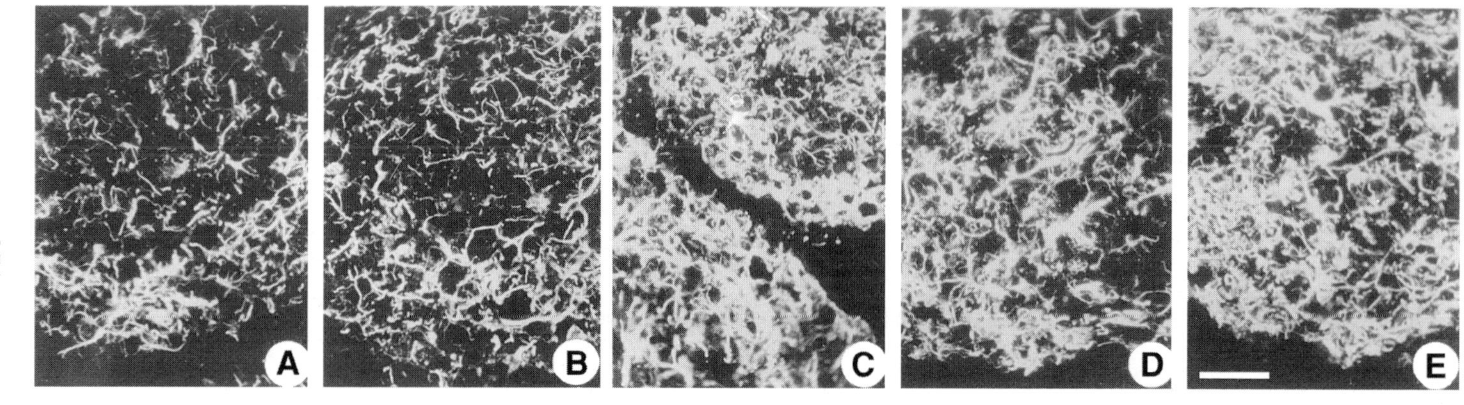

Fig. 3. Effects of TMT on GFAP in immature aggregate cultures. Cultures were treated from DIV 5 to DIV 14 and immunofluorescence staining was examined at DIV 14 with a monoclonal antibody. (**A**) Untreated controls; (**B**) 10^{-9} M TMT; (**C**) 10^{-8} M TMT; (**D**) 10^{-7} M TMT; (**E**) 10^{-6} M TMT. Bar = 50 μm. (Reprinted from ref. *19* with permission from Elsevier Science.)

are known to affect other cell types in the brain by releasing various biologically active molecules. Microglial cells are also highly sensitive to signals emitted by various types of cell. One of the most commonly described characteristics of microglial activation is the alteration in cellular morphology. In response to sublethal neuronal injury, the resting ramified microglial cells become hyperplasic and adopt distinct morphological features such as swollen cell bodies and stouter processes *(26,27)*. In more severe injuries, microglial cells can migrate toward dying neurons and act as phagocytic scavengers. Although primary reactive microglia are able to revert to the resting form, the phagocytic microglia will probably undergo cell death *(25,28–30)*. Because of their polyvalent nature, the role played by microglial cells in the neurotoxic action of chemicals needs to be examined in each case. Microglia are present in the aggregates and have been shown to be highly responsive to trimethyltin treatment *(31)*. The microglial reaction, characterized by an increase in the number and/or clustering of GSI-B4 lectin-positive cells, was elicited by low concentrations of trimethylin (TMT), which caused no detectable changes in either neuronal or astroglial parameters. These results suggested that microglial activation might provide an even more sensitive indicator of TMT neurotoxicity than GFAP measurements. This view is in accord with in vivo observations by McCann et al. *(32)*, who reported that microglial and astroglial reactions following TMT-induced neuronal necrosis were separated in time, with microglial activation clearly preceding astrogliosis. In brain cell aggregate cultures, high sensitivity of microglial cells was found also after treatment with low concentrations of ochratoxin A *(33)* and mercury compounds *(20)* (*see* Fig. 4), the latter in accord with observation in vivo by Charleston et al. *(34)*.

2.4. Use of Aggregating Brain Cell Cultures for Neurotoxicological Studies

2.4.1. Dose–Response Relationships, First Screening

For the initial evaluation of a potential neurotoxicant, our experience has shown that it is useful to establish a dose–response relationship for a wide range of concentrations (generally covering five orders of magnitude) using only a restricted set of criteria. Treatment with the potential neurotoxicant starts at DIV 5, on four replicate cultures for each concentration. Aggregates are treated after each medium change (every 2 d) and are harvested at DIV 15. For each concentration of the toxicant, half of the aggregates contained in each replicate culture are homogenized, aliquoted for different biochemical analyses, and kept at –80°C; the remaining fractions are harvested for morphological analyses.

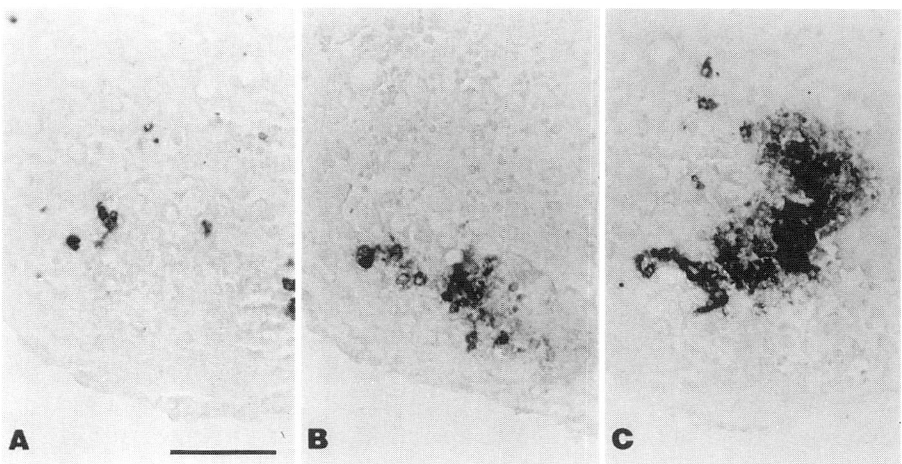

Fig. 4. Representative examples for the histochemical evaluation of microglia stained with the GSI-B4 isolectin bound to horseradish peroxidase. Undifferentiated cultures were treated from DIV 5 to DIV 15 with $HgCl_2$. (**A**) Section of an aggregate from untreated cultures; (**B**) section of an aggregate from cultures treated with $HgCl_2$ (10^{-10} M) shows a characteristic clustering of stained cells; (**C**) section of an aggregate from cultures treated with $HgCl_2$ (10^{-8} M) shows a large clustering of stained cells typically found under these conditions. Bar = 50 μm. (Reprinted from ref. *20* with permission.)

The first series of analyses concerns general cytotoxicity, determined by measuring the remaining LDH activity and total protein content. Test conditions that cause more than 50% decrease of both criteria are considered cytotoxic and are not further analyzed. The remaining samples are assayed for subcytotoxic effects by measuring cell-type-specific parameters as described in Subheading 2.3. If indicated by the results obtained, subsequent analyses involve criteria indicative for astrocytosis (GFAP) and microglial reactivity to determine the lowest concentrations of the neurotoxicant causing an effect. Based on the combined results obtained from this dose–response assay, the concentration range will be adjusted for follow-up studies, for which additional end points, including immunocytochemical and morphological criteria, will be considered.

2.4.2. Maturation-Dependent Toxicity

Screening tests as outlined in Subheading 2.4.1. allow the first rapid evaluation of a series of chemicals for their potential toxicity. The cultures used for this purpose contain brain cells in an early stage of differentiation. However, the sensitivity of cells to a given neurotoxicant can change as a function of cell maturation. Furthermore, certain toxicants can affect developmental processes that occur only at more advanced stage of maturation, such as synaptogenesis and myelination. Thus, for a more complete evaluation of maturation-dependent toxicity, further experiments are required in order to study drug effects on successive developmental events. Aggregating brain cell cultures provide a particularly suitable model for studying the effects of toxicants on developmental processes, because, after the proliferative period, extensive maturation confers on the cells a high degree of differentiation.

To extend the screening approach described previously to the more advanced maturational events, aggregates are treated with toxicants during the late period of differentiation (DIV 25–35) characterized by synaptogenesis and myelination. A first set of criteria, as described in Subheading 2.4.1., is used for a general evaluation of neurotoxicity. Then, according to the results, specific criteria, as described in Subheading 2.3., are applied to evaluate the effects of the toxicant on synaptogenesis and/or myelination.

By the use of this approach, the toxic effects of several metal compounds were found to be maturation dependent. Based on general and cell-type-specific criteria, it was found that several metal compounds (i.e., mercuric chloride, triethyltin chloride, and thallium chloride) were more toxic in immature cultures, whereas bismuth sodium tartrate, dimethylmercury, and nickel chloride were more effective in differentiated cultures *(35)*. Using the same criteria, a typical development-dependent effect was also observed in aggregate cultures treated with diphenylhydantoin (DPH), a commonly used anticonvulsant *(36)*. The results showed that neurons were sensitive to DPH during both developmental periods tested, whereas glial cells were sensitive to DPH only during the early developmental stage. Because most glial cells are mitotically active only during the first 2 wk in culture, this finding suggests that the glia toxicity of DPH was restricted to glioblasts.

The mechanism(s) involved in the higher sensitivity of young animals to organophosporus pesticides (OPs) is still not fully understood. It has been proposed that it might be the result of differences in the maturation of detoxication mechanisms mainly localized in the liver *(37–39)*. Aggregates were used to analyze the intrinsic maturation-dependent sensitivity of brain cells to chronic exposure of the OPs parathion, chlorpyrifos, and their oxygen analogs *(40)*. It was found that OPs exerted toxic effects, although only at concentrations that resulted in a high degree of inhibition of acetylcholinesterase (AChE). In general, neurons were more sensitive to OPs than glial cells. Neurons showed distinct maturation-dependent sensitivities to different OPs. Cholinergic neurons were more affected during an early maturational stage by chlorpyrifos and chlorpyrifos-oxon, whereas differentiated GABAergic neurons showed higher sensitivity to paraoxon. These results are in accord with recent findings of Liu et al. *(41)*, indicating that a group of compounds with similar chemical structure and reactivity could exert different maturation-dependent and cell type-specific effects. Selective neurotoxicity can be further analyzed with respect to glial reactivity and structural changes in neurons.

In case of TMT, a neurotoxicant occurring as a byproduct in the manufacture of plastics, development-dependent effects were observed on glial cells and on neurons *(19,31)*. Detailed analyses showed that at noncytotoxic concentrations, TMT induced astrocytic and microglial reactions and decreased the content of synaptic proteins, whereas the growth cone-associated protein GAP-43 was affected only at cytotoxic concentrations *(31)*.

2.4.3. Long-Term and Delayed Toxicity

The consequences of long-term exposure to low levels of xenobiotics are difficult to assess in the living individual. The effects may not exceed the limits of normality and thus remain undetected. Some neurotoxicants might require cellular accumulation before exerting adverse effects, whereas others might induce very subtle sequential modifications at the molecular and cellular level that will ultimately become pathogenic. At any rate, it can be expected that the mechanism(s) of action underlying chronic drug effects differ from those of acute intoxication. Aggregating cultures provide a unique model to study long-term effects of toxicants because they are able to maintain a highly differentiated state for months in vitro. The following examples illustrate how the prolonged exposure of brain cells to low doses of chemicals might increase the selective toxic effects.

Brain cell aggregates were treated with 6-aminonicotinamide *(42)* at 1–4 μM, for either 9 or 29 d. It was found that 9 d of treatment had very little effect on the cell-type-specific enzyme activities measured (CAT, GAD, GS, and CNP), even at the highest dose (4 μM). In contrast, after 29 d of treatment, CNP was affected at a much lower concentration (1 μM), and at 4 μM, all of the enzymatic activities measured were drastically reduced. These results showed that prolonged exposure to relatively low concentrations of 6-aminonicotinamide increased the toxic action on brain cells. Similarly, aggregates treated with lead acetate at very low concentration (10^{-7} M) showed considerable decrease of enzymatic parameters (GS, CNP, and GAD) after 50 d of treatment, whereas no toxic effects were found after 10 and 30 d of treatment *(43)*. This finding is in line with the work of Tiffany-Castiglioni et al. *(44,45)*, showing that lead accumulates in cells of the nervous system.

A neurotoxicant could selectively affect one or several molecules in the early development of the brain, but the consequences would be manifest only when development is completed. This important aspect of "delayed toxicity" can also be studied in aggregates. After short- or long-term treatment during different stages of differentiation, part of the cultures are harvested immediately at the end of the period of treatment; others are only washed free of toxicant and then kept longer in culture until the harvest. This approach allowed us to observe a delayed degradation of neuronal parameters after an early treatment with lead acetate (unpublished observations). Furthermore, after treatment with OPs, we observed delayed effects on the neuronal parameters ChAT and GAD, in spite of a partial recovery of the activity of acetylcholinesterase (unpublished observations).

2.4.4. Demyelination/Remyelination Studies

In the aggregates, oligodendrocyte proliferation is restricted essentially to the first 2 wk in culture. Thereafter, oligodendrocytes progressively differentiate, and within 3–4 wk in culture, they form compact sheaths of myelin around axons *(46)*. The use of a chemically defined medium enabled the identification of a series of factors that enhance oligodendrocyte maturation and myelination. The three-dimensional structure of the aggregates is not only essential for the myelination of axons, but it also permits oligodendrocytes to undergo cell–cell interactions that have been shown to play an important role in oligodendroglial signal transduction pathways *(47)*.

In highly differentiated cultures, demyelination can be induced by antibodies directed against the myelin/oligodendrocyte glycoprotein (MOG) in the presence of complement. This demyelination is followed by a significant increase in mitotic activity, ultimately leading to remyelination and the formation of compact myelin *(48)*. Demyelination induced by several cytokines, such as interleukin-1α, interferon-γ, and tumor necrosis factor-α has also been investigated *(6)*. These features and the extensive characterization of myelination and demyelination make the aggregate cultures a unique in vitro system to assess the potential effects of toxic agents on these processes. For example, fumonisin B1, a mycotoxin often present in corn-based food products, has been shown to selectively affect glial cells. In particular, fumosin B1 delayed oligodendrocyte development and impaired myelin formation and myelin deposition *(49)* (*see* Table 1). Noncytotoxic concentrations of the organophosphorus insecticide parathion interfered with the myelination process and/or with already deposited myelin *(21)*, whereas protein kinase C (PKC) activators, such as mezerein and phorbol 12-myristate acetate, induced demyelination *(48)*. The potential of remyelination of the aggregate cultures might allow for the identification of toxicants slowing down this process.

Table 1
Radioimmunoassay for MBP After Fumonisin B1 Treatment at Two Developmental Periods

[Fumonisin B1] (μM)	DIV 18–28	DIV 25–35
0	5.4 ± 0.2	5.0 ± 0.4
3	$3.8 \pm 0.1^{**}$	6.6 ± 1.5
10	$1.8 \pm 0.2^{**}$	4.4 ± 0.4
40	$1.8 \pm 0.1^{**}$	3.9 ± 0.7

Note: Aggregate cultures at two developmental periods were treated for 10 d with fumonisin B1. At the end of the treatment, aggregates were homogenized and MBP content was measured by radioimmunoassay. Values represent the mean (μg MBP/flask) of five to six replicate cultures ± SEM. Statistical evaluation was made by analysis of variance followed by Mann–Whitney posttest.
$^{**}p<0.002$.
Source: Reprinted from ref. *49* with permission.

2.4.5. Modulation of Toxic Effects by Cell–Cell Interactions

Signals provided by the cellular environment are recognized as essential complements to genetic determinants for the development of the nervous system (for review, *see* ref. *50*). Some of these extracellular modulatory or regulatory signals, termed "epigenetic factors," are supplied by the circulation, others by neighboring cells. Neurons as well as non-neuronal cells appear to respond to a wide spectrum of signaling molecules, which modulate critical processes in cellular development *(51)* and pattern formation *(52)*. With respect to the development of neurons and glial cells, a wealth of convincing evidence indicates that epigenetic factors, including hormones, trophic factors, extracellular matrix components, secreted proteases or protease inhibitors, neurotransmitters, and cytokines, specifically influence cell proliferation, differentiation, and survival. Furthermore, in analogy with the epigenetic modulation of neuronal development by glia-derived factors, it seems that glial cell development depends on neuronal influence and on glia–glia interactions. In addition to their important role during development, at least part of these epigenetic factors are thought to be essential also for mature cellular functions and maintenance. In this context, it can be expected that a toxic insult to the brain will probably affect not only one single cell type, but will most likely induce perturbations in the entire system by chain reactions. Furthermore, among the various paracrine molecules, some could attenuate the neurotoxicity, whereas others will exacerbate it.

Toxic effects might be modulated by cellular interactions in several ways. For example, a type of cell might provide protection to other cell types by forming a physical barrier, thus limiting toxicant access. Alternatively, signaling factors, such as neurotrophins, growth factors, and cytokines, released by one cell type might modulate the toxic effects on another cell type. Activated astrocytes and microglial cells are well known sources of such factors.

Microglial cells are known to react to several pathological events in the central nervous system and therefore are considered as early markers of toxicity *(28,31,53,54)*. Microglial activation is generally characterized by a gradual transition from a quiescent stellate form to a macrophagelike form, which is accompanied by the upregulation of surface antigens and by the formation of clusters *(27,29,55)*. Lipopolysaccharide is a potent direct activator of microglial cells *(56)*. However, microglia can also be activated by indirect pathways, involving the release of molecules by injured neurons *(54,57)*, dying astrocytes *(58)*, or cell debris occurring during demyelination *(59)*. In turn, activated microglial cells are able to upregulate the formation of several bioactive molecules, including reactive oxygen species and nitrogen intermediates, proteolytic enzymes, glutamate, and cytokines such as interleukins, tumor necrosis factor-α (TNF-α) or transforming growth factor-β (TGF-β) *(28,60,61)*. They were also shown to release neurotrophins such as nerve growth factor (NGF) and brain-derived neurotrophic factor (BDNF) *(62–64)*.

Trimethyltin at a concentration as low as 10^{-9} M was shown to induce microglial reactions in brain cell aggregate cultures, whereas it caused astrocytic reactions at 10^{-8} M and neuronal cell death at 10^{-6} M *(19,31)*. In contrast, the use of isolated cultures did not permit the direct observation of effects of TMT on microglial morphology, proliferation, and viability for concentrations up to 10^{-6} M. In monolayer cocultures, 10^{-6} M of TMT induced morphological changes in microglial cells in the presence of neurons but not in the presence of astrocytes. These results suggest that the presence of neurons is necessary to activate microglial cells under TMT treatment. Furthermore, they show that aggregating brain cell cultures, allowing extensive cell–cell interactions, permitted the observation of microglial activation in response to TMT with a very high sensitivity *(65)*.

Methylmercury (MeHgCl) was shown to induce microglial clustering in the aggregates at concentration as low as 10^{-10} M, astrocytic reactions at 10^{-8} M, and neuronal death at 10^{-6} M *(20)*. In the vicinity of the clusters of microglial cells, astrocytes were prevalent and immunoreactivity for the neuronal cytoskeletal marker MAP-2 was decreased. Addition of interleukin (IL)-6 prevented the decrease in MAP-2 staining and caused an increase in GFAP staining. In isolated cultures, methylmercury directly activated microglial cells at concentrations ranging from 10^{-10} to 10^{-7} M. Furthermore, treatment with MeHgCl increased the release of IL-6 by cocultures of astrocytes with a high proportion of microglial cells. Together, these results suggest that microglial cells are directly activated by methylmercury and that, in a histotypic environment, clusters of these activated microglial cells might interact with neighboring astrocytes leading to local increase of IL-6 release. The released IL-6 can, in turn, induce astrocytic reactions and protect neurons from methylmercury toxicity *(66)*.

2.4.6. Potential Use of Aggregating Brain Cell Cultures in the Risk Assessment Process

Humans are exposed to a multitude of potentially toxic natural and synthetic chemicals. Risk assessment strategies have been developed to address the significance for human health of such exposures, which combine toxicological data with estimated degrees of exposure to evaluate the probability of adverse effects for the human population. Risk assessment is usually divided into four major steps: (1) hazard identification, (2) hazard characterization, (3) exposure assessment, and (4) risk characterization. Hazard characterization assesses the dose–effect relationships and leads to the establishment of safety standards such as the acceptable daily intake (ADI). Up to now, safety standards have relied heavily on animal studies, and in vitro data have not been exploited significantly *(67,68)*. Several aspects of the hazard characterization process could clearly benefit from the application of in vitro test systems such as the aggregating brain cell cultures.

Whereas human safety standards are generally based on animal data, interspecies extrapolation constitutes a key issue. In the food safety domain, it has been suggested that the application of sensitive and diagnostic markers of toxicity in a combination of animal and human test systems could improve the extrapolation process *(68,69)*. In such a complementary approach, the first step would involve animal studies aimed at identifying key toxic effects and appropriate markers for toxicity prediction. The next step should aim at the establishment of in vitro systems able to reproduce the toxicity observed in vivo. This step can be achieved by investigating the effects of the test compound on selected markers in cell cultures prepared from the specific target tissues of the same animal species as that employed in the in vivo study. In the following step, an equivalent human in vitro system would be employed to investigate the species specificity of the toxic effects and to check the relevance to humans of the effects and mechanisms identified in the animal in vivo and in vitro models. If integrated in such an approach, aggregating brain cell cultures might play a significant role in the assessment of neurotoxicological risks. In theory, aggregates can be prepared from any animal species. So far, neurotoxicological studies have been reported in aggregate cultures derived from chick *(70)*, rat *(71–73*; our work), and man *(74–76)*. These studies have covered a wide range of neurotoxic agents, including metals, mycotoxins, organophosphorous insecticides, excitatory amino acids, drugs, and human immunodeficiency virus. These investigations have involved many diagnostic markers of neurotoxicity (e.g., astrogliosis, microglial reaction) that allow a direct comparison of the effects obtained in in vivo and in vitro test systems. In this context, it is worth mentioning that aggregating brain cell cultures can be used as an efficient tool to develop and validate new biochemical markers of neurotoxicity.

Aggregating brain cell cultures can also be used to confirm the suitability of safety standards already established. For example, concerns have been raised about the adequacy of current safety standards (e.g., ADIs) to cover all of the potential neurotoxicological and neurodevelopmental effects of OPs. Usually, it is considered that the ADIs for OPs can be derived on the basis of brain AChE inhibition in mature animals. However, it has been questioned whether brain AChE inhibition is the most sensitive marker of the toxic effects of OPs and whether it should be considered as the critical mechanism for the ADI setting. Moreover, the suitability of data obtained in adult animals to cover risk assessment for infants has been challenged. Studies conducted in aggregating brain cell cultures indicated that the cytotoxic effects of OPs were unrelated to AChE inhibition *(40)* and that other mechanisms of toxicity, which may be compound-specific, are likely to exist. However, all toxic effects on neuronal and glial markers were found at OP concentrations that exceeded the IC_{50} values for AChE inhibition. In addition, age-dependent susceptibility to toxic effects was found to be compound-specific, whereas no maturation-dependent differences were observed for AChE inhibition. Overall, these data support brain AChE inhibition as a suitable and conservative end point to derive human safety standards such as the ADI.

3. CONCLUSIONS

Because of their three-dimensional architecture, aggregating brain cell cultures are unique in their ability to establish a tissue-specific cellular organization and to reproduce very closely the expression of the in vivo phenotype. The large number of replicate cultures that can be prepared in a single batch makes this procedure suitable for routine tests of a whole series of compounds. Both the general cytotoxic effects and cell-type-specific toxicity can be determined by selecting a set of representative diagnostic criteria. Maturation-dependent toxic effects can be examined at well-defined developmental stages of the cultures, such as periods of mitotic activity, synaptogenesis, or myelination, with the help of very sensitive and reliable markers. The ability to maintain the aggregates in a highly differentiated state for prolonged periods in culture also allows long-term observations of toxic drug action, such as the effect of chronic exposure to low concentrations of a given neurotoxicant or the long-term consequences of an acute toxic insult during a critical period of development. In addition to the possibility of testing compounds in a screening approach, aggregating brain cell cultures also offer the possibility of studying mechanisms of action at the cellular and molecular levels. All of these features make the brain cell aggregates a suitable, versatile, and relevant in vitro system for neurotoxicological studies.

REFERENCES

1. Harrison, R.G. (1907) Observations on the living developing nerve fiber. *Anat. Rec.* **1,** 116–118.
2. Moscona, A. A. (1960) Patterns and mechanisms of tissue reconstruction from dissociated cells, in *Developing Cell Systems and their Control* (Rudnick, D., ed.), Ronald, New York, pp. 45–70.
3. Honegger, P., Lenoir, D., and Favrod, P. (1979) Growth and differentiation of aggregating fetal brain cells in a serum-free defined medium. *Nature* **282,** 305–308.
4. Honegger, P. and Monnet-Tschudi, F. (1997) Aggregating neural cell cultures, in *Protocols for Neural Cell Culture* (Fedoroff, S. and Richardson, A., eds.), Humana, Totowa, NJ, pp. 25–49.
5. Honegger, P. and Werffeli, P. (1988) Use of aggregating cell cultures for toxicological studies. *Experientia* **44,** 817–822.
6. Loughlin, A. J., Honegger, P., Woodroofe, M. N., Comte, V., Matthieu, J.-M., and Cuzner, M. L. (1994) Myelination and cytokine-induced demyelination in aggregating rat brain cell cultures: effects of macrophage-enrichment. . *Neurosci. Res.* **37,** 647–653.
7. Honegger, P. (1985) Biochemical differentiation in serum-free aggregating brain cell cultures, in *Cell Culture in the Neurosciences* (Bottenstein, J. E. and Sato, G., eds.), Plenum, New York, pp. 223–243.
8. Riederer, B. M., Monnet-Tschudi, F., and Honegger, P. (1992) Development and maintenance of the neuronal cytoskeleton in aggregated cell cultures of fetal rat telencephalon and influence of elevated K^+ concentrations. *J. Neurochem.* **58,** 649–658.
9. Corthésy-Theulaz, I., Mérillaz, A. M., Honegger, P., and Rossier, B. C. (1990) Na+-K+-ATPase gene expression during in vitro development of rat fetal forebrain. *Am. J. Physiol.* **258,** C1062–C1069.
10. Honegger, P. and Pardo, B. (1999) Separate neuronal and glial Na^+,K^+-ATPase isoforms regulate glucose utilization in response to membrane depolarization and elevated extracellular potassium. *J. Cereb. Blood Flow Metab.* **19,** 1051–1059.
11. Honegger, P. and Matthieu, J.-M. (1990) Aggregating brain cell cultures: a model to study myelination and demyelination, in *Cellular and Molecular*

Biology of Myelination (Jeserich, G., Althaus, H. H., and Waehneldt, T. V., eds.), Springer-Verlag, Berlin, pp. 155–170.

12. Honegger, P. and Richelson, E. (1979) Neurotransmitter synthesis, storage and release by aggregating cell cultures of rat brain. *Brain Res.* **62,** 89–101.

13. Mata, M., Honegger, P., and Fink, D. J. (1997) Modulation of phosphorylation of neuronal cytoskeletal proteins by neuronal depolarization. *Cell. Mol. Neurobiol.* **17,** 129–140.

14. Norton, W. T., Aquino, D. A., Hozumi, I., Chiu, F.-C., and Brosnan, C. F. (1992) Quantitative aspects of reactive gliosis: a review. *Neurochem. Res.* **17 (9),** 877–885.

15. O'Callaghan, J. P. (1991) Assessment of neurotoxicity: use of glial fibrillary acidic protein as a biomarker. *Biomed. Environ. Sci.* **4,** 197–206.

16. McMillian, M. K., Thai, L., Hong, J.-S., O'Callaghan, J. P., and Pennypacker, K. R. (1994) Brain injury in a dish: a model for reactive gliosis. *TINS* **17,** 138–142.

17. Wu, V. W. and Schwartz, J. P. (1998) Cell culture models for reactive gliosis: new perspectives. *J. Neurosci. Res.* **51,** 675–681.

18. Rozovsky, I., Laping, N. J., Krohn, K., Teter, B., O'Callaghan, J. P., and Finch, C. E. (1995) Transcriptional regulation of glial fibrillary acidic protein by corticosterone in rat astrocytes in vitro is influenced by the duration of time in culture and by astrocyte-neuron interactions. *Endocrinology* **136,** 2066–2073.

19. Monnet-Tschudi, F., Zurich, M.-G., Riederer, B. M., and Honegger, P. (1995) Effects of trimethyltin (TMT) on glial and neuronal cells in aggregate cultures: dependence on the developmental stage. *NeuroToxicology* **16,** 97–104.

20. Monnet-Tschudi, F., Zurich, M.-G., and Honegger, P. (1996) Comparison of the developmental effects of two mercury compounds on glial cells and neurons in aggregate cultures of rat telencephalon. *Brain Res.* **741,** 52–59.

21. Zurich, M.-G., Honegger, P., Schilter, B., Costa, L. G., and Monnet-Tschudi, F. (2000) Use of aggregating brain cell cultures to study developmental effects of organophosphorus insecticides. *NeuroToxicology* **21,** 599–606.

22. Aquino, D.A., Chiu, F.-C., Brosnan, C. F., and Norton, W. T. (1988) Glial fibrillary acidic protein increases in the spinal cord of Lewis rats with acute experimental autoimmune encephalomyelitis. *J. Neurochem.* **51,** 1085–1095.

23. Streit, W. J. and Kreutzberg, G. W. (1987) Lectin binding by resting and reactive microglia. *J. Neurocytol.* **16,** 249–260.

24. Giulian, D. (1987) Ameboid microglia as effectors of inflammation in the central nervous system. *J. Neurosci. Res.* **18,** 155–171.

25. Perry, V. H. and Gordon, S. (1991) Macrophage and the nervous system. *Int. Rev. Cytol.* **125,** 203–244.

26. Morioka, T. and Streit, W. J. (1991) Expression of immunomolecules on microglial cells following neonatal sciatic nerve axotomy. *J. Neuroimmunol.* **35,** 21–30.

27. Marty, S., Dusart, I., and Peschanski, M. (1991) Glial changes following an excitotoxic lesion in the CNS-I. Microglia/macrophages. *Neuroscience* **45,** 529–539.

28. Stoll, G. and Jander, S. (1999) The role of microglia and macrophages in the pathophysiology of the CNS. *Prog. Neurobiol.* **58,** 233–247.
29. Streit, W. J., Walter, S. A., and Pennell, N. A. (1999) Reactive microgliosis. *Prog. Neurobiol.* **57,** 563–581.
30. Gehrmann, J. and Kreutzberg, G. W. (1995) Microglia in experimental neuropathology, in *Neuroglia* (Kettenmann, H. and Ransom, B. R., eds.), Oxford University Press, New York, pp. 883–904.
31. Monnet-Tschudi, F., Zurich, M.-G., Pithon, E., van Melle, G., and Honegger, P. (1995) Microglial responsiveness as a sensitive marker for trimethyltin (TMT) neurotoxicity. *Brain Res.* **690,** 8–14.
32. McCann, M. J., O'Callaghan, J. P., Martin, P. M., Bertram, T., and Streit, W. J. (1996) Differential activation of microglia and astrocytes following trimethyl tin-induced neurodegeneration. *Neuroscience* **72,** 273–281.
33. Monnet-Tschudi, F., Sorg, O., Honegger, P., Zurich, M.-G., Huggett, A. C., and Schilter, B. (1997) Effects of naturally occurring food mycotoxin ochratoxin A on brain cells in culture. *NeuroToxicology* **18,** 831–840.
34. Charleston, J.S., Bolender, R.P., Mottet, N.K., Body, R.L., Vahter, M.E. and Burbacher, T.M. (1994) Increases in the number of reactive glia in the visual cortex of *Macaca fascicularis* following subclinical long-term methyl mercury exposure. *Toxicol. Appl. Pharmacol.* **129,** 196–206.
35. Monnet-Tschudi, F., Zurich, M.-G., and Honegger, P. (1993) Evaluation of the toxicity of different metal compounds in the developing brain using aggregating cell cultures as a model. *Toxic. In Vitro* **7,** 335–339.
36. Honegger, P. and Schilter, B. (1992) Serum-free aggregate cultures of fetal rat brain and liver cells: methodology and some practical application in neurotoxicology, in *The Brain in Bits and Pieces. In Vitro Techniques in Neurobiology, Neuropharmacology and Neurotoxicology* (Zbinden, G., ed.), MTC Verlag, Zollikon, Switzerland, pp. 51–79.
37. Benke, G. M. and Murphy, S. D. (1975) The influence of age on the toxicity and metabolism of methyl parathion and parathion in male and female rats. *Toxicol. Appl. Pharmacol.* **31,** 254–269.
38. Mortensen, S. R., Chanda, S. M., Hooper, M. J., and Padilla, S. (1996) Maturational differences in chlorpyrifos-oxonase activity may contribute to age-related sensitivity to chlorpyrifos. *J. Biochem. Toxicol.* **11,** 279–287.
39. Lassiter, T. L., Padilla, S., Mortensen, S. R., Chanda, S. M., Moser, V. C., and Barone, S., Jr. (1998) Gestational exposure to chlorpyrifos: apparent protection of the fetus? *Toxicol. Appl. Pharmacol.* **152,** 56–65.
40. Monnet-Tschudi, F., Zurich, M.-G., Schilter, B., Costa, L. G., and Honegger, P. (2000) Maturation-dependent effects of chlorpyrifos and parathion and their oxygen analogs on acetylcholinesterase and neuronal and glial markers in aggregating brain cell cultures. *Toxicol. Appl. Pharmacol.* **165,** 175–183.
41. Liu, J., Olivier, K., and Pope, C. N. (1999) Comparative neurochemical effects of repeated methyl parathion or chlorpyrifos exposures in neonatal and adult rats. *Toxicol. Appl. Pharmacol.* **158,** 186–196.

42. Honegger, P. and Schilter, B. (1995) The use of serum-free aggregating brain cell cultures in neurotoxicology, in *Neurotoxicology: Approaches & Methods* (Chang, L. W., ed.), Academic, New York, pp. 507–516.

43. Zurich, M.-G., Monnet-Tschudi, F., and Honegger, P. (1994) Long-term treatment of aggregating brain cell cultures with low concentrations of lead acetate. *NeuroToxicology* **15(3)**, 715–720.

44. Tiffany-Castiglioni, E., Zmudzki, J., and Bratton, G. R. (1986) Cellular targets of lead neurotoxicity: in vitro models. *Toxicology* **42**, 303–315.

45. Tiffany-Castiglioni, E., Zmudzki, J., Wu, J. N., and Bratton, G. R. (1987) Effects of lead treatment on intracellular iron and copper concentrations in cultured astroglia. *Metab. Brain Dis.* **2(1)**, 61–79.

46. Guentert-Lauber, B., Monnet-Tschudi, F., Omlin, F. X., Favrod, P., and Honegger, P. (1985) Serum-free aggregate cultures of rat CNS glial cells: biochemical, immunocytochemical and morphological characterization. *Dev. Neurosci.* **7**, 33–44.

47. He, M., Howe, D. G., and McCarthy, K. D. (1996) Oligodendroglial signal transduction systems are regulated by neuronal contact. *J. Neurochem.* **67**, 1491–1499.

48. Pouly, S., Storch, M. K., Matthieu, J.-M., Lassman, H., Monnet-Tschudi, F., and Honegger, P. (1997) Demyelination induced by protein kinase C-activating tumor promoters in aggregating brain cell cultures. *J. Neurosci. Res.* **49**, 121–132.

49. Monnet-Tschudi, F., Zurich, M.-G., Sorg, O., Matthieu, J.-M., Honegger, P., and Schilter, B. (1999) The naturally occuring food mycotoxin fumonisin B1 impairs myelin formation in aggregating brain cell culture. *NeuroToxicology* **20**, 41–48.

50. Arenender, A. T. and De Vellis, J. (1989) *Basic Neurochemistry: Molecular, Cellular, and Medical Aspects*, Raven, New York, pp. 479–506.

51. Hunt, R. K. (1987) *Neural Development, Part IV: Cellular and Molecular Differentiation*, Current Topics in Developmental Biology, Vol. 21, Academic, New York.

52. Steindler, D. A., Faissner, A. and Schachner, M. (1989) Brain "cordones": transient boundaries of glia and adhesion molecules that define developing functional units. *Comments on Developmental Neurobiology* **1**, 29–60.

53. Thomas, W. E. (1992) Brain macrophages: evaluation of microglia and their functions. *Brain Res. Rev.* **17**, 61–74.

54. Kreutzberg, G. W. (1996) Microglia: a sensor for pathological events in the CNS. *TINS* **19**, 312–318.

55. Sawada, M., Kondo, N., and Marunouchi, T. (1989) Production of tumor necrosis factor-alpha by microglia and astrocytes in culture. *Brain Res.* **491**, 394–397.

56. Finsen, B. R., Jorgensen, M. B., Diemer, N. H., and Zimmer, J. (1993) Microglial MHC antigen expression after ischemic and kainic acid lesions of the adult rat hippocampus. *Glia* **7**, 41–49.

57. Beyer, M., Gimsa, U., Eyüpoglu, I. Y., Hailer, N. P., and Nitsch, R. (2000) Phagocytosis of neuronal or glial debris by microglial cells: upregulation of MHC class II expression and multinuclear giant cell formation in vitro. *Glia* **31,** 262–266.
58. Ashwell, K. (1990) Microglia and cell death in the developing mouse cerebellum. *Dev. Brain Res.* **55,** 219–230.
59. Lassmann, H., Schmied, M., Vass, K., and Hickey, W. F. (1993) Bone marrow derived elements and resident microglia in brain inflammation. *Glia* **7,** 19–24.
60. Banati, R. B., Gehrmann, J., Schubert, P., and Kreutzberg, G. W. (1993) Cytotoxicity of microglia. *Glia* **7,** 111–118.
61. Mizuno, T., Sawada, M., Suzumura, A., and Marunouchi, T. (1994) Expression of cytokines during glial differentiation. *Brain Res.* **656,** 141–146.
62. Mallat, M., Houlgatte, R., Brachet, P., and Prochiantz, A. (1989) Lipopolysaccharide-stimulated rat brain macrophages release NGF in vitro. *Dev. Biol.* **133,** 309–311.
63. Miwa, T., Furukawa, S., Nakajima, K., Furukawa, Y., and Kohsaka, S. (1997) Lipopolysaccharide enhances synthesis of brain-derived neurotrophic factor in cultured rat microglia. *J. Neurosci. Res.* **50,** 1023–1029.
64. Elkabes, S., diCicco-Bloom, E. M., and Black, I. B. (1996) Brain microglia/macrophages express neurotrophins that selectively regulate microglial proliferation and function. *J. Neurosci.* **16,** 2508–2521.
65. Eskes, C. (2000) Implication of microglial cells in the cascade of cell–cell interactions following subchronic neurotoxicant treatments: a multiple in vitro study. Thesis dissertation, University of Lausanne.
66. Eskes, C., Honegger, P., Juillerat-Jeanneret, L., and Monnet-Tschudi, F. Microglial reaction induced by non-cytotoxic methylmercury treatment leads to neuroprotection via interactions with astrocytes and IL-6 release. *Glia* **37,** 43–52.
67. Walton, K., Walker, R., van de Sandt, J. J. M., et al. (1999) The application of in vitro data in the derivation of the Acceptable Daily Intake (ADI) of food additives. *Food Chem. Toxicol.* **37,** 1175–1197.
68. Schilter, B., Holzhäuser, D., Cavin, C., and Huggett, A. C. (1996) An integrated in vivo/in vitro strategy to improve food safety evaluation. *Trends Food Sci. Technol.* **7,** 327–332.
69. Huggett, A. C., Schilter, B., Roberfroid, M., Antignac, E., and Koemen, J. H. (1996) Comparative methods of toxicity testing. *Food Chem. Toxicol.* **34,** 183–192.
70. Funk, K. A., Liu, C.-H., Higgins, R. J., and Wilson, B. W. (1994) Avian embryonic brain reaggregate culture system II. NTE activity discriminates between effects of a single neuropathic or nonneuropathic organophosphorus compound exposure. *Toxicol. Appl. Pharmacol.* **124,** 159–163.
71. Atterwill, C. K., Hillier, G., Johnston, H., and Thomas, S. M. (1992) A tiered system for in vitro neurotoxicity testing: a place for neural cell line and organotypic cultures? in *The Brain in Bits and Pieces* (Zbinden, G., ed.), MTC Verlag, Zollikon, Switzerland, pp. 81–114.

72. Fox, R. M., Davenport Jones, J. E., and Atterwill, C. K. (1995) Oxidative stress induces neurotoxicity in rat brain reaggregate cultures that can be prevented by β-tocopherol. *NeuroToxicology* **16,** 558.
73. Fox, R. M., Davenport Jones, J. E., and Atterwill, C. K. (1995) Excitatory amino acids produce toxic glial responses in whole rat brain reaggregate cultures. *NeuroToxicology* **16,** 559.
74. Hayes, G. M., Fox, R. M., Cuzner, M. L., and Griffin, G. E. (2000) Human rotation-mediated fetal mixed brain cell aggregate culture: characterization and N-methyl-D-aspartate. *Neurosci. Lett.* **287,** 146–150.
75. Pulliam, L., Gascon, R., Stubblebine, M., McGuire, D., and McGrath, M. S. (1997) Unique monocyte subset in patients with AIDS dementia. *Lancet* **349,** 692–695.
76. Pulliam, L., Stubblebine, M., and Hyun, W. (1998) Quantification of neurotoxicity and identification of cellular subsets in a three-dimensional brain model. *Cytometry* **32,** 66–69.

11

Use of Complimentary In Vitro and In Vivo Methods for Assessing Neuroendocrine Disruptors

W. Les Dees, Jill K. Hiney, Robert K. Dearth, and Vinod K. Srivastava

1. INTRODUCTION

It is often necessary to use a variety of techniques to more completely assess a specific area of study. In recent years, this has been increasingly true for the field of neuroendocrinology. Anatomical and molecular methodologies are often used in conjunction with in vitro and in vivo physiological approaches to gain meaningful information regarding factors controlling or altering neuroendocrine functions. When used together in a given study, in vitro and in vivo methods can be complimentary to one another and, thus, provide vital information. The focus of this chapter will be to demonstrate how both in vitro and in vivo techniques can be used in this complimentary fashion to provide new and important insights into basic neuroendocrine events and their mechanisms of action. Furthermore, we will demonstrate how these techniques can be used to help better understand the sites of action and the effects of specific toxic substances that alter neuroendocrine function.

2. NEUROENDOCRINE ACTIONS OF INSULIN-LIKE GROWTH FACTOR-1 DURING PUBERTY

2.1. Endocrine Perspective: Initial Basic In Vivo Studies

Dees and Skelley (1) first reported that the ethanol (ETOH)-induced delay in female puberty was associated with depressed growth hormone (GH) and

From: *Methods in Pharmacology and Toxicology: In Vitro Neurotoxicology: Principles and Challenges*
Edited by: E. Tiffany-Castiglioni © Humana Press Inc., Totowa, NJ

luteinizing hormone (LH). Interestingly, the GH levels were depressed prior to LH, suggesting to us that perhaps insulin-like growth factor-1 (IGF-1), a peripheral signal that mediates many of the effects of GH *(2–6)*, might be able to act at the level of the hypothalamus to induce the peripubertal increase in luteinizing hormone-releasing hormone (LHRH) and, hence, play an early role in the initiation of puberty. The localization of the type 1 IGF receptors in the median eminence (ME) region of the hypothalamus provides an anatomical basis to support a potential regulatory action of IGF-1 to elicit LHRH release from the neuron terminals in this area *(7,8)*. Therefore, the first step was to test the hypothesis that IGF-1 could induce the prepubertal release of hypothalamic LHRH.

2.2. *In Vitro Studies: IGF-1-Induced LHRH Release*

To test our above hypothesis, we chose to utilize the static in vitro incubation system first described by Negro-Vilar and Ojeda over 20 yr ago when they reported the stimulatory influence of norepinephrine (NE) on LHRH release *(9)*. Importantly, these initial in vitro results have been validated by in vivo studies over the years, and the involvement of NE in LHRH secretion is now well accepted, hence further demonstrating the usefulness of this technique for assessing factors controlling or altering the secretions of this neuropeptide. A distinct advantage of this protocol is that it allows the investigator to use very small volumes (250–400 µL) of medium, which will allow accurate measurement of picogram amounts of peptide released. Briefly, the in vitro procedure calls for the removal of the ME region from the base of the hypothalamus, then transferring the tissue immediately to an incubation well containing Krebs bicarbonate glucose buffer (pH 7.4) in an atmosphere of 95% O_2 and 5% CO_2. The tissues are preincubated for 30 min to allow for equilibration. Tissues are then incubated for 1–3 h so that basal LHRH release into the medium could be assessed and compared to that release following a challenge with a specific substance that is known or suspected of being able to induce the secretion of the peptide.

Using the above-described static incubation system, we investigated whether IGF-1 could stimulate LHRH release from ME fragments of prepubertal female rats *(10)*. Figure 1 demonstrates that IGF-1 stimulated LHRH release in a dose-dependent manner, suggesting a possible link between somatic development and the activation of the LHRH/LH releasing system. Whether this effect of IGF-1 on LHRH release is the result of a direct effect on the LHRH neuron terminals or an indirect action on glial networks of the ME is not known. Perhaps future studies designed using cell culture methodologies might be able to generate useful information, especially since Duenas et al. *(11)* demonstrated that glial elements localized in the ME have

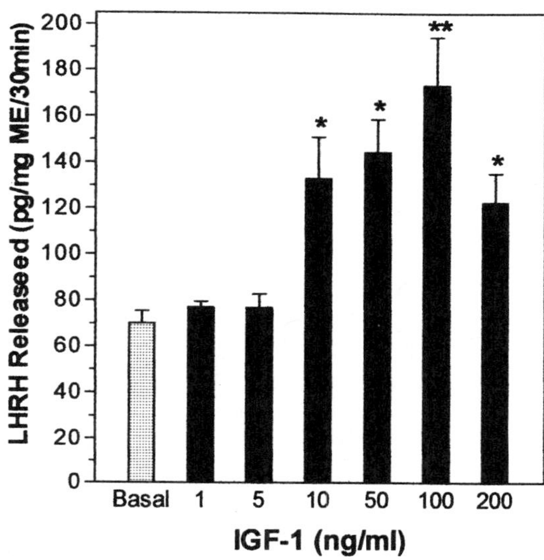

Fig. 1. Effect of IGF-1 on LHRH secretion in vitro. Fragments of median eminence from prepubertal female rats were exposed to IGF-1 in a short-term static incubation system, and the amount of LHRH released into the medium was measured. IGF-1 significantly stimulated LHRH release in a dose-dependent manner. Bars represent the mean values ± SEM; N= 7–25. $^*p<0.05$ and $^{**}p<0.01$ vs basal value.

high levels of IGF-1 immunoreactivity during first proestrus, suggesting this was the result of the uptake of the peptide from the circulation. Whatever the mechanism, it was apparent from our in vitro study that a potentially important physiological action of IGF-1, other than cell differentiation and proliferation, might exist, thus demonstrating a critical need to validate this finding in vivo.

2.3. In Vivo Studies: IGF-1-Induced LH Release

To further test our hypothesis that IGF-1 is involved in the hypothalamic control of LHRH/LH secretion at the time of puberty, we utilized an approach *(12)* that has been used for many years to assess the effects of substances thought to act within the hypothalamus to subsequently influence pituitary hormone secretion. The technique requires a stainless-steel cannula to be implanted into the third ventricle of the brain. After several days of recovery, a cannula is also implanted in the external jugular vein 1– 2 d before the experiment *(13)* in order to take blood samples every 10 min prior to and after the central administration of test substances. This methodology allows for assessing pulsatile hormone secretion from freely moving,

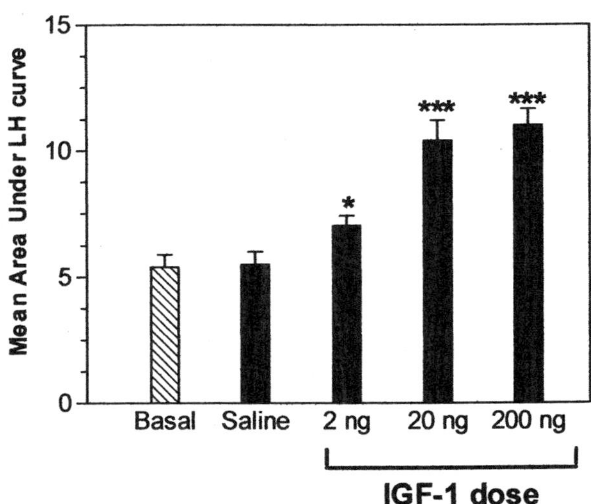

Fig. 2. Effect of IGF-1 on the mean areas under the LH curves of secretion in vivo. Prepubertal female rats were injected with IGF-1 through a cannula into the third ventricle of the brain, and blood was sampled for LH from a jugular cannula in unanethetized, freely moving animals. The hatched bar represents the mean (±SEM) area under the basal segment of the LH curve, and the solid bars represent the arithmetic mean (±SEM) of the area under the postsaline or post-IGF-1 injection segment of the LH curve. Note that saline-injected animals showed no increase in LH secretion, whereas those animals injected with IGF-1 showed significant increases in LH release. $^{*}p<0.05$ and $^{***}p<0.001$; $N= 9$–15.

unanesthetized animals. By utilizinig these techniques, we discovered that intraventricular administration of IGF-1 was capable of stimulating LH release from late juvenile and peripubertal animals *(14)*. Figure 2 demonstrates the combined data from each group of immature female rats showing the arithmetic means of the areas under the LH curves of secretion. In this regard, the 2-, 20-, and 200-ng doses of IGF-1 all caused significant increases in LH levels. In order to determine if this action of IGF-1 was a centrally mediated or a pituitary effect, a similar in vivo study was designed *(14)*. We immunoneutralized hypothalamic LHRH, via third ventricular administration of a LHRH antiserum, further demonstrating the hypothalamic site of action of IGF-1 to induce LH release. Figure 3 depicts that animals that received the normal rabbit serum (NRS) showed a significant increase in LH after IGF-1 stimulation, whereas this increase was blocked in the animals that received the antiserum. These results indicate that immunoneutralization of hypothalamic LHRH inhibits the increase in LH released following the intraventricular injection of IGF-1; thus, demonstrat-

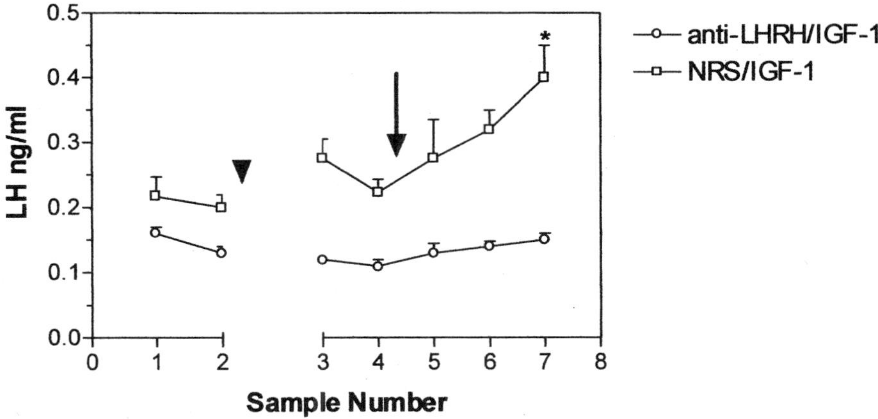

Fig. 3. Effect of in vivo immunoneutralization of LHRH biological activity on IGF-1-induced LH release. Prepubertal animals treated before and after receiving either normal rabbit serum (NRS) (□) plus IGF-1 (200 ng) or anti-LHRH serum (○) plus IGF-1. Each point represents the mean ±SEM LH values. Note that the animals receiving NRS showed a significant post-IGF increase in LH release, whereas this increase was blocked in the animals that received the anti-LHRH serum. The asterisk represents the maximum LH response determined by Prism software. The arrowhead represents the third ventricular injection of NRS or anti-LHRH serum. The arrow denotes the injection of IGF-1 after the fourth sample. *$p<0.05$; $N=8–11$.

ing in vivo that the ability of IGF-1 to stimulate the LH release is a centrally mediated effect.

We continued to use an in vivo approach to determine whether IGF-1 administration could advance the onset of female puberty *(14)*. In order to simulate the enhanced afternoon increase in LH levels that occurs prior to puberty *(15–17)*, we administered IGF-1 into the third ventricle of juvenile animals twice daily at 1300 and 1500 h. This method advanced vaginal opening and first ovulation by 5 d ($p<0.001$) in the animals given IGF-1 (34.0±.36 d of age) compared to animals given saline (38.9±0.4 d of age). These results have been confirmed by in vivo experiments using transgenic mice and primates. Specifically, in the GH receptor knockout mouse, IGF-1 levels are low and puberty is delayed, but administration of IGF-1 increased their IGF-1 levels and advanced puberty *(18)*. In primates, administration of IGF-1 was shown to advance the timing of first ovulation *(19)*.

2.4. In Vitro Assessment of IGF-1's Mechanism of Action

Knowing that IGF-1 plays an important early role in the prepubertal process, questions regarding its mechanism of action to activate LHRH secre-

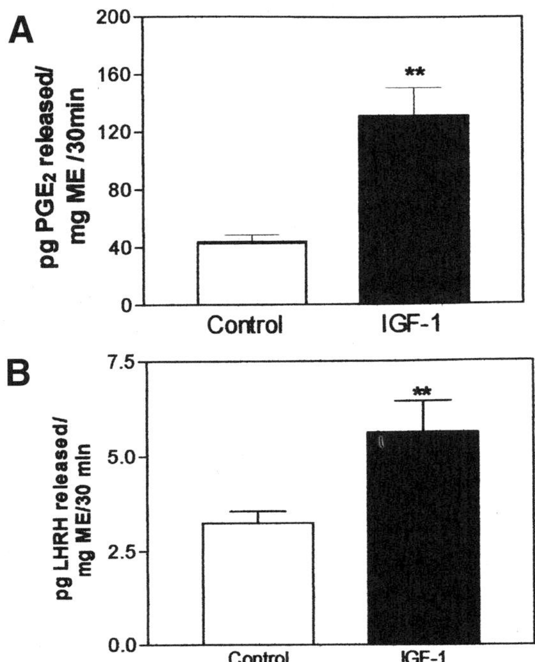

Fig. 4. Induction of PGE$_2$ (**A**) and LHRH (**B**) release by IGF-1 in vitro. Fragments of median eminence from prepubertal female rats were placed in a static incubation system. Fragments were treated with IGF-1, and the secretion of PGE$_2$ and LHRH was assessed. Bars represent the mean ±SEM of the respective hormone released into the medium. Note that IGF-1 significantly stimulated both PGE$_2$ and LHRH release from the same samples. **$p<0.01$; $N=15$.

tion become important. Because our initial in vitro and subsequent in vivo studies were supportive of one another, we felt that additional in vitro studies would allow us to assess mechanistic questions. In this regard, we used the static incubation system to show that IGF-1-induced LHRH release is mediated by prostaglandin E$_2$ (PGE$_2$). Figure 4A,B illustrates that IGF-1 can induce PGE$_2$ and LHRH release from the same ME fragments.

To further demonstrate the necessity of PGE$_2$, we added indomethacin, a prostaglandin synthesis inhibitor, to the incubation media. Figure 5 demontrates that indomethacin blocks IGF-1-induced LHRH release, indicating that PGE$_2$ mediates IGF-1-induced LHRH release.

2.5. Summary of the IGF-1 Influence on Puberty

The results from our initial in vitro study *(10)* led to subsequent in vivo studies in our lab *(14)*, as well as others *(18,19)*, that support the hypothesis

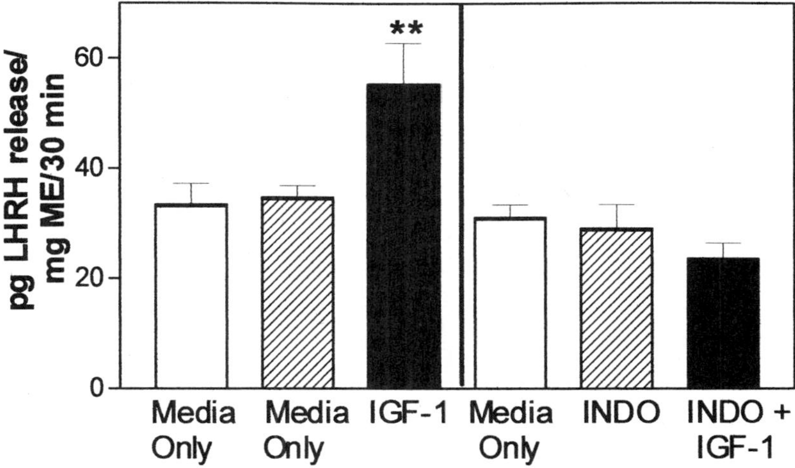

Fig. 5. Effect of indomethacin on IGF-1-induced LHRH release in vitro. This experiment was carried out as described in the legend of Fig. 4. Indomethacin blocked the ability of IGF-1 to stimulate LHRH release, indicating that PGE_2 mediates IGF-1-induced LHRH release. Bars represent mean ±SEM. **$p < 0.01$; $N = 8$–9.

that IGF-1 is a metabolic signal capable of providing the link between the somatotrophic axis and the central activation of the LHRH/LH-releasing system at the time of puberty. Furthermore, those in vivo studies lead us back to additional in vitro studies to begin assessing mechanisms of action. Taken together, these data indicate strongly that IGF-1 plays a crucial, if not pivotal, role in the initiation of the female pubertal process. Importantly, these studies demonstrate that in vitro and in vivo methodologies can be used in an alternative fashion to begin new initiatives, validate their importance in the animal, and begin assessing mechanisms of action. Not only can these techniques be used to advance basic science in specific body systems, but they can also be used to assess the effects of toxic substances that may alter those systems. The remainder of this chapter will address this issue.

3. EFFECTS OF ETOH ON IGF-1 ACTIONS DURING PUBERTY

3.1. Endocrine Perspective

Several different in vitro protocols, such as cell culture *(20–22)* and static incubation of tissue explants *(23–26)*, have been utilized to test the effects of ETOH on different systems. We showed that NE-induced LHRH release was blocked by ETOH, an effect resulting from a decrease in the production of PGE$_2$ *(23)*. Because this was later observed following stimulation with other neurotransmitters that influence LHRH release *(24–26)*, we aimed to determine if prepubertal IGF-1-induced LHRH release could also be blocked by ETOH.

3.2. In Vitro ETOH/IGF-1 Studies

The median eminence region of juvenile female rats were tested in the static incubation system described earlier. The MEs were incubated in medium containing ETOH (50 m*M*), or in buffer only, prior to and along with IGF-1 stimulation. PGE$_2$ and LHRH were measured from the same samples of medium. Figure 6A,B demonstrate that IGF-1 stimulated the release of PGE$_2$ ($p<0.001$) and LHRH ($p<0.01$) from the MEs in the absence of ETOH; however, their respective release was blocked by the drug *(27)*. We showed previously that the addition of PGE$_2$ to the medium overrides the effect of ETOH and induces LHRH release *(23)*. Thus, we have demonstrated that PGE$_2$ is involved in IGF-1-induced LHRH release and contributes to a growing body of evidence suggesting that the principal action of ETOH to block LHRH release is the result of altering PGE$_2$ formation.

3.3. In Vivo ETOH/ IGF-1 Studies

The aforementioned in vitro and in vivo studies demonstrating the influence of IGF-1 on the initiation of puberty and the subsequent in vitro data showing the potential effect of ETOH on IGF-1-induced LHRH release prompted us to conduct in vivo studies to more completely assess the toxic effects of ETOH on the IGF-1 system. Results from earlier studies showing that chronic ETOH exposure delays puberty in the female rat *(1,28)* and that acute ETOH exposure disrupts the pulsatile release of these two hormones *(29–31)* made further in vivo studies assessing potential ETOH/IGF-1 interactions necessary. To begin, we administered ETOH by a specific diet regimen for 5 d to rats as they approached puberty *(32)*. Results demonstrated ETOH's ability to suppress expression of IGF-1 mRNA in the liver, but not in the hypothalamus. This hepatic effect was subsequently associated with significant depressions in the serum levels of IGF-1 and LH. Thus, we suggested that the detrimental effects exerted by ETOH on growth rates, LH levels, and the female pubertal process are associated, at least in part, with this drug's ability to alter the peripheral synthesis of IGF-1. Consequently, suppressed circulating levels of the peptide cause an insufficient amount of the peptide to stimulate LHRH release from the nerve terminals in the ME. We have recently showed that suppressed serum IGF-1 and LH levels also occur in primates following chronic exposure to ETOH *(33)*.

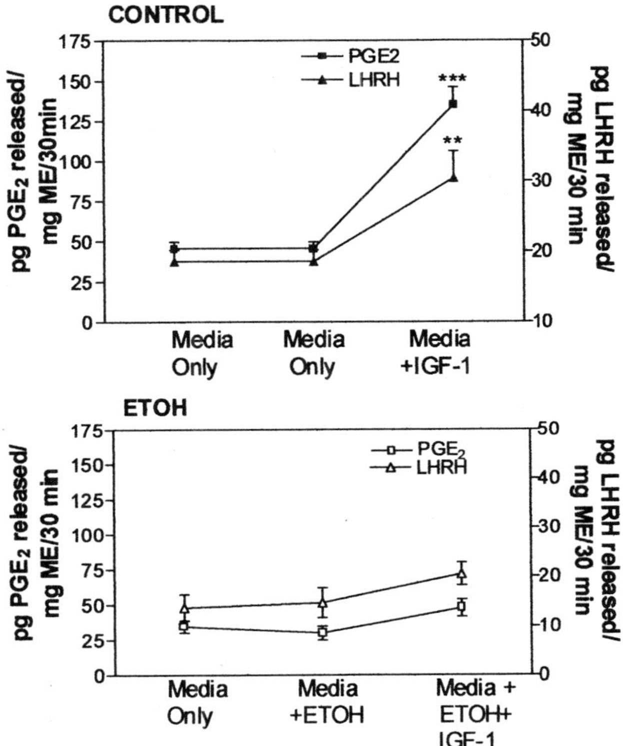

Fig. 6. Effects of ETOH on IGF-1-induced PGE_2 and LHRH release from the MEs of prepubertal female rats in vitro. (**A**) The corelease of PGE_2 and LHRH from the ME tissue incubated without ETOH. (**B**) The corelease of the two substances from ME tissues incubated in the presence of ETOH (50 m*M*). Note that in the control vials, IGF-1 stimulated significant increases in both PGE_2 (***p<0.001) and LHRH (**p<0.01). In test vials, ETOH did not alter basal release of either substance, but it blocked the IGF-1 induced release of both PGE_2 and LHRH. N=8–10.

Although the above-described in vivo studies provided important information, based on our earlier in vitro study showing that ETOH blocked IGF-1-induced LHRH release *(27)*, it was still necessary to assess this potential effect more directly, by measuring the effect of ETOH on the in vivo release of LH after intraventricular administration of IGF-1. In this regard, we demonstrated that IGF-1-induced prepubertal LH secretion and this release was blocked by a single, moderate dose of ETOH *(27)*.

3.4. Summary of ETOH/IGF-1 Interactions

The combined use of in vivo and in vitro approaches have shown that ETOH can acutely block IGF-1-induced LH release during late prepubertal development. Furthermore, this is a centrally mediated action that is the result of decreased PGE_2 formation resulting in suppressed release of LHRH. Importantly, by using in vitro and in vivo techniques together, as well as assessing both the chronic and acute effects of ETOH, we determined that the drug appears to have more than one effect to alter LH release and the subsequent progression of the pubertal process. This depends on the timing of exposure relative to the phase of pubertal development and the duration of exposure. For example, studies assessing the acute effects of ETOH demonstrated the central action of ETOH to alter IGF-1-induced LHRH/LH release at the transition between juvenile and peripubertal phases of development *(27)*, and studies assessing effects of chronic ETOH exposure showed delayed entry into the peripubertal period *(32)*. Importantly, this action was associated with the ability of the drug to decrease peripheral IGF-1 synthesis and subsequent release of the peptide into systemic circulation *(32)*.

4. EFFECTS OF ETOH ON NMDA-RECEPTOR ACTIVATION DURING PUBERTY

4.1. Endocrine Perspective: Initial Basic In Vivo and In Vitro Studies

Activation of hypothalamic *N*-methyl-DL-aspartic acid (NMDA) receptors (NMDA-R) causes the stimulation of LH secretion via a hypothalamic action to release LHRH and not by any direct action on the pituitary *(34–41)*. Also, NMDA was shown to effectively induce LHRH release in vitro *(24,41–43)* and caused precocious puberty in rats *(34)* and primates *(35)* when given systemically, suggesting its involvement in the pubertal process. Because of these actions and because of the known effects of ETOH on the NMDA-R in the brain *(24,44–46)*, we decided to determine if ETOH could (1) alter prepubertal NMDA-induced LHRH release in vitro and (2) alter the ability of NMDA to advance puberty in vivo *(47)*.

4.2. In Vitro ETOH/NMDA Studies

The in vitro incubations were identical to those described earlier in this chapter except for two methodological differences. First, the tissue fragment used included the arcuate nucleus (AN) still attached to the ME. Using this AN–ME fragment is important because the AN contains the NMDA-R and, thus, it must be left attached to the ME for NMDA to stimulate LHRH release in vitro. Second, the $MgSO_4$ content of the medium was reduced to 0.4 m*M*, because it has been shown that concentrations above 1 m*M* can

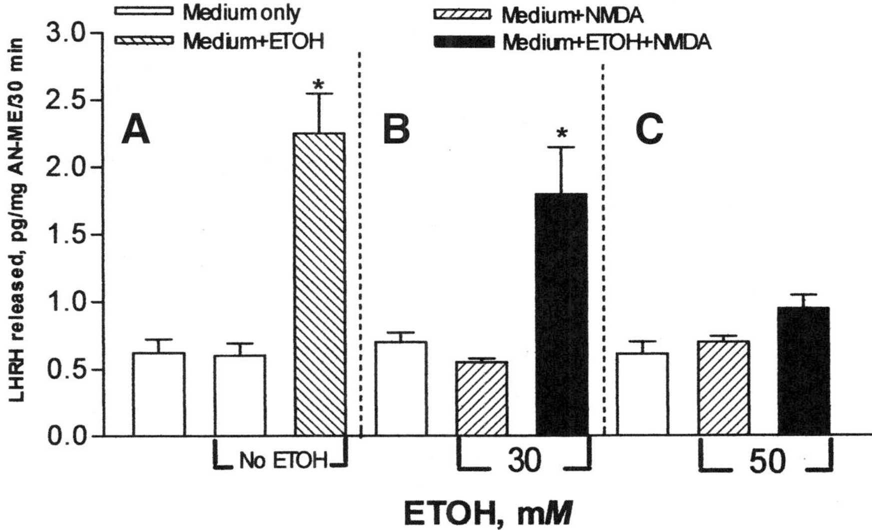

Fig. 7. Effects of ETOH on basal and NMDA-induced LHRH release from the AN–ME tissue of prepubertal female rats in vitro. Note that basal LHRH levels were similar in both control (**A**) and test (**B,C**) vials. Media containing ETOH had no effect on basal secretion. During the challenge period, the addition of NMDA (20 m*M*) significantly elicited LHRH release in the control vials and those AN–ME's exposed to 30 m*M* ETOH (**B**). However, the 50-m*M* dose of ETOH blocked the NMDA-induced release of LHRH. *$p<0.01$; *N*=32 for control vials, *N*= 12 for 30-m*M* ETOH vials; *N*=23 for 50-m*M* ETOH vials.

block the stimulatory effects of NMDA *(41)*. Our results *(24)* as depicted in Fig. 7 demonstrated that an ETOH dose of 50 m*M* blocked NMDA-R-activated LHRH release from prepubertal female rats, thus further suggesting that ETOH might alter the timing of puberty.

4.3. In Vivo ETOH/NMDA Studies

For the initial experiment *(24)*, prepubertal female rats began receiving saline or saline–ETOH (3 g/kg) solution by gastric gavage daily at 1230 h. Each day at 1400 and 1600 h, the animals received subcutaneous injections of saline or NMDA in saline. The timing of puberty was assessed in all animals by monitoring vaginal opening and subsequent cytology. Figure 8 demonstrates that NMDA advanced vaginal opening and the acute exposure to ETOH significantly attenuated this response. Additionally, first ovulation was also delayed in those animals. This combination of in vitro and in vivo

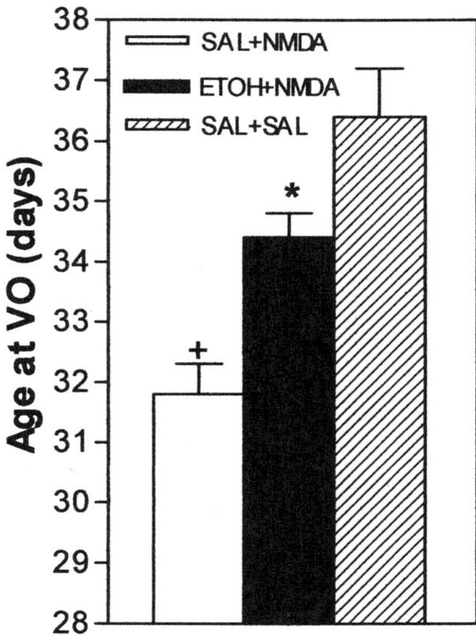

Fig. 8. Effects of ETOH on NMDA-induced puberty in vivo. Bars represent mean age (±SEM) at vaginal opening (VO). Note that NMDA injections advanced the onset of puberty, whereas exposure to ETOH significantly attenuated NMDA's ability to advance puberty. N=10; [+]p <0.01, [*]p <0.01.

methods shows that ETOH exposure of rats during late prepubertal development clearly alters NMDA-R-activated events associated with the progression of puberty. In a later study *(47)*, we showed that there was an increase in NMDA-R mRNA in the preoptic area of the brain at the time of first proestrus (Fig. 9). Importantly, this is the brain region containing most of the LHRH neurons and the increased mRNA at this time was associated with an increased ability for NMDA to stimulate LH release in vivo. It was also shown *(47)* that ETOH can block this NMDA-induced responsiveness during proestrus (*see* Fig. 10).

4.4. Summary of ETOH/NMDA-R Interactions

Initial in vivo and in vitro studies demonstrated that NMDA-R activation could induce mammalian puberty by an action at the hypothalamic level to stimulate LHRH release. The continued use of these methods enabled us to demonstrate that ETOH is a toxin that detrimentally affects the function of these receptors, causing depressed LHRH secretion and thereby altering the progression of puberty.

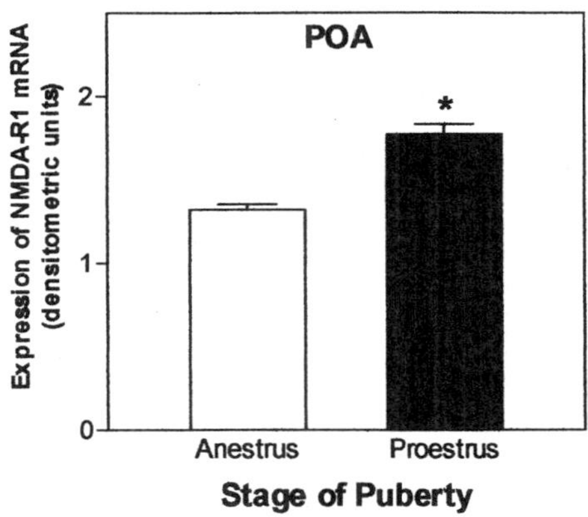

Fig. 9. NMDA-R1 mRNA in the POA of 34- to 36-d-old peripubertal female rats, as assessed by densitometric analysis. In the POA region, NMDA-R1 mRNA expression increased significantly on the day of first proestrus. *$p<0.05$; bars represent the mean (±SEM) of four determinations.

5. EFFECTS OF ETOH ON LEPTIN ACTIONS DURING PUBERTY

5.1. Endocrine Perspectives: Initial Basic In Vitro and In Vivo Studies

Leptin, a peptide derived from adipose tissue, is an important metabolic signal involved in maintaining reproductive function. Mutant mice unable to produce leptin (*ob/ob*) or its receptor (*db/db*) are obese, infertile, and unable to secrete sufficient amounts of gonadotropin *(48–51)*. Leptin administration to mutant animals restores reproductive function and stimulates gonadotropin secretion *(52–54)*. In normal rodents, leptin administration has been shown to induce precocious puberty *(55,56)*. Because the adult *ob/ob* mouse has a gonadotropin secretory pattern similar to that of prepubertal animals, investigators hypothesized that leptin might play a role in the control of gonadotropin secretion.

Initial studies *(57)* used adult male rats and found that leptin induced the release of LHRH from the hypothalamic AN–ME explants and LH release from anterior pituitaries in vitro. Furthermore, the peptide stimulated LH release in vivo following delivery into the third ventricle. These results clearly depicted a central action of leptin to induce LH secretion in adult animals. About this same time, it was shown that leptin is a metabolic signal

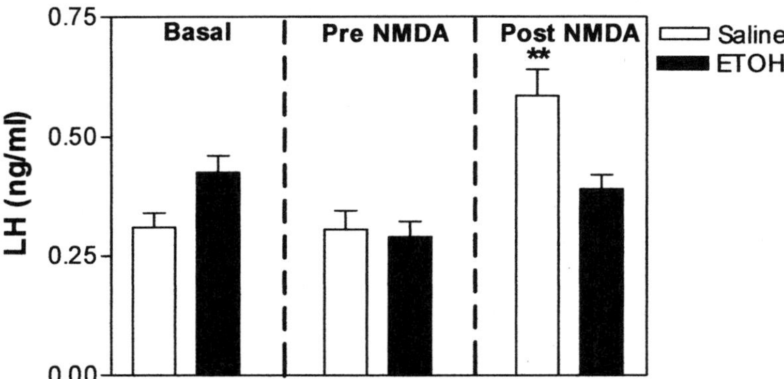

Fig. 10. In vivo effect of NMDA on LH secretion during first proestrus after intragastric administration of saline (open bar) or ETOH (solid bar). Mean basal LH was not altered by saline nor was the ability of NMDA to induce a marked increase in LH release (post-NMDA). In contrast, ETOH blocked the ability of NMDA to stimulate LH release (post-NMDA). Basal represents the mean (±SEM) basal secretion derived using the means of the first three samples taken from each animal. Pre-NMDA represents the mean (±SEM) of the single blood sample taken from each animal 90 min after saline or ETOH treatment. Post-NMDA represents the mean (±SEM) peak LH response in each animal 10 or 20 min post-NMDA treatment. $^{**}p<0.001$; N=16–24.

necessary for puberty *(58,59)*; however, the timing and site of action were not known. Therefore, we conducted in vivo studies to address these issues *(60)*. The ability of leptin to act centrally to induce LH secretion was observed in late juvenile rats (*see* Fig. 11), an effect not observed during later phases of pubertal development. Importantly, this effect in late juvenile rats was paralleled by an increase in serum leptin levels (*see* Fig. 12). Thus, we suggested the main effect of this peptide was early in the pubertal process.

5.2. In Vivo and In Vitro ETOH/Leptin Studies

Based on the above early action of leptin and because reproductive problems associated with leptin deficiency are similar to those that occur in the prepubertal female rat after chronic ETOH exposure *(1)*, we assessed the potential effects of ETOH on leptin *(61)*. When administered chronically, ETOH significantly lowered serum leptin (*see* Fig.13), IGF-1, and LH levels. Leptin replacement to ETOH-treated animals did not restore serum IGF-1 levels. However, leptin effectively restored LH levels to normal, but did not advance the timing of puberty. When administered acutely, ETOH blocked leptin-induced LH release following central administration of the peptide (*see* Fig. 14). Conversely, halved anterior pituitaries removed from

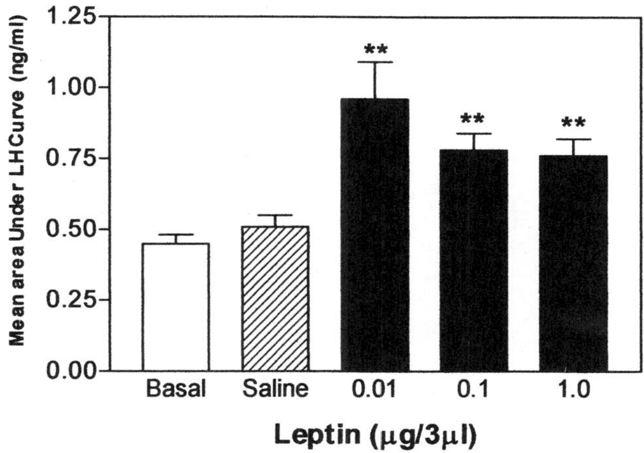

Fig. 11. Effect of leptin on the mean areas under the respective LH curves of secretion from prepubertal rats in vivo. Open bar represents the arithmetic mean (±SEM) of the area under the basal or preinjection segment of the LH curve. The solid bar represents the arithmetic mean (±SEM) of the area under the postsaline or postleptin injection segment of the LH curve. Note that leptin, not saline, induced postinjection increases in the areas under the respective LH curves. $**p<0.01$; N=9–13.

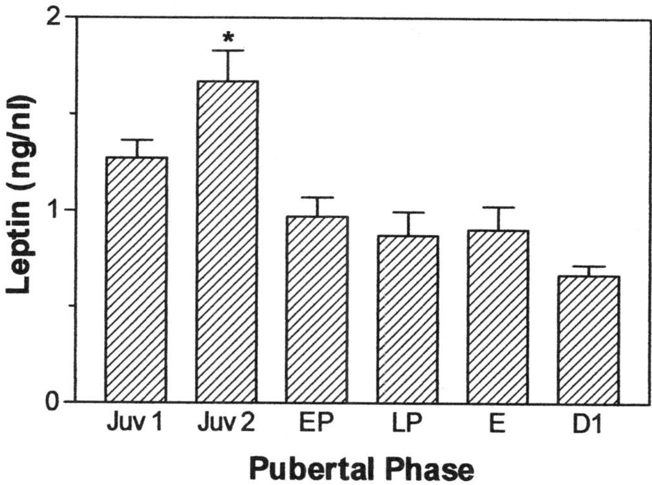

Fig. 12. Serum leptin levels during the phases of the pubertal development. Note the increased levels of leptin in the older juvenile (late prepubertal) animals when compared to the younger juvenile and the peripubertal aged animals. Bars indicate the mean (±SEM) levels of the peptide. Juv-1, juvenile animals 28–30 d old; Juv-2, juvenile animals 32–34 d old; EP, early proestrus; LP, late proestrus; E, estrus; D1, first diestrus. $*p<0.05$; N=7–23.

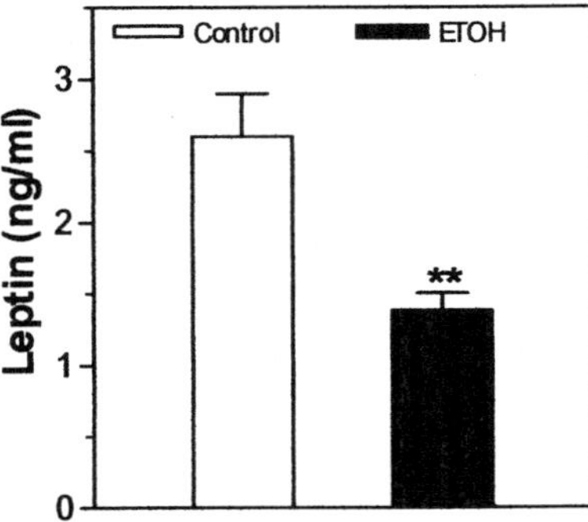

Fig. 13. Effect of ETOH administration on mean prepubertal levels of leptin in vivo. Note that serum leptin levels were significantly decreased in the ETOH-treated group when compared to the control group. **$p<0.01$; $N=22$ for controls, $N=11$ for ETOH treated rats.

control and 5-d ETOH-treated animals were incubated in vitro in the same static system used for hypothalamic incubation, and significantly released equal amounts of LH in response to leptin (*see* Fig. 15).

5.3. Summary of ETOH/Leptin Interactions

This combination of in vivo and in vitro experiments showed that ETOH acts not only to suppress peripheral levels of leptin, but also to block its central action to facilitate LH secretion. Leptin replacement can reverse the ETOH-induced suppression of LH by a direct action at the level of the pituitary, but it cannot elevate serum IGF-1, a peripheral signal that acts centrally to stimulate LHRH/LH release during the juvenile–peripubertal transition period and thus accelerate the initiation of female puberty. Together, these in vivo and in vitro methods allowed us to further dissect out the complex actions and interactions of multiple hormones and sites of their actions involved in the pubertal process, as well as the vulnerability of their actions to the toxic effects of ETOH.

6. IMPACT OF IN VITRO STUDIES TO ASSESS MECHANISMS OF ACTION

Once initial in vitro results are confirmed by in vivo observations, in vitro methods can again be used to isolate and characterize mechanisms of action. It is known that NE, NMDA-R activation, leptin, and IGF-1 all stimulate LHRH release by increasing PGE_2 synthesis/release *(10,23,24,58)*. In 1991, we showed that ETOH blocked PGE_2 release in vitro *(23)*. Subsequent in vitro studies have shown *(62,63)* that NE and NMDA-R activation result in

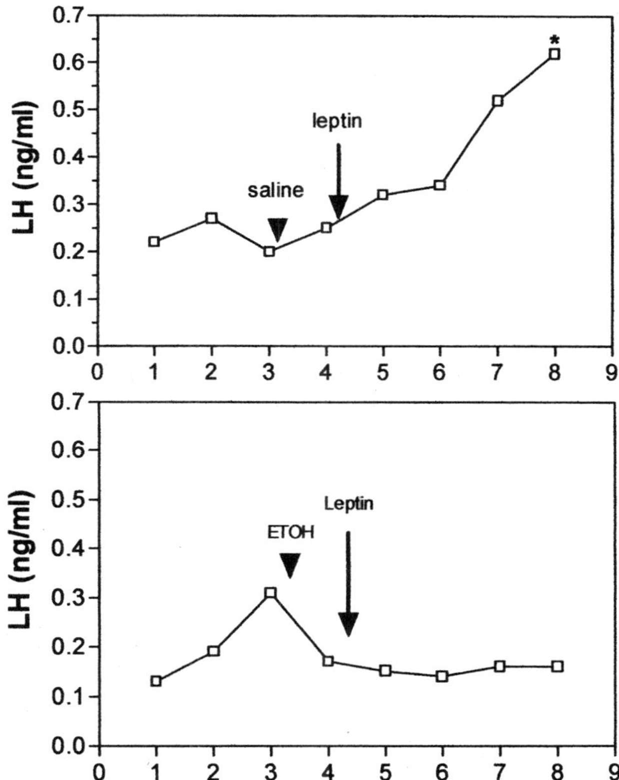

Fig. 14. Acute effects of ETOH on leptin-induced LH release in vivo. Representative LH secretory profiles from prepubertal rats before and after receiving saline or ETOH. Note that the animal receiving saline had a significant increase in LH following leptin stimulation, whereas the animal that received ETOH did not respond to the leptin. Arrowheads denote the administration of saline or ETOH by gastric gavage after the third sample. Arrows denote the injection of leptin after the fourth sample. Animals were allowed a 90-min absorption phase between the third and fourth samples. The asterisk (*) denotes the maximum LH response over basal determined by Prism software.

the release of nitric oxide (NO). Once NO is released, it diffuses into the LHRH terminals in the ME where it causes activation of cyclo-oxygenase and the conversion of arachidonate into PGE_2, which then induces release of LHRH *(62)*. Whether ETOH acts to inhibit formation of PGE_2 directly or first acts to alter the production of NO is still unclear. One in vitro study showed that ETOH did not affect NO production by AN–ME explants or the increased release of NO induced by NE *(26)*. However, those same authors later showed that ETOH might have increased release of two hypothalamic

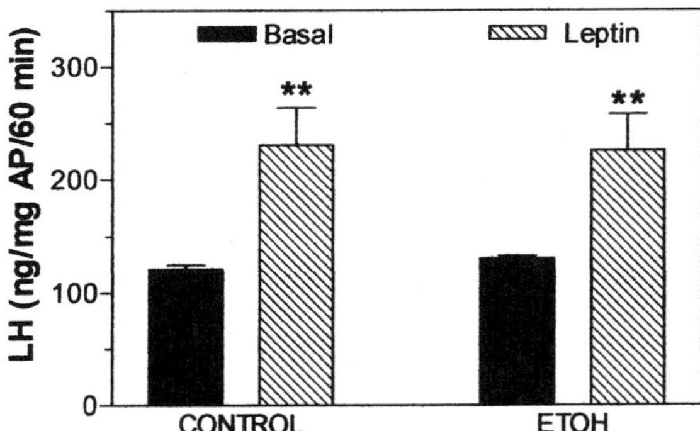

Fig. 15. The effect of leptin on LH release from prepubertal anterior pituitaries of control and ETOH-treated rats incubated in vitro. The solid bar represents the basal secretion of LH; the hatched bar represents the leptin-induced secretion of LH from the anterior pituitaries of the respective control and ETOH-treated groups. Note that control and ETOH-treated pituitaries showed the same increase in LH release in response to leptin, indicating that pituitary responsiveness was unaltered by ETOH. ***p*<0.01; *N*=7 control, *N*=11 ETOH-treated rats.

inhibitory peptides that then caused a decrease in NO production *(63)*. Regardless of the specific action on NO, it is clear that the overall effect of ETOH to decrease PGE_2 formation is responsible for the drug's ability to diminish LHRH release. Taken together, the above results demonstrate the usefulness and importance of in vitro methodology in discerning mechanisms of hormone action, as well as mechanisms by which toxic substances, such as ETOH, can alter hormone actions.

7. CONCLUSIONS

In this chapter, we have illustrated using the neuroendocrine system that in vitro and in vivo methodologies can be used in a complimentary fashion to investigate specific scientific questions. We have provided several examples depicting the alternating use of these methods to address basic neuroendocrine responses, as well as more mechanistic questions. For example, not only have we described the use of this approach to initiate a new area of study (i.e., central actions of IGF-1 at puberty) and to advance our basic understanding of the neuroendocrinology of puberty but also to assess neuroendocrine influences of both acute and chronic ETOH exposure. We suggest that experimental designs using these techniques in a complimentary fashion would also be beneficial to other studies assessing potential neuroendocrine deficits that might be caused by toxins such as lead, 2,3,7,8-

tetrachlorodibenzo-*p*-dioxins, polychlorinated biphenyls, and organophosphate compounds.

REFERENCES

1. Dees, W. L. and Skelley, C. W. (1990) Effects of ethanol during the onset of female puberty. *Neuroendocrinology* **51,** 64–69
2. Tannenbaum, G. S., Guyda, H. J., and Posner, B. I. (1983) Insulin-like growth factors: a role in growth hormone negative feedback and body weight regulation via brain. *Science* **220,** 77–79
3. Schoenle, E., Zapf, J., Hauri, C., Steiner, T., and Froesch, E. R. (1985) Comparison of in vivo effects of insulin-like growth factor I and II and of growth hormone in hypophysectomized rats. *Acta Endocrinol.* **108,** 167–174
4. Philipps, A. F., Persson, B., Hall, K., et al. (1988) The effects of biosynthetic insulin-like growth factor 1. Supplementation of somatic growth, maturation, and erthropoiesis on neonatal rat. *Pediatr. Res.* **23,** 298–305
5. Hizuka, N., Takano, K., Shizume, K., et al. (1986) Insulin-like growth factor I stimulates growth in normal growing rats. *Eur. J. Pharmacol.* **125,** 143–146
6. Behringer, R. R., Lewin, T. L., Quaife, C. J., Palmiter, R. D., Brinster, R. L., and D‘Ercole, A. J. (1990) Expression of insulin-like growth factor 1 stimulates normal somatic growth in growth hormone deficient transgenic mice. *Endocrinology* **127,** 1033–1040
7. Bohannon, N. J., Figlewicz, D. P., Corp, E. S., Wilcox, J., Porte, C. D., Jr., and Baskin, D G. (1986) Identification of binding sites for an insulin-like growth factor (IGF-1) in the median eminence of the rat brain by quantitative autoradiography. *Endocrinology* **119,** 943–945
8. Marks, J. L., Porte, D., Jr., and Baskin, D. G. (1991) Localization of type 1 insulin-like growth factor receptor messenger RNA in the adult rat brain by in situ hybridization. *Mol. Endocrinol.* **5,** 1158–1168
9. Negro-Vilar, A., Ojeda, S. R., and McCann, S. M. (1979) Catecholaminergic modulation of luteinizing hormone-releasing hormone release by median eminence terminals in vitro. *Endocrinology* **128,** 1749–1757.
10. Hiney, J. K., Ojeda, S. R., and Dees, W. L. (1991) Insulin-like growth factor-1: a possible metabolic signal involved in the regulation of female puberty. *Neuroendocrinology* **54,** 420–423
11. Duenas, M., Luquin, S., Chowen, J. A., Torres-Aleman, I., Naftolin, F., and Garcia-Segura, L. M. (1994) Gonadal hormone regulation of insulin-like growth factor-1-like immunoreactivity in hypothalamic astroglia of developing and adult rats. *Neuroendocrinology* **59,** 528–538.
12. Antunes-Rodrigues, J. and McCann, S. M. (1970) Water, sodium chloride, and food intake induced by injections of cholinergic and adrenergic drugs into the third ventricle of the rat brain. *Proc. Soc. Exp. Biol. Med.* **133,** 1464–1469.
13. Harms, P. G. and Ojeda, S. R. (1974) Methods for cannulation of the rat jugular vein. *J. Appl. Physiol.* **309,** 261–263.

14. Hiney, J. K., Srivastava, V., Nyberg, C. L., Ojeda, S. R., and Dees, W. L. (1996) Insulin-like growth factor-1 of peripheral origin acts centrally to accelerate the initiation of female puberty. *Endocrinology* **137,** 3717–3727.

15. Andrews, W. W. and Ojeda, S. R. (1981) A detailed analysis of the serum LH secretory profile in conscious, free-moving female rats during the time of puberty. *Endocrinology* **109,** 2032–2039.

16. Terasawa, E., Bridson, W. E., Nass, T. E., Noonan, J. J., and Dierschke, D. J. (1984) Developmental changes in the luteinizing hormone secretory pattern in peripubertal female rhesus monkeys: comparisons between gonadally intact and ovariectomized animals. *Endocrinology* **115,** 2233–2240.

17. Urbanski, H. F. and Ojeda, S. R. (1985) The juvenile peripubertal transition period in the female rat: Establishment of a diurnal pattern of pulsatile LH secretion. *Endocrinology* **117,** 644–649.

18. Danilovich, N., Wernsing, D., Coschigano, J. J., Kopchick, J. J., and Bartke, A. (1998) Deficits in female reproductive function in GH-R-KO mice; role of IGF-1. *Endocrinology* **140,** 2637–2640.

19. Wilson, M. E. (1998) Premature elevation in serum insulin-like growth factor-1 advances first ovulation in rhesus monkeys. *J. Endocr.* **158,** 247–257.

20. Xiaowei, X., Ingram, R. L., and Sonntag, W. E. (1995) Ethanol suppresses growth hormone-mediated cellular responses in liver slices. *Alcoholism: Clin. Exp. Res.* **19,** 1246–1251.

21. De, A., Boyadjieva, N. I., and Sarkar, D. K. (1999) Effects of ethanol on alpha-adrenergic and beta-adrenergic agonist-stimulated beta endorphin release and cAMP production in hypothalamic cells in primary cultures. *Alcoholism: Clin. Exper Res.* **23,** 46-51.

22. Frasor, J. M., Anderson, R. A., and Russell, L. D. (1992) Ethanol impairs secretory activity of Sertoli celss in conventional and bicameral culture. *Biol. Reprod.* **46(Suppl. 1),** 171.

23. Hiney, J. K. and Dees, W. L. (1991) Ethanol inhibits luteinizing hormone-releasing hormone from the median eminence of prepubertal female rats in vitro: Investigation of its actions on norepinephrine and prostaglandin-E2. *Endocrinology* **128,** 1404–1408.

24. Nyberg, C. L., Hiney, J. K., Minks, J. E., and Dees, W. L. (1993) Ethanol alters *N*-methyl-DL-aspartic acid -induced LH secretion of luteinizing hormone releasing hormone and the onset of puberty in the female rat. *Neuroendocrinology* **57,** 863–868.

25. Rettori,, V., Kamat, A., and McCann, S. M. (1994) Nitric oxide mediates the stimulation of luteinizing-hormone releasing hormone release induced by glutamic acid in vitro. *Brain Res. Bull.* **33,** 501–503.

26. Canteros, G., Rettori, V., Franchi, A., et al. (1995) Ethanol inhibits luteinizing hormone-releasing hormone (LHRH) secretion by blocking the response of LHRH neuronal terminals to nitric oxide. *PNAS* **92,** 3416–3420.

27. Hiney, J. K., Srivastava, V., Lara, T., and Dees, W. L. (1998) Ethanol blocks the central action of IGF-1 to induce luteinizing hormone secretion in the prepubertal female rat. *Life Sci.* **62,** 301–308.

28. Dees, W. L., Skelley, C. W., Hiney, J. K., and Johnston, C. A. (1990) Actions of ethanol on hypothalamic and pituitary hormones in prepubertal female rats. *Alcohol* **7,** 21–25

29. Soszynski, P. A. and Frohman, L. A. (1992) Inhibitory effects of ethanol on the growth hormone (GH)-releasing hormone-GH-Insulin-like growth factor-I axis in the rat. *Endocrinology* **131,** 2603–2608.

30. Dees, W. L., Rettori, V., Kozlowski, G. P., and McCann, S. M. (1985) Ethanol and the pulsatile release of luteinizing hormone, follicle stimulating hormone and prolactin in ovariectomized rats. *Alcohol* **2,** 641–646.

31. Dees, W. L., Skelley, C. W., Rettori, V., Kentroti, M. S., and McCann, S. M. (1988) Influence of ethanol on growth hormone secretion in adult and prepubertal female rats. *Neuroendocrinology* **48,** 495–499.

32. Srivastava, V., Hiney, J. K., Nyberg, C. L., and Dees, W. L. (1995) Effect of ethanol on the synthesis of insulin-like growth factor 1 (IGF-1) and the IGF-1 receptor in late prepubertal female rats: a correlation with serum IGF-1. *Alcoholism: Clin. Exp. Res.* **19,** 1467–1473.

33. Dees, W. L., Dissen, G. A., Hiney, J. K., Lara, F., and Ojeda, S. R. (2000) Alcohol ingestion inhibits the increased secretion of puberty-related hormones in the developing female Rhesus monkey. *Endocrinology* **141,** 1325–1331.

34. Urbanski, H. F. and Ojeda, S. R. (1987) Activation of luteinizing hormone-releasing hormone release advances the onset of female puberty. *Neuroendocrinology* **46,** 273–276.

35. Gay, V. L. and Plant, T. M. (1987) *N*-Methyl-D,L-aspartate elicits hypothalamic gonadotropin-releasing hormone release in prepubertal male rhesus monkeys (Macaca mulatta). *Endocrinology* **120,** 2289–2296.

36. Claypool, L. E. and Terasawa, E. (1989) *N*-Methyl-DL-aspartate (NMDA) induces LHRH release as measured by in vivo push-pull perfusion in the stalk-median eminence of pre and peripubertal female rhesus monkeys. *Biol. Reprod.* **40(Suppl.),** 83.

37. Price, M. T., Olney, J. W., and Cicero, T. J. (1978) Acute elevations of serum luteinizing hormone induced by kainic acid, N-methyl-aspartic acid or homosysteic acid. *Neuroendocrinology* **26,** 352–358.

38. Ondo, J. G., Wheeler, D. D., and Dom, R. M. (1988) Hypothalamic site of action for *N*-methyl-D-aspartate (NMDA) on LH secretion. *Life Sci.* **43,** 2283–2286.

39. Wilson, R. C. and Knobil, E. (1982) Acute effects of *N*-methyl-DL-aspartate on the release of pituitary gonadotropins and prolactin in the adult female rhesus monkey. *Brain Res.* **248,** 177–179.

40. Tal, J., Price, M T., and Olney, J. W. (1983) Neuroactive amino acids influence gonadotropin output by a suprapituitary mechanism in either rodents or primates. *Brain Res.* **273,** 170–182.

41. Bourgiuignon, J. P., Gerard, A., and Franchimont, P. (1989) direct activation of gonadotropin-releasing hormone secretion through different receptors to neuroexcitatory amino acids. *Neuroendocrinology* **49,** 402–408

42. Donoso, A. O., Lopez, F. J., and Negro-Vilar, A. (1990) Glutamate receptors of the non-*N*-methyl-D-aspartic acid type mediate the increase in luteinizing hormone-releasing hormone release by excitatory amino acids in vitro. *Endocrinology* **126**, 414–420.

43. Lopez, F. J., Donoso, A. O., and Negro-Vilar, A. (1990) Endogenous excitatory amino acid neurotransmission regulates the estradiol-induced LH surge in ovariectomized rats *Endocrinology* **126**, 1771–1773.

44. Lovinger, D. M., White, G., and Weight, F. F. (1989) Ethanol inhibits NMDA-activated ion current in hippocampal neurons. *Science* **128**, 1541–1547.

45. Leslie, S. W., Brwon, L. M., Dildy, J. E., and Sims, J. S. (1990) Ethanol and neuronal calcium channels. *Alcohol* **7**, 233–236.

46. Simson, P. E., Criswell, H. E., Johnson, K. B., Hicks, R. E., and Breese, G. R. (1991) Ethanol inhibits NMDA-evoked electrophysiological activity in vivo. *J. Pharmacol. Exp. Ther.* **257**, 225–231.

47. Nyberg, C. L., Srivastava, V., Hiney, J. K., Lara, F., and Dees, W. L. (1995) *N*-Methyl-aspartic acid receptor messenger ribonucleic acid levels and luteinizing hormone release in immature female rats. Effects of stage of pubertal development and exposure to ethanol. *Endocrinology* **136**, 2874–2880.

48. Swerdloff, R., Batt, R., and Bray, G. (1976) Reproductive hormonal function in the genetically obese (*ob/ob*) mouse. *Endocrinology* **103**, 542–547.

49. Swerdloff, R. S., Peterson, M., Vera, A., Batt, R. A. L., Heber, D., and Bray, G. (1978) The hypothalamic–pituitary axis in genetically obese (ob/ob) mice: Response to luteinizing hormone-releasing hormone. *Endocrinology* **103**, 542–547.

50. Johnson, L. M. and Sidnam, R. L. (1979) A reproductive endocrine profile in the diabetes (db) mutant mouse. *Biol. Reprod.* **20**, 552–559.

51. Batt, R., Everard, D., Gillies, G., Wilkinson, M., Wilson, C., and Yeo, T. (1982) Investigation into the hypogonadism of the obese mouse (genotype *ob\ob*). *J. Reprod. Fertil.* **64**, 363–371.

52. Chehab, F. F., Lim, M. E., and Ronghua, L. (1996) Correction of the sterility defect in homozygous obese female mice. *Nature Genet.* **12**, 318–320.

53. Barash, I. A., Cheung, C. C., Weigle, D. S., et al. (1996) Leptin is a metabolic signal to the reproductive system. *Endocrinology* **137**, 3144–3147.

54. Mounzith, K., Ronghua, L., and Chehab, F. F. (1997) Leptin treatment rescues the sterility of genetically obese ob/ob males. *Endocrinology* **138**, 1190–1193.

55. Chehab, F. F., Mounzih, K., Ronghua, L., and Lim, M. E. (1997) Early onset of reproductive function in normal female mice treated with leptin. *Science* **275**, 88–90.

56. Ahima, R. S., Dushay, J., Flier, S. N., Prabakaran, D., and Flier, J. S. (1997) Leptin accelerates the onset of puberty in normal female mice. *J. Clin. Invest.* **99**, 391–395.

57. Yu, W. H., Kimura, M., Walczewska, A., Karanth, S., and McCann, S. M. (1997) Role of leptin in hypothalamic-pituitary function. *Proc. Natl. Acad. Sci. USA* **94**, 1023–1028.

58. Carro, E., Pinilla, L., Seoane, L. M., et al. (1997) Influence of endogenous leptin tone on the estrous cycle and luteinizing hormone pulsatility in female rats. *Neuroendocrinology* **66,** 375–377.
59. Cheung, C. C., Thornton, J. E., Kuijper, J. L., Weigle, D. S., Clifton, D. K., and Steiner, R. A. (1997) Leptin is a metabolic gate for the onset of puberty in the female. *Endocrinology* **138,** 855–858.
60. Dearth, R. K., Hiney, J. K., and Dees, W. L. (2000) Leptin acts centrally to induce the prepubertal secretion of luteinizing hormone in the female rat. *Peptides* **21,** 387–392.
61. Hiney, J. K., Dearth, R. K., Lara, F., Wood, S., Srivastava, V., and Dees, W. L. (1999) Effects of ethanol on leptin secretion and the leptin-induced luteinizing hormone (LH) release from the late juvenile female rats. *Alcoholism: Clin. Exp. Res.* **23,** 1785–1792.
62. Rettori, V., Gimeno, M., Lyson, K., and McCann, S. M. (1992) Nitric oxid mediates norepinephrine-induced prostaglandin E_2 release from the hypothalamus. *Proc. Natl. Acad. Sci. USA* **89,** 11,543–11,546.
63. Lomniczi, A., Mastronardi, C. A., Faletti, A. G., et al. (2000) Inhibitory pathways and the inhibition of luteinizing hormone-releasing hormone release by alcohol. *Proc. Natl. Acad. Sci. USA* **97,** 2337-2342.

12

Establishing In Vitro Models
to Study Endogenous Neurotoxicants

Heather D. Durham

1. INTRODUCTION

Advances in molecular genetics over the last decade have resulted in the identification of genetic mutations responsible for several inherited neurological diseases. Not only has cloning of these genes led to methods for diagnosis of patients and identification of carriers but also to the establishment of animal and cell culture models to study mechanisms by which mutant proteins induce toxicity in vulnerable cell types. Early neuropathological studies of autopsy tissue from patients with degenerative neurological diseases commonly revealed the presence of inclusion bodies in affected neuronal populations (*see* Table 1; *1–44*). These include tangles and plaques in Alzheimer's disease, Lewy bodies in Parkinson's disease, and nuclear or cytoplasmic aggregates in the trinucleotide repeat diseases (spinal bulbar muscular atrophy, Huntington's disease, spinocerebellar ataxia 1 and 3, dentato-pallidoluysian atrophy) and cytoplasmic inclusions in familial and sporadic motor neuron diseases *(45,46)*. That similar inclusions are observed in both sporadic and hereditary forms of neurological diseases suggested that similar pathways might be involved in pathogenesis whether protein abnormalities result from inherited sequence differences, DNA damage, or posttranslational modifications. The presence in inclusions of ubiquitin, a stress protein required for targeting abnormal proteins for degradation, suggested failure of proteolytic processing to rid cells of aberrant proteins. However, the primary or secondary role of these inclusions in the pathogenesis of disease could not be surmised from studies of postmortem tissue at end-stage disease. Once genes responsible for familial forms were cloned, gene

From: *Methods in Pharmacology and Toxicology: In Vitro Neurotoxicology: Principles and Challenges*
Edited by: E. Tiffany-Castiglioni © Humana Press Inc., Totowa, NJ

Table 1
Examples of Proteotoxicants Resulting in Genetic Mutations Responsible for Human Neurological Disease

Mutant protein	Human disease	Inclusion bodies	Cells most affected	Ref.
Amyloid precursor protein	Alzheimer's	Extracellular β-amyloid in plagues, neurofibrillary tangles	Limbic and association cortices, hippocampus	*1–4*
Tau	Frontotemporal dementias Multisystem atrophy	Paired helical filaments in neurofibrillary tangles	Frontotemporal cortical neurons	*5–7*
Presenilin 1 and 2	Alzheimer's	Amyloid plaques	Limbic and association cortices, hippocampus	*3,4,8–10*
α-Synuclein	Parkinson's Lewy body dementia	Lewy bodies	Substantia nigra Cortical pyramidal neurons	*6,11*
Cu/Zn-superoxide dismutase (SOD-1)	Chromosome 21-linked amyotrophic lateral sclerosis (ALS)	Cytoplasmic inclusions	Upper and motor motor neurons, astrocytes	*12–15*
High-molecular-weight neurofilament protein (NF-H)	Rare cases of familial ALS	Hyaline and skeinlike inclusions, Bunina bodies	Upper and lower motor neurons	*16*
*Huntingtin	Huntington's	Nuclear and cytoplasmic inclusions	Striatum, cerebral cortex	*17–20*
*Androgen receptor	Kennedy's disease	Nuclear and cytoplasmic inclusions	Lower motor neurons, dorsal root ganglia	*18–22*

Protein	Disease	Pathology	Region affected	Refs
*Ataxin-1	Spinocerebellar ataxia (SCA1)	Eosinophillic spheroids, nuclear inclusion body	Cerebellar Purkinje, dentate nucleus, brainstem	18–20,23
*Ataxin-2	SCA2	Increased mutant protein, but no inclusions	Cerebellar Purkinje, brain-stem, fronto- temporal lobes	18–20,24–26
*Ataxin-3	SCA3 / Machado–Joseph disease	Nuclear inclusions	Cerebellar dentate neurons, basal ganglia, brainstem, spinal cord	18–20,27
$8\alpha_{1A}$-subunit of voltage-dependent calcum channel	SCA6	Cytoplasmic inclusions	Cerebellar Purkinje and granule neurons, dentate nucleus, inferior olive	18–20,28,29
*Ataxin-7	SCA7	Nuclear inclusion	Cerebellum, brainstem, macula, visual cortex	18–20,30
*Atrophin-1	Dentorubropallidoluysian atrophy	Nuclear inclusion	Cerebellum, cerebral cortex, basal ganglia	18–20,31,32
**Poly(A) binding protein 2	Oculopharyngeal dystrophy	Nuclear inclusion	Skeletal muscle	33
Neuroserpin	Familial dementia/progressive myoclonus epilepsy	Collins bodies	Cortical neurons, subcortical nuclei	34–36
Prion protein	Creutzfeld-Jacob (CJD), Gerstmann-Stäussler–Scheinker disease	PrP[Sc] deposition in plaques	Cortex, basal ganglia Cerebellum, cerebrum, brainstem	2,37–39
Fatal familial insomnia	Kuru	Multiple	Cerebellum, cerebrum, brainstem	
PMP22, P0	Charcot-Marie-Tooth	Accumulation in endoplasmic reticulum	Schwann cells	40–44

Note: Trinucleotide repeat diseases with expansion of *polyglutamine or **polyalanine tracts.

transfer and gene knockout technologies could be used to examine the progression of toxicity in cell culture and animal models. These studies have also extended our knowledge about how cells handle proteins with inherited or acquired structural abnormalities.

This chapter will focus on the challenges of establishing and interpreting data from cell culture models to study proteotoxicity, an emerging field of toxicology. The discussion commences with a review of the types of proteotoxicants in the nervous system, then turns to issues of modeling genetic disorders in cell culture, including choice of cell lines or primary cultures, methodology for gene transfer, and technological developments that are facilitating studies of toxicity in cultured neural tissue. Specific examples of in vitro studies will be used to illustrate general concepts, but the reference list will focus on recent review articles as a means of referring the reader to the literature relevant to specific proteins.

2. PROTEINACEOUS NEUROTOXICANTS

Toxic proteins can be expressed in cells as a result of genetic mutation or generated through posttranslational modification. Recessively inherited or X-linked diseases are usually the result of loss of function resulting from interference with synthesis, transport, stability, or enzymatic activity of the product. Although initial misfolding might be responsible for failure of protein stability or proper targeting to its site of action, normal expression from one allele is sufficient to render heterozygotes free of disease.

On the other hand, dominantly inherited diseases result when a toxic gain of function is conferred to the protein by the genetic mutation. Examples are presented in Table 1 and include mutations in amyloid precursor protein and presenilins in Alzheimer's disease, mutations in Cu/Zn-superoxide dismutase (SOD-1) in familial amyotrophic lateral sclerosis, and expansion of a polyglutamine repeat domain in huntingtin in Huntington's disease. In such cases, normal function may or may not be compromised in the mutant protein, but toxicity is not abrogated by expression of the normal allele or experimentally by gene knockout. However, a dominantly inherited loss of function disease can result when protein derived form the mutant allele exerts a dominant negative effect on normal protein. This occurs in the peripheral sensory-motor neuropathy, Charcot-Marie Tooth disease type 1A (CMT1A) and the more severe Déjérine–Scottas syndrome resulting from mutations in the gene encoding a peripheral myelin protein, PMP22. The so-called *Trembler-J* (*Tr*J) and *Trembler* (*Tr*) point mutations result in interruption of trafficking through the endoplasmic reticulum, but transport of the wild-type protein is also prevented by heterodimer formation with mutant proteins *(40)*. In the case of prion diseases (Creutzfeld–Jacob, spongiform encephalopathies), prion protein transitions from a primarily helical structure to a β-pleated sheet. The abnormal conformation can occur spontaneously as a result of genetic mutation or by conversion through association with other abnormally transformed prion molecules, which may even be transmitted from other hosts in the case of bovine spongiform encephalopathy. Finally, exposing cells to chemical toxicants can induce modifications to normal proteins (e.g., carbonylation, peroxidation, nitrosylation, glycoxidation). The requirement to catabolize and replace these modified proteins could stress cells and contribute to toxicity.

What these dominantly inherited mutant proteins have in common is the propensity to adopt altered conformations and to self-associate and aggregate. The terms "conformation diseases" or "protein folding diseases" have been coined to categorize these disorders. Theories on the toxic properties conferred by such mutations include enhancement of alternate enzymatic properties, binding and sequestering wild-type protein or other key cellular proteins, and disrupting the function of proteasomes, the major effectors of proteolysis of abnormal proteins as well as turnover of most normal cytosolic proteins. For information about mechanisms of toxicity for specific mutant proteins, the reader is referred to the references provided in Table 1.

3. STUDY OF PROTEOTOXICANTS IN CULTURE MODELS

The same considerations apply to the choice of culture model to study proteotoxicants as chemical toxicants (discussed in other chapters of this volume) with the added considerations of the methods to be used for gene transfer and detection of gene expression. The major types of culture preparations used in neurotoxicological investigations are listed in Table 2 along with the advantages and disadvantages for experimental investigation and the techniques of gene transfer that can be applied to express mutant proteins. Because toxic proteins act in a dominant fashion regardless of expression of normal alleles, 'proteinopathies' can be modeled simply by expressing a cDNA encoding the mutant protein in cells from normal organisms.

3.1. Vectors for Gene Transfer to Neural Cells

3.1.1. Delivery of Plasmid DNA

In general, plasmid DNA can be delivered into cells chemically (by cationic lipid or cationic polymer-mediated transfection), physically (microinjection or biolistics/gene gun), or by electroporation. Primary cultures of neural tissue more closely replicate the conditions in the intact animal relative to dividing tumor cell lines; however, primary cells, particularly those

Table 2
Culture Models Used in Neurotoxicity Studies

Culture type	Advantages	Disadvantages	Methods for gene transfer
Whole-embryo cultures	Cytoarchitecture preserved Metabolic activity preserved Excellent to study fetal development and teratogenicity	Large numbers of animals required Limited microscopic visualization in living state Limited duration of culture	Plasmid DNA • Biolistics (gene gun) • Electroporation Viral vectors • Local injection
Organotypic/ explant/slice cultures	Reasonable preservation of cytoarchitecture (neural networks) Extension of nerve tracts to appropriate targets Good myelination Cultures viable for months Electrophysiological recordings possible Microscopic visualization of peripheral explant	Microscopy of individual cells difficult in living cultures Limited material for biochemical analysis Time-consuming to maintain	Plasmid DNA • Biolistics (gene gun) • Electroporation Viral vectors • Local injection
Reaggregate cultures	Large number per animal General cell–cell interactions develop Myelination Longevity Material for biochemical analysis	Cytoarchitecture not normal Difficult to visulaize microsopically in the living state	Plasmid DNA • Biolistics • Electroporation
Dissociated monolayer cultures	Excellent visualization in living state Variety of cell types and physiological processes Multiple assessments in the same cell or culture Large number per animal Maintained in culture for weeks/months Subject to morphological, neurophysiological and biochemical analyses	Normal cytoarchitecture not preserved Myelination poor	Viral vectors Plasmid DNA • Microinjection • Biolistics • Electroporation • Limited transfection with calcium phosphate or cationic lipids

Embryonic stem cell/ immortalized neuronal lines	Both proliferative and differentiated phenotypes Express neuronal properties Suitable for morphological, neurophysiological, and biochemical analyses	Difficult to establish lines initially Require special culture conditions to differentiate Many cell–cell interactions missing	Plasmid DNA • Cationic lipid/DNA transfection • Receptor ligand-lipid/ DNA complexes • Biolistics • Electroporation • Microinjection Viral vectors
Other cell lines (tumor lines, hybrid lines)	Proliferate to large numbers Ease of culture Material for biochemical analyses Many can be differentiated to neuronal phenotype	Limited representation of cell types and properties *in situ* Loss of normal cytoarchitecture Cellular properties may not be stable over time	Plasmid DNA • Cationic lipid/DNA transfection • Biolistics • Electroporation • Microinjection Viral vectors
Neural tissue from transgenic animals	Control of cells expressing protein of interest Can be analyzed ex vivo or placed in culture Architectural integrity, viability, ease of manipulation depending on preparation	Expensive and labor intensive to generate transgenic mice and maintain colonies	Gene of interest is integrated into genome

that are postmitotic, are difficult to transfect with plasmid DNA. This condition results from the various barriers that must be crossed for DNA to penetrate the nuclear compartment and be transcribed *(47,48)*. The basis of transfection is the condensation of negatively charged plasmid DNA with cationic lipids or cationic polymers; the resulting positively charged complexes have affinity for anionic cell membranes, which facilitates the interaction and uptake through endocytosis. This process can be assisted by incorporating a surface-receptor ligand (e.g., transferrin) into the complex [(e.g., transferrin–polylysine *(49)* or transferrin–polyethylenimines *(47)*] such that endocytosis becomes receptor mediated. Whether taken up by bulk or receptor-mediated endocytosis, the DNA must then escape endosomal/lysosomal compartments, which varies with the physico-chemical properties of the complex. Coexposure to lysosomotropic agents, [e.g., chloroquine *(50)*, peptides *(51)*, or replication-deficient viruses *(52)*], has been used to facilitate plasmid release, but toxicity can be an issue, particularly in neuronal cultures.

The greatest impediment to transfection of postmitotoic cells is the nuclear membrane. When cells are dividing, this barrier is removed and the cDNA can integrate into the host genome to produce stable transfectants. Even when plasmid DNA is microinjected into the cytoplasm of motor neurons in long-term culture, no expression is detected (Durham, unpublished observations). Other studies have shown that nuclear import of linear DNA is limited to less than 1.5 kb *(48)*. Transport of linear DNA is facilitated by non-covalent attachment to nuclear localization amino acid sequences, but this has not improved transfection efficiency of plasmid DNA *(48)*. For the above reasons, transfection efficiencies have typically been low (a few percent) in primary cultured neurons, although this has been sufficient in many laboratories to obtain results in specific neuronal populations, particularly hippocampal neurons, cortical neurons, and dorsal root ganglion neurons. A recent study reports transfection efficiencies of 20–25% in cortical neurons and 25–30% in hippocampal neurons with LIPOFECT-AMINE2000™ *(53)*. In our hands, this and other transfecting agents have failed to transfect motor neurons in spinal cord cultures that have been maintained several weeks in vitro (*see* Fig. 1A). Use of commonly employed cationic lipids, calcium phosphate precipitation, and transferrin–polylysine–DNA complexes led to expression of a CMV*lac*Z plasmid in some glial cells, but not in neuronal cells (*see* Fig. 1).

Alternative physical methods for bypassing the membranous barriers to gene transfer are biolistics (gene gun) and intranuclear microinjection. Particle-mediated gene transfer or biolistic transfection has been used for gene transfer into several different culture preparations of nervous tissue, includ-

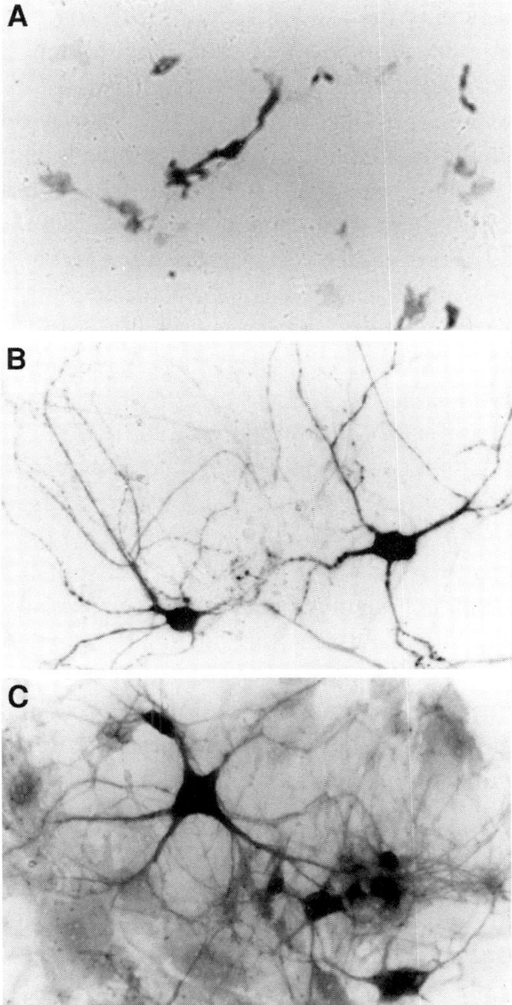

Fig. 1. Comparison of three methods of transferring a reporter gene construct (*lacZ*) into spinal motor neurons in dissociated cultures of embryonic murine spinal cord. (**A**) Liposome-mediated transfection of plasmid DNA (CMVlacZ) by lipofectamine. Only background glial cells express β-galactosidase 3 d following transfection. (**B**) Expression of β-galactosidase following microinjection of CMVlacZ plasmid DNA into nuclei of motor neurons. Concentration of plasmid is adjusted to result in expression in 80–100% of injected cells. (**C**) Replication-deficient adenoviral recombinant (AdCMVlacZ) transduces all cell types in the spinal cord culture with high efficiency. Both percentage of cells transduced and level of expression are proportional to viral titer, but can be limited by toxicity of the vector and nonspecific toxicity of protein product, particularly in long-term experiments. (From ref. *54.*) For additional information, *see* ref. *54.*

ing dissociated, organotypic, and slice cultures *(55–57)*. Plasmid DNA-coated gold or tungsten particles are "shot" into cultures at high velocity. Usually, compressed helium is used for particle acceleration. Transfection efficiency is determined by the number of particles entering the cell, but limited by the cellular damage inflicted by membrane disruption. Although better than conventional transfection, efficiency in neurons is still in the order of less than 10% in most studies, but 34% was achieved in cerebellar organotypic slice cultures under optimized conditions *(58)*.

In our laboratory, we have had success using intranuclear microinjection of plasmid expression vectors for gene transfer into primary cultured neurons *(12,59,60)* (*see also* Fig. 1B). Glass micropipets with inner filaments for quick filling, the same as used for electrophysiological recording, are pulled and a small amount of plasmid DNA in TRIS/EDTA is placed in the bottom of the shank with Eppendorf microloaders. Pressure injection is used to force the solution out of the pipet tip and, when the microelectrode tip is micromanipulated into the cell nucleus, into the nucleoplasm. Suppliers of pressure microinjectors include Eppendorf, Narashige, World Precision Instruments, and Applied Scientific Instrumentation. The procedure requires that cultures be maintained outside of the incubator on the microscope stage. Because neural cultures are particularly sensitive to pH changes, they are placed in minimum essential medium without bicarbonate, pH adjusted to 7.2, for the period of manipulation and transferred at the end of the procedure to fresh culture medium containing 0.75% gentamycin, pre-equilibrated in the incubator to 37°C, pH 7.2–7.4. The disadvantages of microinjection are that considerable training is required to develop expertise; a certain number of cells will be killed by the procedure depending on the skill of the personnel performing the injections; it is time-consuming, and the number of cells injected is too small for conventional biochemical analyses. On the other hand, the number of micromethods available to analyze ion concentrations, activity of signaling pathways, and gene expression in single cells is rapidly growing. These include activity-dependent antibodies, optical probes for microfluorometric assays, fluorescence resonance energy transfer (FRET), and single cell reverse transcription–polyacrylamide gel electrophoresis (RT-PCR). In addition, with laser capture microdissection, specific cells can be removed from cultures for analysis of gene expression and correlation with morphological markers.

3.1.2. Gene Transfer Using Viral Vectors

The ability of viruses to penetrate membranous barriers in cells and utilize the host to express viral genes has been exploited for transferring foreign DNA into cells. The most commonly used viruses include replication-defective adenovirus (ADV), herpes simplex virus (HSV), and adeno-associated virus (AAV). For a comprehensive discussion of the properties, advantages, and disadvantages of various viral vectors, the reader is referred to refs. *61–63*. High efficiency of transduction of neuronal and glial cells is achievable by viral vector-mediated gene transfer (*see* Fig. 1C). However, the titer or multiplicity of infection (MOI) that can be used is limited by direct toxicity of the vector's lysosomotropic effect and over-expression of gene product in cells transduced with high copy number *(54)*. Preliminary experiments are required with each culture system, recombinant, and experimental duration to optimize protocols.

The major inconveniences with viral vectors are the effort and time required for production and limitations on the size of cDNA that can be inserted. ADV was initially rendered replication defective by removal of the E1 region of the viral genome, allowing a maximal cDNA insert size of 7.5 kb. This size can be extended somewhat by deletion of other "E" regions. Insert size can be increased to 36 kb by use of a gutted vector containing cis-acting DNA sequences necessary for viral replication and packaging but no viral coding sequences *(64)*. However, replication of gutted vectors requires a helper virus to provide the necessary viral proteins in trans and it can be difficult to obtain high titres. For most purposes, in vitro E1- or E1/E3-deleted ADV is adequate. To produce recombinants, the expression cassette containing the cDNA of interest is introduced by homologous recombination and the virus is replicated in mammalian packaging lines, usually HEK293 cells, that stably express the viral genes required for replication that have been deleted from the vector. The recombinant ADV must be plaque purified and verified not to have incorporated genes of replication by recombination events in the packaging line. A simplified method for generating recombinant ADV has been developed that eliminates the need for plaque purification. A recombinant adenoviral plasmid is generated by homologous recombination in bacteria rather than eukaryotic cells *(65)*. After transfection of this plasmid into the mammalian packing line, viral production is followed with green fluorescent protein encoded by a gene incorporated into the viral backbone. This system is available as the Stratagene AdEasy kit.

Two types of HSV1-derived vectors are recombinant nonlytic HSV1, which can accommodate up to 30 kb of cDNA, and plasmid-based amplicons *(66)*. Although slightly more toxic than ADV, HSV1-expression vectors have been utilized considerably in primary neuronal cultures. AAV is a non-pathogenic human parvovirus that can integrate into the genome of dividing cells and is relatively nontoxic *(67)*. Although requiring helper virus for replication, AAV recombinants can be purified free of helper virus. The major insert size is limited (about 5 kb).

3.1.3. RNA Delivery Methods

Messenger RNA can be transfected into nondividing cells with cationic lipids or peptide-modified low-molecular-weight polycations, overcoming the nuclear membrane barrier to gene transfer *(68)*. The major disadvantages over plasmid DNA transfection are the difficulty of mRNA production and susceptibility to degradation, both prior to and following transfer into cells. Intracellular stability is increased by incorporating a 5' cap and a substantial 3' poly(A) tail *(68)*. Only recently have studies been carried out to optimize delivery methods. An alternative is Simian Forest virus, a self-replicating and self-transcribing RNA molecule *(69)*. However, cytotoxicity is a limiting factor. Few studies have utilized RNA-based transfection to express proteins, given the relative ease of DNA-based methodologies.

3.1.4. Culture of Neural Tissue from Transgenic Mice

Studies of proteotoxicity in vivo are conducted by producing mice transgenic for the mutant gene of interest, or for experimental controls, the wild-type gene. Gene knockout can confirm whether mutations confer a toxic gain of function to the protein or loss of function is the mechanism of toxicity. Any of the in vitro preparations listed in Table 2 can be produced from transgenic mice and can be valuable for mechanistic studies or screening of potential therapeutic agents if a mutant phenotype can be defined. For preparations requiring culture of embryonic tissue, individual embryos must be cultured separately and the embryonic tissue subsequently genotyped unless the transgenic mice have been bred to homozygosity. Examples include the demonstration of increased vulnerability to glucose deprivation and chemical hypoxia in cortical neurons cultured from presenilin 1 mutant mice *(70)*, increased glutamate sensitivity of motor neurons cultured from G93A mutant SOD-1 mice *(71)*, and analysis of Ca^{2+} handling in Purkinje cells of cerebellar slices prepared from spinocerebellar ataxia type 1 (SCA1) transgenic mice overexpressing ataxin 1 with an expanded polyglutamine repeat *(72)*.

3.2. Dosimetry

For cells undergoing mitosis, levels of short-term expression will be proportional to the strength of the promotor element utilized to drive gene expression, the number of copies of plasmid or viral vector accessing the nuclear compartment, and the turnover of the specific mRNA and protein. However, maintenance of expression for more than a few days depends on integration of plasmid or viral DNA into the genome of the host cell or use of self-replicating plasmid (e.g., pCEP4, Invitrogen). Retroviral and AAV viral vectors can integrate, whereas ADV and HSV recombinants do not. In postmitotic cells, integration is neither possible nor an issue because the cells do not divide to dilute out the copies of vector. We have found that expression persists for several weeks in cultured neurons following micro-injection of plasmid DNA or transduction with viral vectors.

In the case of plasmid transfection or transduction of viral vectors, proto-cols must be optimized for the amount of plasmid or titer of viral recombi-nant to add to the culture and for how long. In the case of microinjection, the major determinant is concentration of plasmid DNA in the injectate because the volume of fluid injected is restricted and should be minimized. To moni-tor the efficiency of transfer of plasmid DNA by microinjection, we include 70-kDa dextran (neutral or anionic) conjugated to fluorescein or rhodamine in the injectate at 20 mg/mL as a nontoxic marker of injected cells (conju-gates to other epifluorescent tags are also available; Molecular Probes). The number of neurons containing the marker can be counted easily in living cultures under epifluorescence microscopy and compared to the number of cells expressing the protein of interest by immunocytochemistry. The lowest concentration of plasmid DNA giving detectable protein expression in 80–100% of the surviving injected cells is determined in preliminary studies. Our fixation protocol is 8 min in 3% paraformaldehyde, followed by 1-min permeabilization in 0.5% Nonidet P-40 and subsequent fixation for 2 min in paraformaldehyde. With this protocol some of the 70-kDa dextran marker usually persists in the nuclear compartment after fixation. Lysine-fixable dextrans are not recommended because they precipitate plasmid DNA into oligomeric complexes incompatible with the microinjection procedures.

For studies of proteotoxicity, the issues of dosimetry are similar to those important for studies of chemical toxicity. Toxicity will be proportional to the dose (level of gene expression) and duration of the exposure. How does the scientist model experimentally low levels of expression of a mutant pro-tein over decades and are the same mechanisms responsible for toxicity with high-level expression over a short-term experiment as in the disease? Most studies have utilized gene transfection in short-term studies (i.e., 24 h to a few days). Commercially available expression systems have incorporated viral gene promoters such as cytomegalovirus (CMV) to achieve high-level gene expression. However, most proteins will be toxic if highly overexpressed (just as any chemical is toxic if administered at a sufficiently high concentration) and viral promoters might be too strong if the experi-ment is to be conducted in a time frame of weeks rather than a few days. If lower levels of expression are required, this can be achieved by use of eukaryotic promoters (e.g., neuron-specific enolase [NSE], neurofilament-L, phosphoglycerokinase [PGK], glial fibrillary acidic protein elongation factor 1B [EF1B], or tubulin). On the other hand, the duration of experiments in culture is limited by their viability and lower-level expression might not be sufficient to achieve a phenotype, depending on the end points being measured. Preliminary studies with the appropriate controls are necessary to identify the appropriate conditions for each case. For example, in our laboratory, expression and toxicity of mutant SOD-1 proteins in motor neurons of dissociated spinal cord cultures was examined over a 1- to 2-wk period following intranuclear microinjection of plasmid expression vectors *(12,59)*. In this case, either pCEP4 or pcDNA3 plasmids, which contain the CMV promoter could be utilized because expression of wild-type SOD-1 from these vectors was not toxic (*see* Fig. 2B). However, in recent experiments to establish a similar model of Kennedy's disease resulting from trinucleotide repeat expansion in the androgen receptor gene, it was necessary to utilize a weaker promoter (PGK) to drive expression because the CMV-driven level of androgen-receptor protein with a normal number of glutamine repeats was toxic and resulted in inclusion formation (unpublished observations). A caveat of overexpression is that nonspecific protein aggregation can occur that is not related to the disease-causing mechanism.

In many toxic gain-of-function neurological diseases, clinical onset is delayed into adulthood and certain neural cell populations are preferentially vulnerable to toxicity. This indicates that aging effects and exposure to other stresses are important in the development of the disease phenotype and has implications for modeling these diseases in vitro. Manifestations of toxicity will be different with acute expression of the mutant gene product than with long-term stable expression in cell lines or neural tissue cultured from transgenic mice. In the former, toxicity eventually manifests in lethality (as illustrated in Fig. 2), whereas cells stably expressing the mutant gene must either express lower levels of the toxic protein or have mustered protective mechanisms in order to remain viable. For example, motor neurons in dissociated spinal cord cultures prepared from transgenic mice overexpressing the G93A mutant human SOD-1 remain viable, but are more sensitive to additional toxic stresses and have altered calcium homeostasis *(59,71)*. Upregulation of heat shock proteins correlates with the ability of NIH 3T3 cells to survive stable expression of mutant SOD-1 *(60)*. To overcome the difficulty in establishing stable cell lines that express toxic proteins, inducible expression systems have been used, including Tet-On *(73)* and ecdysone-inducible *(74)* mammalian expression systems.

Thus, the context of mutant protein expression must be considered in design and interpretation of experiments. Paradigms of acute expression (transient transfection, inducible expression systems, microinjection) prejudice the outcome to the toxic gain-of-function of the mutant protein, whereas long-term,

A

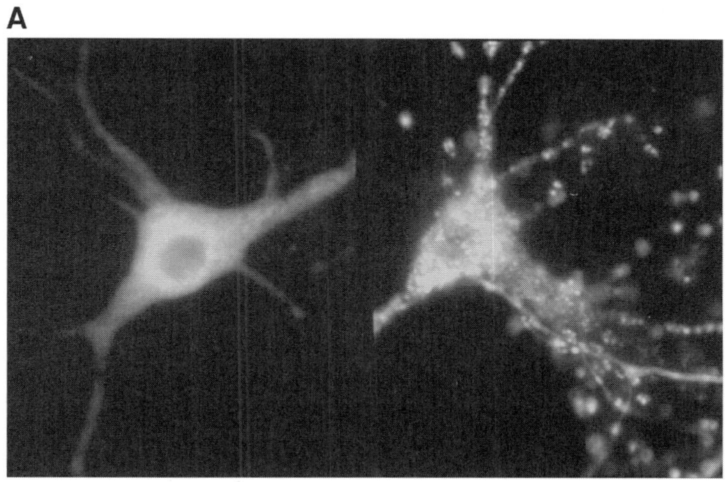

B

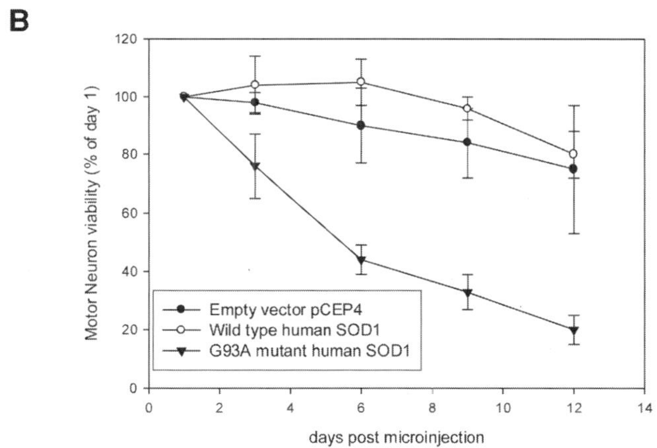

Fig. 2. Monitoring expression and toxicity of neurotoxic proteins following gene transfer by intranuclear microinjection. (**A**) Postfixation immunolabeling provides qualitative analysis of protein expression and detects changes in trafficking and distribution. Wild-type human SOD-1 (*left*) and G93A mutant SOD-1 (*right*) detected by immunolabeling with antibody specific for human SOD-1 (SD-G6; Sigma-Aldrich) 3 d following microinjection of *SOD-1* pCEP4 expression vector (200 µg/mL). Mutant SOD-1 is detected in cytoplasmic inclusions in approx 30% of expressing motor neurons, whereas wild-type protein is always distributed diffusely. (**B**) Monitoring viability of motor neurons following microinjection of SOD-1 expression vectors. Seventy kilo-Daltons dextran–FITC (20 mg/mL) was coinjected with *SOD-1* expression vector. Motor neurons containing the marker were counted under epifluorescence microscopy and the number expressed as a percentage of those present the day after microinjection. For further methodological details, see ref. *12*.

stable expression provides a better opportunity to study interactions with other physiological and environmental stressors.

3.3. Controls

Mandatory controls for transfer of mutant genes are (1) wild-type cDNA in the same vector to control for nonspecific toxicity resulting from overexpression, (2) "empty" vector to control for toxicity of the vector or gene transfer protocol, and (3) cultures that have not been subjected to gene transfer to control for normal attrition. Once a gene transfer protocol has been optimized, the latter might not be necessary because a general culture condition will be manifested in the "empty" vector control. Many studies also incorporate transfer of an additional reporter gene such as *lacZ* or green fluorescent protein (GFP); however, potential toxicity of the reporter protein is a consideration, particularly in longer-term studies. When cotransferred with the gene of interest, either as a separate vector, as a fusion tag, or bicistronic with the gene of interest in the same construct, expression of these sequences monitors the efficiency of gene transfer. Transfer of the reporter construct alone provides an additional control for overexpression; however, given the difference in toxicity and turnover rates of proteins, we consider the latter unnecessary when the wild-type counterpart to the cDNA of interest is being investigated as the control for mutants. Following gene transfer, the levels of protein expression should be monitored at various times over the duration of the experiment. Monitoring expression of other housekeeping genes controls for nonspecific suppression of endogenous gene expression.

3.4. Monitoring Gene Expression and Toxicity

3.4.1. Detecting Transfected Cells

The most conventional method of monitoring gene expression is postfixation by immunocytochemistry using antibody specific to the transgenic protein. An example is illustrated in Fig. 2B. Plasmid expression vector for the G93A mutant of human SOD-1, responsible for a familiar form of motor neuron disease *(13)*, was microinjected into nuclei of motor neurons of dissociated cultures of murine spinal cord. Antibody specific to human SOD-1 (Sigma-Aldrich) was used to visualize expression of human SOD-1. In most cases, species-specific antibodies are not available or the transferred gene encodes the sequence from the same species as the cultured cells. In such cases, antibody labeling of the protein produced from the transferred gene is superimposed upon the endogenous gene product. Coexpression of a reporter gene or coinjection of a fluorescent dextran aids in identifying transfected cells. An alternative is to incorporate sequences encoding epitope tags (e.g., HA, Flag, his) or GFP (or its derivatives) as a fusion tag in the cDNA sequence inserted into the expression vector. The advantage of GFP is that the distribution of the protein can be visualized by epifluorescence microscopy in living cells, providing information on trafficking and changes in distribution over time in the same cell. In the example illustrated in Fig. 2, aggregation of mutant human SOD-1 protein into inclusions was detected by immunocytochemistry after fixation in some neurons expressing mutant protein, but never in those expressing wild-type human SOD-1. To quantitate this manifestation of toxicity, the number of neurons containing aggregates was counted and expressed as a percentage of the total number of cells expressing the mutant protein *(12,59)*. In those experiments, different cultures were evaluated at each time period following microinjection of expression vectors. If a GFP fusion tag were to be incorporated into the vector, the time-course of aggregate formation could be followed over time in a single neuron. GFP and enhanced GFP (EGFP) tags have been utilized to study formation of intracellular inclusions of disease-causing polyglutamine repeat expansions (e.g., constructs of EGFG-exon 1 of huntingtin containing the trinucleotide repeat sequence) and their association with heat shock proteins *(73)*.

With the use of GFP fusion tags or comicroinjection of fluorescent dextran, precise viability studies can be conducted in each culture over time, because these markers leak out from dead cells. This is illustrated for the mutant SOD-1 example in Fig. 2B; the number of cells containing the marker were counted under epifluorescence microscopy, expressed as a percentage of those present on the day following microinjection (to exclude cells dying of the procedure) and plotted against time. Viable morphology can be verified under phase contrast microscopy. Viability curves are particularly useful to assess the effectiveness of potential neuroprotective therapies *(59)*. A possible disadvantage of fusion tags, which must be controlled for, is that they could alter conformation of the protein in ways that significantly affect turnover, activity, and toxicity. However, HA and Flag epitope tags and GFP fusion tags have been used successfully in numerous studies of polyglutamine-expanded proteins. The disadvantage of fluorescent dextran markers is that they are slowly phagocytosed over time and cleared from the cell, limiting the time they can be detected microscopically for screening purposes to less than 2 wk.

3.4.2. Monitoring Toxicity in Specific Neural Cell Types in Mixed Neural Cultures

Important aspects of neurotoxicity include the differences in susceptibility of specific neural cell populations to toxicity and the importance of cell–cell interactions in determining the physiological conditions responsible for this preferential vulnerability. To reproduce the mechanisms of neurotoxicity operating in the intact organism, more and more attention is being paid to assessing the effects of toxicants on neuron–neuron and neuron–glial interactions. In organotypic and even in dissociated cultures of nervous tissue, many of these cellular interactions can be preserved and evaluated; however, this requires analysis at the single-cell level. There have been many recent advances in the ability to assess gene expression and biochemical pathways in individual cells. These studies will be important in understanding why expression of mutant proteins is differentially toxic to cell types.

With laser capture microdissection, cells with a particular morphology can be removed from cultures and tissues for quantitiation of mRNA expression. Using DNA microarray technology, analysis of gene expression from a few, or even single, cells is possible *(75)*. Analysis of protein expression in single cells is only possible *in situ* at this time, but considerable information on protein trafficking and signaling can be obtained with currently available antibodies, particularly antibodies recognizing specific phosphorylated epitopes or cleavage products. Advances in microfluidics, two-dimensional gel electrophoresis detection systems, and antibody microarrays are reducing the sample size required for detection of proteins using proteomic approaches. Two-dimensional gel electrophoresis can be performed on material captured by laser microdissection, but thousands of cells are required *(76)*.

Microfluorometric assays of membrane potential, pH, calcium ion concentrations, and so forth are routinely as vital end points for toxicity. In standard methods, cell-permeant esterified indicators are added to culture medium, cross the plasma membrane, and are trapped within cells following cleavage by intracellular esterases. Long-term and repeated measures are difficult because the indicators distribute widely and often alter cell physiology (e.g., calcium indicators are powerful calcium chelators). Techniques have been developed to incorporate the indicators into nanosphere matrices, which greatly improves compatibility with long-term and repeated measures. Once nanospheres are introduced into the cell by transfection, ballistics, or microinjection, they can serve as bystanders to monitor parameters without significantly interfering with the biology of the cell *(77)*.

Green fluorescent protein fusion tags can be used to monitor changes in cellular compartmentalization that may coincide with activation [e.g., nuclear translocation of transcription factors, retention of protein kinase C isoforms at cell membranes in response to activation by diacylglycerol *(78)*]. With the generation of GFP mutants with different excitation and emission spectra, more specific assays have been developed based on FRET, a technique that permits the study of protein–protein interactions and protein conformation changes in vivo *(79)*. FRET can occur between two fluorophores in nanometer proximity. Excitation of a donor fluorophore can transfer energy to and excite an acceptor fluorophore with a longer wavelength of emission. Events increasing the distance between the donor and acceptor fluorophores or that bring fluorophores together can be monitored by measuring changes in FRET. Activity-based assays have been developed by incorporating both donor and acceptor fluorophores in the same construct separated by a linker containing, for example, protease cleavage, calcium/calmodulin binding, or phosphorylation domains of specific proteins in proteolytic or signaling cascades (intramolecular FRET) *(79–81)*. When expressed in cells by gene transfer, such designer macromolecules can be used to assess dynamic effects of neurotoxicants. Donor and acceptor fluorophores are incorporated into different expression constructs to study protein–protein interactions. Mutant proteins have a propensity to adopt abnormal conformations and to aggregate and localize to inclusion bodies along with normal proteins such as heat shock proteins and ubiquitin. Intermolecular FRET analysis can be used to test how closely these proteins interact.

4. CONCLUDING REMARKS

During the past decade there has been an explosion in identifying genetic mutations that result in synthesis of toxic proteins in cells. Considerable progress has been made in applying in vitro culture systems to model and study proteotoxicity. Although the same principles apply as with the study of chemical toxicants, specific challenges include controlling the dosage and quantitating gene expression over time. New technologies are improving our capability to monitor the effect of both chemical and protein toxicants on gene expression, morphology, and biochemical pathways in postmitotic, adherent cells in mixed cultures or tissue slices. These will extend the capability to examine how expression of proteotoxicants affects complex interactions between neural cell types that are integral to neural function.

REFERENCES

1. Fidani, L. and Goate, A. (1992) Mutations in APP and their role in β-amyloid deposition. *Prog. Clin. Biol. Res.* **379,** 195–214.
2. Carrell, R. W. and Gooptu, B. (1998) Conformational changes and disease—serpins, prions and Alzheimer's. *Curr. Opin. Struct. Biol.* **8,** 799–809.
3. Selkoe, D. J. (2001) Alzheimer's disease: genes, proteins, and therapy. *Physiol. Rev.* **81,** 741–766.
4. Tanzi, R. E. and Bertram, L. (2001) New frontiers in Alzheimer's disease genetics. *Neuron* **32,** 181–184.

5. Goedert, M., Crowther, R. A., and Spillantini, M. G. (1998) Tau mutations cause frontotemporal dementias. *Neuron* **21,** 955–958.

6. Spillantini, M. G. and Goedert, M. (2000) The alpha-synucleinopathies: Parkinson's disease, dementia with Lewy bodies, and multiple system atrophy. *Ann. NY Acad. Sci.* **920,** 16–27.

7. Spillantini, M. G. and Goedert, M. (2001) Tau gene mutations and tau pathology in frontotemporal dementia and parkinsonism linked to chromosome 17. *Adv. Exp. Med. Biol.* **487,** 21–37.

8. Sherrington, R., Rogaev, E. I., Liang, Y., et al. (1995) Cloning of a gene bearing missense mutations in early-onset familial Alzheimer's disease. *Nature* **375,** 754–760.

9. Levy-Lahad, E., Wasco, W., Poorkaj, P., et. al. (1995) Candidate gene for the chromosome 1 familial Alzheimer's disease locus. *Science* **269,** 973–977.

10. Mattson, M. P., Chan, S. L., and Camandola, S. (2001) Presenilin mutations and calcium signaling defects in the nervous and immune systems. *BioEssays* **23,** 733–744.

11. Polymeropoulos, M. H., Lavedan, C., Leroy, E., et al. (1997) Mutation in the alpha-synuclein gene identified in families with Parkinson's disease. *Science* **276,** 2045–2047.

12. Durham, H. D., Roy, J., Dong, L., and Figlewicz, D. A. (1997) Aggregation of mutant Cu/Zn superoxide dismutase proteins in a culture model of ALS. *J. Neuropathol. Exp. Neurol.* **56,** 523–530.

13. Rosen, D. R., Siddique, T., Patterson, D., et al. (1993) Mutations in Cu/Zn superoxide dismutase gene are associated with familial amyotrophic lateral sclerosis. *Nature* **362,** 59–62.

14. Bruijn, L. I., Becher, M. W., Lee, M. K., et al. (1997) ALS-linked SOD1 mutant G85R mediates damage to astrocytes and promotes rapidly progressive disease with SOD1-containing inclusions. *Neuron* **18,** 327–338.

15. Verbeke, P., Fonager, J., Clark, B. F., and Rattan, S. I. (2001) Heat shock response and ageing: mechanisms and applications. *Cell Biol. Int.* **25,** 845–57. 845–857.

16. Figlewicz, D. A., Krizus, A., Martinoli, M. G., et al. (1994) Variants of the heavy neurofilament subunit are associated with the development of amyotrophic lateral sclerosis. *Hum. Mol. Genet.* **3,** 1757–1761.

17. The Huntington's Disease Collaborative Research Group (1993) A novel gene containing a trinucleotide repeat that is expanded and unstable on Huntington's disease chromosomes. *Cell* **72,** 971–983.

18. Zoghbi, H. Y. and Orr, H. T. (2000) Glutamine repeats and neurodegeneration. *Annu. Rev. Neurosci.* **23,** 217–247.

19. Orr, H. T. (2001) Beyond the Qs in the polyglutamine diseases. *Genes Dev.* **15,** 925–932.

20. Fischbeck, K. H. (2001) Polyglutamine expansion neurodegenerative disease. *Brain Res. Bull.* **56,** 161–163.

21. La Spada, A. R., Wilson, E. M., Lubahn, D. B., Harding, A. E., and Fischbeck, K. H. (1991) Androgen receptor gene mutations in X-linked spinal and bulbar muscular atrophy. *Nature* **352,** 77–79.

22. Merry, D. E. (2001) Molecular pathogenesis of spinal and bulbar muscular atrophy. *Brain Res. Bull.* **56,** 203–207.

23. Orr, H. T., Chung, M. Y., Banfi, S., et al. (1993) Expansion of an unstable trinucleotide CAG repeat in spinocerebellar ataxia type 1. *Nature Genet.* **4,** 221–226.
24. Imbert, G., Saudou, F., Yvert, G., et al. (1996) Cloning of the gene for spinocerebellar ataxia 2 reveals a locus with high sensitivity to expanded CAG/glutamine repeats. *Nature Genet.* **14,** 285–291.
25. Pulst, S. M., Nechiporuk, A., Nechiporuk, T., et al. (1996) Moderate expansion of a normally biallelic trinucleotide repeat in spinocerebellar ataxia type 2. *Nature Genet.* **14,** 269–276.
26. Sanpei, K., Takano, H., Igarashi, S., et al. (1996) Identification of the spinocerebellar ataxia type 2 gene using a direct identification of repeat expansion and cloning technique, DIRECT. *Nature Genet.* **14,** 277–284.
27. Kawaguchi, Y., Okamoto, T., Taniwaki, M., et al. (1994) CAG expansions in a novel gene for Machado-Joseph disease at chromosome 14q32.1. *Nature Genet.* **8,** 221–228.
28. Zhuchenko, O., Bailey, J., Bonnen, P., et al. (1997) Autosomal dominant cerebellar ataxia (SCA6) associated with small polyglutamine expansions in the alpha 1A-voltage-dependent calcium channel. *Nature Genet.* **15,** 62–69.
29. Frontali, M. (2001) Spinocerebellar ataxia type 6: channelopathy or glutamine repeat disorder? *Brain Res. Bull.* **56,** 227–231.
30. David, G., Abbas, N., Stevanin, G., et al. (1997) Cloning of the SCA7 gene reveals a highly unstable CAG repeat expansion. *Nature Genet.* **17,** 65–70.
31. Koide, R., Ikeuchi, T., Onodera, O., et al. (1994) Unstable expansion of CAG repeat in hereditary dentatorubral-pallidoluysian atrophy (DRPLA). *Nature Genet.* **6,** 9–13.
32. Nagafuchi, S., Yanagisawa, H., Sato, K., et al. (1994) Dentatorubral and pallidoluysian atrophy expansion of an unstable CAG trinucleotide on chromosome 12p. *Nature Genet.* **6,** 14–18.
33. Brais, B., Bouchard, J. P., Xie, Y. G., et al. (1998) Short GCG expansions in the PABP2 gene cause oculopharyngeal muscular dystrophy. *Nature Genet.* **18,** 164–167.
34. Davis, R. L., Holohan, P. D., Shrimpton, A. E., et al. (1999) Familial encephalopathy with neuroserpin inclusion bodies. *Am. J. Pathol.* **155,** 1901–1913.
35. Davis, R. L., Shrimpton, A. E., Holohan, P. D., et al. (1999) Familial dementia caused by polymerization of mutant neuroserpin. *Nature* **401,** 376–379.
36. Takao, M., Benson, M. D., Murrell, J. R., et al. (2000) Neuroserpin mutation S52R causes neuroserpin accumulation in neurons and is associated with progressive myoclonus epilepsy. *J. Neuropathol. Exp. Neurol.* **59,** 1070–1086.
37. Knight, R. (2001) Creutzfeldt–Jakob disease: a protein disease. *Proteomics* **1,** 763–766.
38. Chiesa, R. and Harris, D. A. (2001) Prion diseases: what is the neurotoxic molecule? *Neurobiol. Dis.* **8,** 743–763.
39. Lovestone, S. and McLoughlin, D. M. (2002) Protein aggregates and dementia: is there a common toxicity? *J. Neurol. Neurosurg. Psychiatry* **72,** 152–161.

40. Tobler, A. R., Notterpek, L., Naef, R., Taylor, V., Suter, U., and Shooter, E. M. (1999) Transport of Trembler-J mutant peripheral myelin protein 22 is blocked in the intermediate compartment and affects the transport of the wild-type protein by direct interaction. *J. Neurosci.* **19,** 2027–2036.

41. Roa, B. B., Garcia, C. A., Suter, U., et al. (1993) Charcot–Marie–Tooth disease type 1A. Association with a spontaneous point mutation in the PMP22 gene. *N. Engl. J. Med.* **329,** 96–101.

42. Notterpek, L., Ryan, M. C., Tobler, A. R., and Shooter, E. M. (1999) PMP22 accumulation in aggresomes: implications for CMT1A pathology. *Neurobiol. Dis.* **6,** 450–460.

43. Notterpek, L., Ryan, M. C., Tobler, A. R., and Shooter, E. M. (1999) PMP22 accumulation in aggresomes: implications for CMT1A pathology. *Neurobiol. Dis.* **6,** 450–460.

44. Tobler, A. R., Liu, N., Mueller, L., and Shooter, E. M. (2002) Differential aggregation of the Trembler and Trembler J mutants of peripheral myelin protein 22. *Proc. Natl. Acad. Sci. USA* **99,** 483–488.

45. Goedert, M., Spillantini, M. G., and Davies, S. W. (1998) Filamentous nerve cell inclusions in neurodegenerative diseases. *Curr. Opin. Neurobiol.* **8,** 619–632.

46. Paulson, H. L. and Fischbeck, K. H. (1998) Trinucleotide repeats in neurogenetic disorders. *Annu. Rev. Neurosci.* **19,** 79–107.

47. Kircheis, R., Wightman, L., and Wagner, E. (2001) Design and gene delivery activity of modified polyethylenimines. *Adv. Drug Deliv. Rev.* **53,** 341–358.

48. Cartier, R. and Reszka, R. (2002) Utilization of synthetic peptides containing nuclear localization signals for nonviral gene transfer systems. *Gene Ther.* **9,** 157–167.

49. Wagner, E., Zenke, M., Cotten, M., Geug, H., and Birnstiel, M. L. (1990) Transferrin–polycation conjugates as carriers for DNA uptake into cells. *Proc. Natl. Acad. Sci. USA* **87,** 3410–3414.

50. Ciftci, K. and Levy, R. J. (2001) Enhanced plasmid DNA transfection with lysosomotropic agents in cultured fibroblasts. *Int. J. Pharm.* **218,** 81–92.

51. Plank, C., Oberhauser, B., Mechtler, K., Koch, C., and Wagner, E. (1994) The influence of endosome-disruptive peptides on gene transfer using synthetic virus-like gene transfer systems. *J. Biol. Chem.* **269,** 12,918–12,924.

52. Curiel, D. T., Agarwal, S., Wagner, E., and Cotten, M. (1991) Adenovirus enhancement of transferrin–polylysine-mediated gene delivery. *Proc. Natl. Acad. Sci. USA* **88,** 8850–8854.

53. Ohki, E. C., Tilkins, M. L., Ciccarone, V. C., and Price, P. J. (2001) Improving the transfection efficiency of post-mitotic neurons. *J. Neurosci. Methods* **112,** 95–99.

54. Durham, H. D., Lochmüller, H., Jani, A., Acsadi, G., Massie, B., and Karpati, G. (1996) Toxicity of replication-defective adenoviral recombinants in dissociated cultures of nervous tissue. *Exp. Neurol.* **140,** 14–20.

55. Biewenga, J. E., Destree, O. H., and Schrama, L. H. (1997) Plasmid-mediated gene transfer in neurons using the biolistics technique. *J. Neurosci. Methods* **71,** 67–75.
56. Wellmann, H., Kaltschmidt, B., and Kaltschmidt, C. (1999) Optimized protocol for biolistic transfection of brain slices and dissociated cultured neurons with a hand-held gene gun. *J. Neurosci. Methods* **92,** 55–64.
57. Usachev, Y. M., Khammanivong, A., Campbell, C., and Thayer, S. A. (2000) Particle-mediated gene transfer to rat neurons in primary culture. *Pflugers Arch.* **439,** 730–738.
58. Murphy, R. C. and Messer, A. (2001) Gene transfer methods for CNS organotypic cultures: a comparison of three nonviral methods. *Mol. Ther.* **3,** 113–121.
59. Roy, J., Minotti, S., Dong, L., Figlewicz, D. A., and Durham, H. D. (1998) Glutamate potentiates the toxicity of mutant Cu/Zn-superoxide dismutase in motor neurons by postsynaptic calcium-dependent mechanisms. *J. Neurosci.* **18,** 9673–9684.
60. Bruening, W., Roy, J., Giasson, B., Figlewicz, D. A., Mushynski, W. E., and Durham, H. D. (1999) Upregulation of protein chaperones preserves viability of cells expressing toxic Cu/Zn-superoxide dismutase mutants associated with amyotrophic lateral sclerosis. *J. Neurochem.* **72,** 693–699.
61. Karpati, G., Lochmüller, H., Nalbantoglu, J., and Durham, H. (1995) The principles of gene therapy for the nervous system. *TINS* **19,** 49–54.
62. Slack, R. S. and Miller, F. D. (1996) Viral vectors for modulating gene expression in neurons. *Curr. Opin. Neurobiol.* **6,** 576–583.
63. Janson, C. G., McPhee, S. W., Leone, P., Freese, A., and During, M. J. (2001) Viral-based gene transfer to the mammalian CNS for functional genomic studies. *TINS* **24,** 706–712.
64. Hartigan-O'Connor, D., Barjot, C., Salvatori, G., and Chamberlain, J. S. (2002) Generation and growth of gutted adenoviral vectors. *Methods Enzymol.* **346,** 224–246.
65. He, T. C., Zhou, S., da Costa, L. T., Yu, J., Kinzler, K. W., and Vogelstein, B. (1998) A simplified system for generating recombinant adenoviruses. *Proc. Natl. Acad. Sci. USA* **95,** 2509–2514.
66. Simonato, M., Manservigi, R., Marconi, P., and Glorioso, J. (2000) Gene transfer into neurones for the molecular analysis of behaviour: focus on herpes simplex vectors. *TINS* **23,** 183–190.
67. Grimm, D., Kern, A., Rittner, K., and Kleinschmidt, J. A. (1998) Novel tools for production and purification of recombinant adenoassociated virus vectors. *Hum. Gene Ther.* **9,** 2745–2760.
68. Bettinger, T., Carlisle, R. C., Read, M. L., Ogris, M., and Seymour, L. W. (2001) Peptide-mediated RNA delivery: a novel approach for enhanced transfection of primary and post-mitotic cells. *Nucleic Acids Res.* **29,** 3882–3891.
69. Simons, M., De Strooper, B., Multhaup, G., Tienari, P. J., Dotti, C. G., and Beyreuther, K. (1996) Amyloidogenic processing of the human amyloid pre-

cursor protein in primary cultures of rat hippocampal neurons. *J. Neurosci.* **16,** 899–908.

70. Mattson, M. P., Zhu, H., Yu, J., and Kindy, M. S. (2000) Presenilin-1 mutation increases neuronal vulnerability to focal ischemia in vivo and to hypoxia and glucose deprivation in cell culture: involvement of perturbed calcium homeostasis. *J. Neurosci.* **20,** 1358–1364.

71. Kruman, I. I., Pedersen, W. A., Springer, J. E., and Mattson, M. P. (1999) ALS-linked Cu/Zn-SOD mutation increases vulnerability of motor neurons to excitotoxicity by a mechanism involving increased oxidative stress and perturbed calcium homeostasis. *Exp. Neurol.* **160,** 28–39.

72. Inoue, T., Lin, X., Kohlmeier, K. A., Orr, H. T., Zoghbi, H. Y., and Ross, W. N. (2001) Calcium dynamics and electrophysiological properties of cerebellar Purkinje cells in SCA1 transgenic mice. *J. Neurophysiol.* **85,** 1750–1760.

73. Wyttenbach, A., Carmichael, J., Swartz, J., et al. (2000) Effects of heat shock, heat shock protein 40 (HDJ-2), and proteasome inhibition on protein aggregation in cellular models of Huntington's disease. *Proc. Natl. Acad. Sci. USA* **97,** 2898–2903.

74. Wang, G. H., Mitsui, K., Kotliarova, S., et al. (1999) Caspase activation during apoptotic cell death induced by expanded polyglutamine in N2a cells. *Neuroreport* **10,** 2435–2438.

75. Mills, J. C., Roth, K. A., Cagan, R. L., and Gordon, J. I. (2001) DNA microarrays and beyond: completing the journey from tissue to cell. *Nature Cell Biol.* **3,** E175–E178.

76. Craven, R. A. and Banks, R. E. (2001) Laser capture microdissection and proteomics: possibilities and limitation. *Proteomics* **1,** 1200–1204.

77. Clark, H. A., Barker, S. L. R., Basuel, M., et al. (1998) Subcellular optochemical nanobiosensors: probes encapsulated by biologically localised embedding (PEBBLEs). *Sensors Actuators B* **51,** 12–16.

78. Ng, T., Squire, A., Hansra, G., et al. (1999) Imaging protein kinase Calpha activation in cells. *Science* **283,** 2085–2089.

79. Truong, K. and Ikura, M. (2001) The use of FRET imaging microscopy to detect protein–protein interactions and protein conformational changes in vivo. *Curr. Opin. Struct. Biol.* **11,** 573–578.

80. Mere, L., Bennett, T., Coassin, P., et al. (1999) Miniaturized FRET assays and microfluidics: key components for ultra-high-throughput screening. *Drug Discov. Today* **4,** 363–369.

81. Zacharias, D. A., Baird, G. S., and Tsien, R. Y. (2000) Recent advances in technology for measuring and manipulating cell signals. *Curr. Opin. Neurobiol.* **10,** 416–421.

Appendix

Annotated Reading List

**Evelyn Tiffany-Castiglioni, Lucio G. Costa,
Marion Ehrich, William R. Mundy, Gerald J. Audesirk,
Michael Aschner, Prasada R. S. Kodavanti,
and Stephen M. Lasley**

This appendix contains a critically reviewed list of works related to in vitro neurotoxicology. The list has been carefully selected and annotated by the contributors to include reference books on neurotoxicology, books and essays on in vitro neurotoxicology, books and chapters on related methods, and important review articles that have appeared in the past 10 yr.

BOOKS ON NEUROTOXICOLOGY

Aschner, M. and Kimelberg, H. K. (eds.) (1996) *The Role of Glia in Neurotoxicity*, CRC, New York

This is the first book to focus exclusively on the roles of neuroglia in neurotoxicity. Contributors review and explore potential sites for neurotoxic action in glial–neuronal interactions in both the central and peripheral nervous systems. Individual chapters address methodologies and concepts of neurotoxicology, including many examples of in vitro approaches. This publication was intended to fill a gap in the literature. With the increasing importance of glia, a journal, *Glia*, has been dedicated to studies on these cells. In addition, many recent textbooks have included discussion of glia, encompassing neurophysiology, neuroanatomy, neuroscience, neurochemistry, and neuropharmacology. None, however, included the role of glia in neurotoxicity, a timely topic and a subject in its own right.

Chang, L.W. (ed.) (1994) *Principles of Neurotoxicology*, Marcel Dekker, New York

This standard reference provides a comprehensive overview of principles and modern concepts of neurotoxicology. The work contains major sections on the central nervous system, behavioral neurotoxicology, biochemical and molecular neurotoxicology, and developmental neurotoxicology.

From: *Methods in Pharmacology and Toxicology: In Vitro Neurotoxicology: Principles and Challenges*
Edited by: E. Tiffany-Castiglioni © Humana Press Inc., Totowa, NJ

Costa, L. and Manzo, L. (eds.) (1998) *Occupational Neurotoxicology*, CRC, New York
This book provides a concise overview of important concerns of the relatively new specialty of occupational neurotoxicology. Among them are commonly encountered workplace neurotoxicants, signs and symptoms of neurotoxicity, detection and monitoring of human exposure by biomarkers, epidemiology, and diagnostic methods.

Harry, G. J. (ed.) (1994) *Developmental Neurotoxicology*, CRC, New York
This book examines the biological characteristics of the developing nervous system that increase its vulnerability to damage by exposure to environmental toxicants. Contributing authors discuss functional alterations that occur at exposure levels too low to produce structural teratogenesis.

Massaro, E. J. (ed.) (2002) *Handbook of Neurotoxicology, Volumes I and II*, Humana, Totowa, NJ
This two-volume set provides a current overview of important topics in contemporary neurotoxicology. In Volume I, 28 topics are covered under 4 sections: pesticides, metals, microbial toxins, and animal toxins (venoms). In Volume II, 21 topics are covered under 4 sections: developmental neurotoxicology, drugs of abuse, imaging, and neurobehavioral assessment methods. Section editors and chapter contributors are international experts from academia, industry, and government agencies. Volume I, in particular, offers excellent further reading on topics relevant to in vitro neurotoxicology, such as pesticide effects on ion channels, mechanisms of lead neuronal toxicity, interactions of metals with the zinc-finger motif, and the blood–brain barrier in metal toxicity.

Slikker, W. B. and Chang, L. W. (eds.) (1998) *Handbook of Developmental Neurotoxicology*, Academic Press, New York
This highly comprehensive multidisciplinary reference addresses the mechanisms and relevance of the developmental toxicity of chemicals. The subject is divided into seven major sections on cellular and molecular morphogenesis, developmental biology and toxicology, synaptogenesis and neurotransmission, nutrient and chemical disposition, behavioral assessment, clinical assessment and epidemiology, specific neurotoxic syndromes, and risk assessment.

Tilson, H. A. and Harry, G. J. (1999) *Neurotoxicology*, 2nd ed., Target Organ Toxicology Series, Taylor & Francis, Philadelphia
The major focuses of this edition are the discovery of sites and mechanisms of neurotoxicity and their value in improving risk assessment. The text focuses primarily on the neurobiological basis underlying neurotoxic sites and modes of action. Contributing authors provide 15 chapters on topics spanning molecular biological approaches in neurotoxicology, in vitro neurotoxicology, specific cellular and biochemical processes damaged by toxicants, effects on learning and behavior, and emerging concepts in risk assessment.

BOOKS AND POSITION PAPERS ON IN VITRO NEUROTOXICOLOGY

Aschner, M., Allen, J. W., Kimelberg, H. K., LoPachin, R. M., and Streit, W. J. (1999) Glial cells in neurotoxicity development. *Annu. Rev. Pharmacol. Toxicol.* **39,** 151–173

> Experts on each of the major classes of neuroglia (astrocytes, oligodendrocytes, microglia, and Schwann cells) present models for neurotoxic sites of action that involve glia. Glial interactions with neurons and other glia that underlie nervous system development and function are examined. The work described is based on in vitro and in vivo models.

Aschner, M. and Kerper, L. E. (2000) Transport of metals in the nervous system, in *Molecular Biology and Toxicology of Metals* (Koropatnick, D.J. and Zalups, R. K., eds.), Taylor & Francis, London, pp. 276–299

> The blood–brain barrier (BBB) is a specialized structure responsible for the maintenance of the neuronal microenvironment. A pivotal function of the endothelial cells comprising the blood–brain barrier is to regulate the selective transport and metabolism of substances from blood to brain, as well as their transport in the opposite direction. This chapter addresses the development of the blood–brain barrier, with emphasis on the crosstalk between astrocytes and endothelial cells, as well as known mechanisms of metal transport by endothelial cells.

Audesirk, G. J. (1997) *In vitro* systems in neurotoxicological studies, in *Nervous System and Behavioral Toxicology, Comprehensive Toxicology, Volume 11* (Lowndes, H. E. and Reuhl, K. R., eds.), Elsevier Science, Amsterdam, pp. 431–446

> This chapter focuses on complementarity between in vitro and in vivo approaches. A concise overview of in vitro systems is provided. Of special interest are discussions of acute versus semichronic neurotoxicity and the problem of concentration and duration of exposure in vitro.

Costa, L. G. (1998) Neurotoxicity testing: a discussion of in vitro alternatives. *Environ. Health Perspect.* **106(Suppl.),** 505–510.

> In addition to briefly discussing the advantages and disadvantages of in vitro systems, the author thoughtfully discusses in vitro systems for mechanistic studies and neurotoxicity screening. Tiered approaches are suggested, because no single invitro system can reliably detect all possible end points.

Costa, L. G. (1998) Biochemical and molecular neurotoxicology: relevance to biomarker development, neurotoxicity testing and risk assessment, *Toxicol. Lett.* **102–103,** 417–421

> Biomarkers are generally divided into three categories: biomarkers of exposure, effect, and susceptibility. This commentary addresses biomarkers of effect and their cross-disciplinary use in animal toxicity studies, epidemiology, and in vitro toxicity testing. The example of organophosphorus insecticide neurotoxicity is explored.

Deng, W. and Poretz, R. D. (2003) Oligodendroglia in developmental neurotoxicity. *Neurotoxicology* **24**, 161–178

> This is the first contemporary review to address the roles of oligodendroglia in developmental neurotoxicity. Topics covered are the developmental lineage of oligodendrocytes, maturational characteristics in vivo and in vitro, and modulation of differentiation in cell culture models. The well-defined oligodendrocyte lineage is presented as an advantageous system for investigations of developmental neurotoxicity. Recent work from the authors' laboratory on lead neurotoxicity is reviewed.

Ehrich, M. and Veronesi, B. (1998) In vitro neurotoxicology, in *Neurotoxicology* (Tilson, H. A. and Harry, G. J., eds.), Taylor & Francis, Philadelphia, pp. 37–50

> This chapter provides a general review of methods and examples of their use for neurotoxicology. The biological basis underlying neurotoxic sites and modes of action is addressed.

Harry, G. J., Billingsley, M., Bruinink, A., Campbell, I. L., Classen, W., Dorman, D. C., Galli, C., Ray, D., Smith, R. A., and Tilson, H. A. (1998) In vitro techniques for the assessment of neurotoxicity. *Environ. Health Perspect.* **106(Suppl.),** 131–158

> This work is an extensive review and discussion of the topic prepared as a document for the International Program on Chemical Safety (IPCS) and cosponsored by the United Nations Environment Program, World Health Organization, and International Labor Organization. The focus of this review is the usefulness of in vitro techniques for the identification of neurotoxic hazards. End points receive particular attention because of their use in distinguishing between a pharmacologic and neurotoxic response. This work is also valuable as an introductory resource for the reader new to culture techniques, as several common techniques, cell lines, and problems encountered in culture are discussed.

Harry, G. J. and Tilson, H. A. (ed.) (1999) *Neurodegeneration Methods and Protocols*, Humana, Totowa, NJ

> The objective of this book is to develop an understanding of and technical ability in various cellular and molecular techniques for studying many aspects of nervous system cell biology. The protocols in this book span a multidisciplinary range of cellular and molecular approaches and should allow investigators to address research questions directed toward understanding nervous system function, injury, degeneration, and the repair/regenerative process.

Pentreath, V. W. (ed.) (1999) *Neurotoxicology In Vitro*, Taylor & Francis, Philadelphia

> This excellent work is suggested as a companion volume to the current book. The book contains concise reviews of principles of neurobiology, commonly used cell lines, and selected in vitro techniques. The uses of in vitro methods for mechanisms versus screening studies are also thoughtfully addressed.

Philbert, M. A. and Aschner, M. (1997) Glial cells, in *Nervous System and Behavioral Toxicology, Comprehensive Toxicology, Volume 11* (Lowndes, H. E. and Reuhl, K. R., eds.), Elsevier Science, Amsterdam, pp. 217–236

> The dynamic role of glia in the maintenance of normal neural tissues and their potential involvement in degenerative disease processes and following exposure to xenobiotics are discussed. This review provides a general overview of glia as targets and mediators of neurotoxicity in the nervous system.

Tiffany-Castiglioni, E. and Qian, Y. (2001) Astroglia as metal depots: molecular mechanisms for metal accumulation, storage and release. *Neurotoxicology* **22,** 577–592

> This review extends the lead-sink hypothesis for astroglia to other metals. In vivo and in vitro evidence that mercury, manganese, and copper might be selectively accumulated by astroglia is examined.

Tiffany-Castiglioni, E., Ehrich, M., Dees, W. L, Costa, L.G., Kodavanti, P. R. S., Lasley, S. M., Oortgiesen, M., and Durham, H. D. (1999) Bridging the gap between in vitro and in vivo models for neurotoxicology. *Toxicol. Sci.* **51,** 178–183

> The authors wrote this commentary as a result of their participation as panelists in a poster-discussion session on the complementarity and usefulness of in vitro and in vivo approaches to neurotoxicity testing. The session was held in the 1998 meeting of the Society for Toxicology. This paper served as a catalyst for the present volume.

Trotti, D., Danbolt, N. C., and Volterra, A. (1998). Glutamate transporters are oxidant-vulnerable: a molecular link between oxidative and excitotoxic neurodegeneration? *Trends Pharmacol. Sci.* **19,** 328–334

> The authors discuss the idea that glutamate transporters in the brain can be oxidized by biological agents, leading to decreased glutamate uptake and extracellular accumulation of neurotoxic glutamate. This phenomenon is of interest to neurotoxicologists in that a similar process can occur when cells are exposed to chemical oxidants. The possible involvement of oxidative alterations of specific glutamate transporters in pathologies (amyotrophic lateral sclerosis, Alzheimer's disease, brain trauma, and ischaemia) is reviewed.

METHODS AND MODEL SYSTEMS APPLICABLE TO IN VITRO NEUROTOXICOLOGY

Aschner, M., Kimelberg, H. K., and Vitarella, D. (1995) Selective techniques designed to evaluate neurotoxicity, in *Neurotoxicology: Approaches and Methodologies* (Chang, L. W., ed.), Academic, New York, pp. 439–444

> This chapter presents a new version of an available technique for dynamic measurement of changes in cell volume of substratum-attached monolayer cell cultures. When combined with release measurements of endogenous cell markers, it affords a powerful tool for rapid measurements of cytotox-

icity and, potentially, a high throughput screening method for various neurotoxicants.

Banker, G. and Goslin, K. (eds.) (1998) *Culturing Nerve Cells*, 2nd ed., MIT Press, Cambridge, MA

> This manual, now in its second edition, offers an outstanding resource for culture of vertebrate neural tissue and cells. It contains several eloquently written chapters on underlying principles, as well as detailed recipes and protocols for culturing specific cell types and mixed cultures. Contributors provide first-hand tutorials on the techniques developed in their laboratories, including advantages, limitations, and troubleshooting.

Boulton, A. A., Baker, G. B., and Bateson, A. N. (eds.) (1999) *In Vitro Neurochemical Techniques*, Humana, Totowa, NJ

> This collection of contemporary techniques for neurochemical and molecular neurobiology research includes assays that are useful for the measurement of cell injury and cell death.

Buznikov, G. A., Nikitina, L. A., Bezuglov, V. V., Lauder, J. M., Padilla, S., and Slotkin, T. A. (2001) An invertebrate model of the developmental neurotoxicity of insecticides: effects of chlorpyrifos and dieldrin in sea urchin embryos and larvae. *Environ. Health Perspect.* **109,** 651–661.

> This article describes an interesting new approach to in vitro developmental neurotoxicity testing that utilizes an invertebrate model.

Ehrich, M. (1998) Human cells as *in vitro* alternatives for toxicological research and testing: neurotoxicity studies. *Comments Toxicol.* **6,** 189–197

> Sources of cells as well as advantages and disadvantages of the use of cells of human origin are discussed.

Freshney, R. I. (2000) *Culture of Animal Cells: A Manual of Basic Technique*, 4th ed., Wiley–Liss, New York

> This book well deserves its common aphorism as the bible of tissue culture users. It is thorough, clearly written, well and generously illustrated, and frequently updated. Included are theoretical and practical considerations of cell, tissue, and organ culture, as well as detailed protocols of common procedures, such as sterile technique, preparation of medium, cytotoxicity assays, and cryopreservation. Detailed protocols are provided for two types of nervous system culture (cerebellar granule neurons and olfactory bulb ensheathing cells), but more specialized works would need to be consulted for other culture protocols.

Gad, S. C. (2000) Neurotoxicology *in vitro*, in *In Vitro Toxicology*, 2nd ed., (Gad, C. G., ed.), Taylor & Francis, New York, pp. 188–221

> This article surveys the tools of in vitro neurotoxicology, including types of cell culture preparation used, specific examples of their use, methods of tissue culture, morphological and functional toxicity assays, and the design of neurotoxicant screening systems. Specific neurotoxicologic studies are briefly discussed as examples to illustrate the problems and potential advantages of in vitro approaches. the subjects selected are anticonvulsants, heavy metals, and excitoxins, mostly from articles published in the 1980s.

Gilbert, M. E. (2000) *In vitro* systems as simulations of in vivo conditions: the study of cognition and synaptic plasticity in neurotoxicology. *Ann. NY Acad. Sci.* **919,** 119–13.

> The effects of regional brain stimulation and ablation on behavior have led to inferences on the impact of these manipulations on psychological constructs of "learning" and "memory." This review describes how an electrophysiological property, long-term potentiation (LTP), greatly expanded the ability to probe cellular aspects of the representation of memories in the brain. The study of plasticity in this manner is an excellent example of how in vivo phenomena translate to more simplified in vitro test systems to directly address cellular and biochemical mechanisms of information storage in the brain.

Maines, M., Costa, L. G., and Reed, D. J. (eds.) (2002) *Current Protocols in Toxicology* Wiley, New York

> This two-volume collection offers detailed laboratory procedures for the assessment of toxicity at multiple levels of biological complexity ranging from whole organisms to biochemical pathways. It is available in updatable looseleaf, CD-ROM, and Web-based formats. Chapter 12, "Biochemical and Molecular Neurotoxicology," contains units written by authorities in their fields on several in vitro topics, including the development of an in vitro blood–brain barrier, culture of rat hippocampal neurons and rat cortical astrocytes, and analytical techniques for cytology and imaging.

O'Hare, S. and Atterwill, C. K. (eds.) (1995) *In Vitro Toxicity Testing Protocols*, Humana, Totowa, NJ

> This collection of detailed protocols includes the preparation and use of cultured astrocytes for assays of gliotoxicity, as well as several chapters on general and topical toxicity.

Tyson, C., Witschi, H., and Frazier, J., (1994) *In Vitro Toxicity Indicators*, Methods in Toxicology Vol. 1B, Academic, New York

> This book contains detailed testing procedures for assessing cell injury and cell death. The chapters do not specifically address neural cells, but protocols can be adapted for use in neurotoxicity testing.

Zurich, M. G., Honegger, P., Schilter, B., Costa, L. G., and Monnet-Tschudi, F. (2000) Use of aggregating brain cell cultures to study developmental effects of organophosphorus insecticides. *Neurotoxicology* **21,** 599–606

> This experimental study shows how aggregating cultures of brain cells can be used to assess developmental neurotoxicity.

REVIEWS ON NEUROTOXIC SUBSTANCES STUDIED IN VITRO

Costa, L. G., Guizzetti, M., Lu, H., Bordi, F., Vitalone, A., Tita, B., Palmery, M., Valeri, P., and Silvestrini, B. (2001) Intracellular signal transduction pathways as targets for neurotoxicants. *Toxicology* **160,** 19–26

This review focuses on the interactions of lead, ethanol, and polychlorinated biphenyls with signal transduction pathways, especially protein kinase C isoenzymes. The potential importance of such pathways in neurotoxic processes is discussed.

Gilbert, M. E. and Lasley, S. M. (2002) Long-term consequences of developmental exposure to lead or polychlorinated biphenyls: synaptic transmission and plasticity in the rodent CNS. *Environ. Toxicol. Pharmacol.* **12,** 105–117

The authors review current evidence concerning the effects of exposure to lead or polychlorinated biphenyls (PCBs) on hippocampal synaptic transmission and use-dependent plasticity, particularly effects that persist long after exposure has ended. Long-term potentiation (LTP) is thought to represent a physiological substrate for memory, and during ontogeny, this type of plasticity guides the establishment and maintenance of synaptic connections in cortical structures. It is proposed that in the developing nervous system PCB or lead perturb activity-dependent plasticity leading to organizational changes in brain. The aberrant connectivity resulting during development is manifested as impaired LTP and cognitive ability in the mature organism.

Guerri, C., Pascual, M., and Renau-Piqueras, J. (2001) Glia and fetal alcohol syndrome. *Neurotoxicology* **22,** 593–559

The article reviews evidence obtained in vivo and in culture that ethanol directly damages astrocytes and radial glia, impairing neuronal migration in the developing brain.

Kodavanti, P. R. S., and Tilson, H. A. (2000). Neurochemical effects of environmental chemicals: *in vitro* and *in vivo* correlations on second messenger pathways. *Ann. NY Acad. Sci.* **919,** 97–105

This article focuses on correlating changes in second-messenger pathways following in vitro and in vivo exposure to persistent environmental chemicals such as polychlorinated biphenyls (PCBs). Second messengers, including calcium, protein kinase C, and inositol phosphates, are critical for nervous system development and function. This article reports changes in these pathways in in vitro neuronal cultures at concentrations that are biologically relevant.

Tiffany-Castiglioni, E., Legare, M. E., Schneider, L.A., Hanneman, W.H., Zenger, E., and Hong, S. (1996) Astroglia and lead neurotoxicity, in *The Role of Glia in Neurotoxicity* (Aschner, M. and Kimelberg, H. K., eds.), CRC, Boca Raton, FL, pp. 175–200

This chapter reviews in vivo and in vitro work on the effects of lead on mammalian astroglia dating from 1993 to 1996. Topics include calcium homeostasis, glutathione metabolism, morphology, and cytoskeletal proteins.

Tiffany-Castiglioni, E. (1993) Cell culture models for lead toxicity in neuronal and glial cells. *Neurotoxicology* **14,** 513–536

This article critically reviews most of the work to 1993 on the effects of lead on astroglia, oligodendroglia, Schwann cells, and neurons in culture.

Mammalian and invertebrate models are included. The work reviewed is organized historically into three phases: the exploratory, expansion, and intensification stages of in vitro lead neurotoxicology. These phases are characterized by progressive refinement of end points from lethal responses at millimolar doses to physiologically relevant molecular responses at submicromolar doses. The article also contains a still timely detailed discussion on problems with lead concentrations and exposure protocols in in vitro.

Veronesi, B., Ehrich, M., Blusztain, J. K., Oortgiesen, M., and Durham, H. (1996) Cell culture models of interspecies selectivity to organophosphorus insecticides. *Neurotoxicology* **18,** 283–298

The article presents an integrated summary of studies by the authors in which interspecies differences in responses of nervous tissue to organophosphorus insecticides were examined in vitro. By the use of human and mouse cell lines, as well as homogenized tissue, the underlying mechanisms for interspecies differences were shown to include targets not previously recognized in vivo, including cellular metabolism, target enzyme baseline activities, and receptor-medicated cell-signaling pathways.

Index